# afoot&afield

# Los Angeles

## A comprehensive hiking guide

### THIRD EDITION

*Jerry Schad*

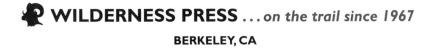
**WILDERNESS PRESS** ...*on the trail since 1967*

**BERKELEY, CA**

*This book is affectionately dedicated to my parents, Jack and Marion, whose support of my eclectic interests from an early age resulted in a life-long fascination with the world*

**Afoot & Afield Los Angeles: A Comprehensive Hiking Guide**

1st Edition 1991
2nd Edition 2000
3rd Edition 2010

Copyright © 2010 by Jerry Schad

Front cover photo copyright © 2010 by Jerry Schad
Interior photos by author
Cover design: Larry B. Van Dyke
Book design and layout: Larry B. Van Dyke
ISBN 978-0-89997-499-6

Manufactured in the United States of America

Published by:  **Wilderness Press**
**1345 8th Street**
**Berkeley, CA 94710**
**(800) 443-7227; FAX (510) 558-1696**
**info@wildernesspress.com**
**www.wildernesspress.com**

Visit our website for a complete listing of our books and for ordering information.

*Cover photos:*   *Top:* Devil's Punchbowl Natural Area in winter; *Left:* Atop Mount Lee in Griffith Park; *Right:* Oak woodland in the Santa Monica Mountains

**SAFETY NOTICE:** Although Wilderness Press and the author have made every attempt to ensure that the information in this book is accurate at press time, they are not responsible for any loss, damage, injury, or inconvenience that may occur to anyone while using this book. You are responsible for your own safety and health while in the wilderness. The fact that a trail is described in this book does not mean that it will be safe for you. Be aware that trail conditions can change from day to day. Always check local conditions, know your own limitations, and consult a map.

# Acknowledgments

Many people have offered their time, talents, and knowledge during the various phases of producing this book. I would like to thank Ralph and Beth Davis, John Elwin, Ellen Feeney, Mike Fry, Rosalind Gold, Jerry Herring, Dan McNeill, Jane Rauch, Nick Soroka, Pamela Stricker, Gene and Emily Troxell, Charles Wilken, and René Schad for sharing adventures with me on the trail, and for helping with transportation during my field work for this project. Several people associated with local parks and preserves and Angeles National Forest have been of assistance too, among them Margie Behm, Donald Gilliland, Gerald Reponen, and Larry Walters. Tom Winnett, the founder of Wilderness Press, in his characteristic meticulous way, superbly edited the first-edition text. I would also like to thank Tom for his sound advice and guidance during this and previous "Afoot and Afield" projects.

Prior to the publication of both the second edition and the third edition of this book, I received many helpful and much-appreciated field reports from M.A. Durrin and John Strauch. I also wish to acknowledge the following persons who joined me for further explorations in Los Angeles County or who informed me of various changes on its trails: Simone Arias, Hugh Blanchard, Chris Brennen, Tom Chester, Sandy Dininger, Ronald Hanke, William Johnston, Paul Lara, Sean McFeely, Ted McGivern, Rachel Rifat, Tom Schad, Bruce and Anita Stoll, Linda Therrien, Laura Thompson, and Linh Trieu.

Jerry Schad
San Diego, California
January 2010

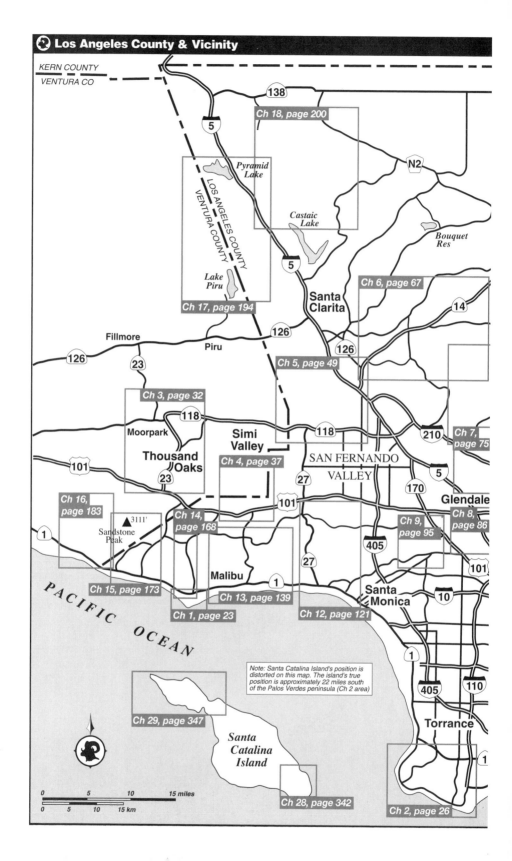

KERN COUNTY
VENTURA CO

138

Ch 18, page 200

N2

5

*Pyramid Lake*

*Castaic Lake*

*Bouquet Res*

LOS ANGELES COUNTY / VENTURA COUNTY

*Lake Piru*

5

Santa Clarita

Ch 6, page 67

14

Ch 17, page 194

126

Fillmore

Piru

126

Ch 5, page 49

126

23

126

Ch 3, page 32

118

Moorpark

Simi Valley

118

210

Ch 7, page 75

Thousand Oaks

Ch 4, page 37

SAN FERNANDO

5

23

27

VALLEY

170

101

Glendale

101

Ch 16, page 183

▲3111'
Sandstone Peak

Ch 14, page 168

Ch 9, page 95

Ch 8, page 86

1

405

101

27

Ch 15, page 173

Malibu

1

Santa Monica

10

Ch 13, page 139

Ch 1, page 23

Ch 12, page 121

1

P A C I F I C   O C E A N

Note: Santa Catalina Island's position is distorted on this map. The island's true position is approximately 22 miles south of the Palos Verdes peninsula (Ch 2 area)

Ch 29, page 347

405

110

*Santa Catalina Island*

Torrance

1

Ch 28, page 342

Ch 2, page 26

| 0 | 5 | 10 | 15 miles |
| 0 | 5 | 10 | 15 km |

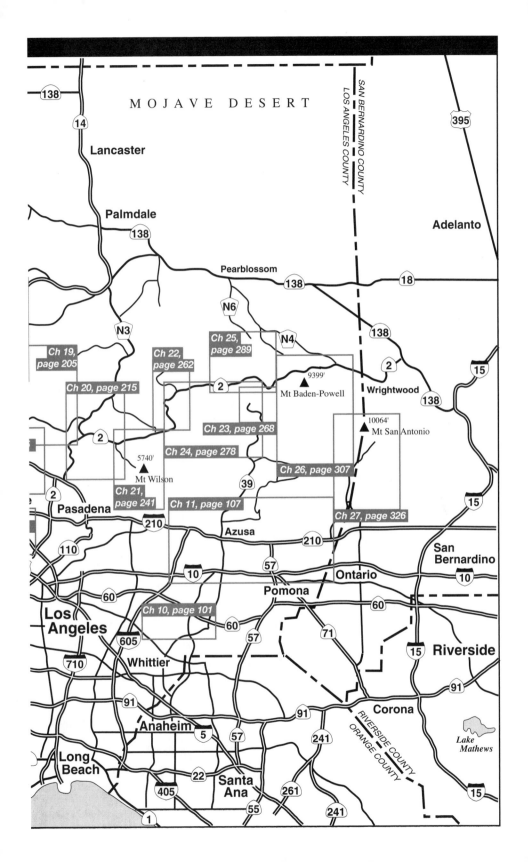

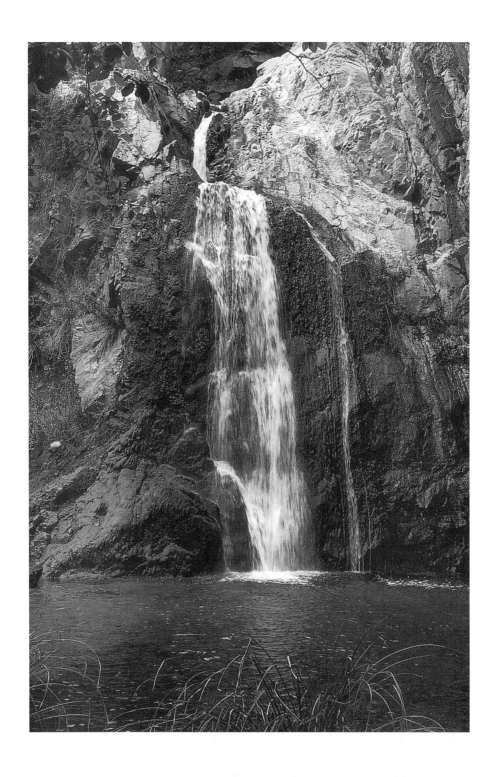

# Contents

Fish Canyon Falls

# SANTA CATALINA ISLAND

# Preface

Pummeled by great heavings of the earth's crust, desiccated by drought, torn by flood, tortured by fire, and pestered by the threat of human intervention, L.A.'s wild spaces are nonetheless *not* the wastelands they may appear to be when viewed through a brown veil of smog or haze. In fact, if you take the time to venture almost anywhere beyond the sprawling metropolitan borders, you'll discover Nature is not only alive out there, it's often triumphant.

While doing field research for this book I've clambered over sandstone boulders the size of trucks, cooled off in the spray of frothing waterfalls, and trekked down a "wild and scenic" river. In the high country of the San Gabriel Mountains, I stood in stunned silence as a herd of two dozen bighorn sheep scooted across a rocky pass just below me. From a chaparral-clad slope above Glendale, I witnessed the strange juxtaposition of a deer's silhouette against the Oz-like towers of downtown L.A.

With friends I've admired sea stars in crystalline tidepools on the Malibu coast, scuffed through powdery snow in the San Gabriels, and inhaled the nectar-rich air of the Mojave Desert in bloom. From the Angeles Crest we've spotted white sails in Santa Monica Bay, and watched the sun sink toward a blue horizon dimpled by four offshore islands. Alone at dawn on the mile-high rim of the L.A. Basin, I've watched the glare of a million lights succumb to the pink twilight.

In all my field trips for this book (totaling more than 1000 miles of walking), never have I needed to venture more than 20 air-miles from the fringe of Los Angeles or its populous satellite cities. Yet once on the trail, I've seldom felt the weight of the teeming millions all around me; indeed in a few places I've walked all day without seeing another person.

Amazingly enough, only on a couple of occasions did I have to put up with the noxious clouds of smog trapped low over the city or borne into the backcountry by the winds. A careful reading of weather conditions and judicious and timely choices among the many possible places to visit in the county often yielded for me the special treat of pristine air and hundred-mile vistas.

This wide-ranging guidebook covers an equally wide-ranging county—a kingdom in itself with elements of coast, foothill, mountain, and desert rolled into a 4083-square-mile space. Remove the urbanized coastal plain and the semi-developed western Mojave from the county's area and you're still left with nearly 2000 square miles of wild or lightly developed land.

Most of L.A. County's publicly accessible open spaces lie north and west of the heavily populated coastal plain. Angeles National Forest, encompassing most of the San Gabriel Mountains, sprawls across 652,000 acres (1019 square miles), about one-quarter of the county's land area. In spite of Southern California's dry climate, the Angeles Forest supports about 240 miles of perennial streams and in some areas a forest cover resembling parts of the high Sierra Nevada. About 600 miles of trail (including a segment of the Pacific Crest National Scenic Trail) connect high and low points within the Forest and link together such disparate locations as the L.A. Basin and the Mojave Desert.

Tucked into the southwestern corner of the county and spilling over into Ventura County are the Santa Monica Mountains. This coastal range includes a patchwork of private and public lands, the latter under the jurisdiction of the National Park Service (Santa Monica Mountains National Recreation Area) and various state and local agencies. The pace of park-land acquisition in the Santa Monicas has quickened in recent years, and the trail network is continually expanding

Close to the heart of the county's urban core are scattered islands of open space—the Santa Susana and Verdugo Mountains bordering the San Fernando Valley, the Puente Hills in the San Gabriel Valley and, of course, venerable Griffith Park.

Rounding out the list of better places to explore in the county are some more-or-less natural stretches of Pacific coastline, the rim of the western Mojave Desert, and Santa Catalina Island.

Despite extensive coverage in this book of all the areas mentioned above, I will refer you to additional sources for more information on specific areas: John Robinson's classic *Trails of the Angeles* in many respects complements my coverage of the San Gabriel Mountains. The most recent (8th edition) of this book contains revisions by Doug Christiansen.

*The Pacific Crest Trail: Southern California,* 6th edition (Jeffrey P. Schaffer, et. al.) contains a complete log and maps of the trail's route through the San Gabriel Mountains. *Walking L.A.,* by Erin Mahoney Harris, takes an entirely different (urban) approach to exploring the city. My two other volumes in the "Afoot & Afield" series, *Afoot & Afield San Diego County* and *Afoot & Afield Orange County,* cover regions that are not within the scope of this book, but are still within a short drive of Los Angeles. More reading resources can be found in Appendix 2 of this book.

Every trip in this book was hiked by me at least once, and every effort has been made to ensure that the information herein is current as of the day of publication. Road access and trailheads do change, however. New acreage is being acquired for public use, and the near future will doubtless see the construction of more trails.

As the third edition of this book was about to go to press in August 2009, the Station Fire erupted in the San Gabriel Mountains. The 160,000-acre fire eventually burned about one-quarter of the entire Angeles National Forest, damaging roads, trails, campgrounds, and picnic grounds. Many hikes covered in the Angeles Forest section of this book will be unavailable for public use for a variable and undetermined amount of time. References to the Station Fire are given where appropriate within this edition.

Updates and new editions of this book are planned for the future. You can keep me apprised of recent developments and/ or changes by writing me in care of Wilderness Press, or send an e-mail to info@ wildernesspress.com Your comments will be appreciated.

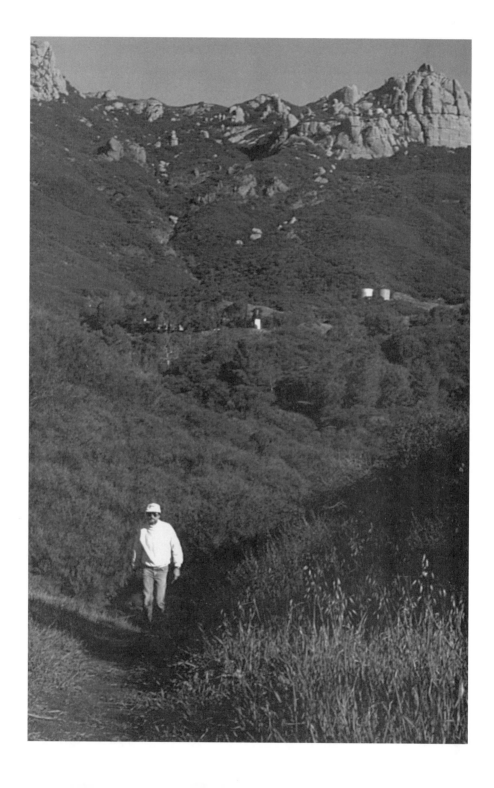

# Introducing
# Los Angeles County

Los Angeles County sits astride one of the earth's most significant structural features—the San Andreas Fault. For more than 10 million years, earth movements along the San Andreas and neighboring faults have shaped the dramatic geology and topography evident throughout the region today. The very complexity of the shape of the land has in turn spawned a variety of localized climates. The varied climates, along with the diverse topography and geology, have resulted in a remarkably diverse array of plant and animal life.

Exploring all this wonderful variety right in L.A.'s backyard is not hard to do. Conveniently enough, many of the best hiking opportunities start right on the edge of town—right off the freeway. Other trailheads can be quickly reached by way of lesser roads such as Pacific Coast Highway, Mulholland Highway, and Angeles Crest Highway. Fewer than a dozen of the hikes described in this book involve any kind of dirt-road driving to reach, and every trip (except for those on Santa Catalina Island) lies within 90 minutes drive of downtown L.A.—assuming light traffic.

In the next few pages of this book, we'll examine Los Angeles County's several climates, its spectacular geology, and its native plants and animals. In the short sections that follow, you'll find some important notes about safety and appropriate behavior on the trail; some useful tips on how to use this book effectively; and finally some helpful advice on how to choose and time your visits so as to avoid smog, excessive heat, and other discomforts that can detract from an otherwise pleasant outing. After perusing that material, you can dig into the heart of this book—descriptions of 200 hiking routes from the coast to the moun-tains, from sea level to 10,000 feet. Happy reading—and happy hiking!

## Land of Many Climates

A fairly accurate and succinct summary of Los Angeles County's climate might take the form of just two phrases: "warm and sunny," and "winter-wet, summer-dry." In the worldwide range of climates, this pattern is called a Mediterranean-type climate, typical of less than 3 percent of the world's landmass.

Actually, a lot of variation exists, a fact readily apparent to anyone traveling almost any direction through the county. Inland, away from the moderating influence of the ocean, temperatures usually climb higher in the day and usually drop lower at night. Also, higher elevations mean cooler temperatures and more rainfall. Since both of these influences are at work in the L.A. area, it's helpful to picture the county as divided into several climate zones, each zone characterized by particular combination of weather characteristics. Informally, let's divide the county into five climate zones: coastal, inland valley, transitional, mountain, and high desert.

The **coastal** (or "maritime fringe") **zone** extends only a few miles inland across the coastal slopes of the Santa Monica Mountains, but about 15 miles across the flat, central urban basin of Los Angeles. Moist air from over the cool Pacific waters sweeps into this zone with some regularity during the daytime hours, while at night the "marine layer" often turns into fog or low overcast. Average Fahrenheit temperatures range from the 60s/40s (daily high/low) in winter, to the 70s/60s in summer. Rainfall averages about 12–15 inches annually, except in the Santa Monicas. The higher

On the trail to The Grotto, with Sandstone Peak in the background profile of this coastal range snags extra moisture from rain-bearing winter storms, yielding an extra 10–15 inches.

The **inland valley zone** encompasses such corners of urban L.A. as the San Gabriel and San Fernando valleys, plus the north slope of the Santa Monica Mountains and the lower foothills of the San Gabriel Mountains. This area, only partly under the influence of moderating sea breezes, experiences more extreme temperatures, both daily and seasonally: typically 60s/30s in winter and 90s/50s in summer. Precipitation averages about 15 inches annually, somewhat more in the foothills.

Higher lands even more removed from coastal influences are classified as having either **transitional** or **mountain climates**. Both these zones are found in interior mountain ranges and are characterized by somewhat lower average temperatures. The subtle difference between the two involves rainfall. Annual rainfall in the semiarid transition zone, which encompasses the northwest corner of Angeles National Forest and the desert-facing slopes of the San Gabriel Mountains, is typically about 15–20 inches. The mountain climate zone, including most of the "Front Range" of the San Gabriels (facing the San Gabriel Valley) and the higher country along Angeles Crest

Highway, receives upwards of 30 inches—enough to support large areas of coniferous and broadleaf forest. Mount Wilson, in the Front Range, for example, gets about 35 inches of precipitation, including about 4 feet of snow, annually. Average temperatures there range from 50s/30s in winter to 80s/50s in summer. Mount Wilson's hilltop position spares it from the effects of cold-air drainage at night; so the day-night thermometer change is rather small. Not so for the canyon bottoms, especially in winter, when temperatures can plummet more than 40°F as the sun sinks out of sight.

In the "High Country" of the San Gabriel Mountains, enough snow falls and remains on the ground during the winter to permit skiing for about four months a year in a few areas. Several small but thriving winter-sports facilities exist here. Still higher, Mount San Antonio (10,064′) lies very near timberline, where the climate verges on alpine.

North of the San Gabriels, 50 or more miles inland, lies the county's driest climate zone, the **high desert,** which encompasses the westernmost Mojave Desert—the Antelope Valley. This area is almost completely cut off from the moderating influence of the ocean, and it experiences a relatively extreme "continental" type of climate. Temperatures typically range from 50s/20s

Grassy slopes, Oat Mountain

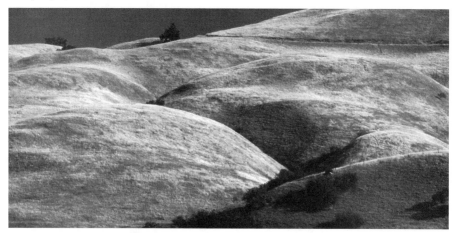

in winter to 90s/60s in summer. The coastal mountains serve as a barrier to rain-bearing clouds moving inland, so annual precipitation amounts to only about 7 inches—somewhat more at the western tip of the valley near Interstate 5, and somewhat less at the county's northeast corner near Edwards Air Force Base.

It's worth noting that the precipitation figures mentioned in the paragraphs above, which are long-term averages, should be taken with a grain of salt. The last 25 years or so have featured a drying trend locally and throughout much of the Western states. (For evidence of this, examine any freshly cut tree stump in the local mountains, and note that the tree rings are crowded together toward the outside edge.) We may or may not be in the beginning stages of a long-term drought.

Also, it's worth noting that "average" statistics tell only part of the story. Hot spells, for example, descend upon the county with some regularity, especially in the fall when searing Santa Ana winds come roaring down through the mountain passes toward the coast. This condition occurs when dry air moves southwest from a high-pressure area in the interior U.S. out toward southern California. Flowing across low gaps in the mountains (notably Cajon Pass on the east flank of the San Gabriels, and Soledad Pass south of Palmdale), this air sometimes reaches the coastline or even Santa Catalina Island. As the air moves downward, it compresses and warms about 5°F for every 1000 feet of descent. At Malibu or Santa Monica, daytime highs can soar to 90–100°, rivaling the hottest temperatures recorded nationwide that day. High in the mountains, Santa Anas are much cooler, but they can assume gale and even hurricane force. Mount Wilson has experienced more than a hour of steady winds in the 80–90-mile-per-hour range.

Santa Ana winds spread wildfires easily. Early Santa Anas (October and November) often coincide with the tail end of months of summer drought. Most wildfires in L.A. County are quickly controlled, but the combination of hot winds, dry chaparral, and flammable hillside homes has set the stage time and time again for disasters of monstrous magnitude.

In a similar way, the generally bland average statistics for rainfall fail to reveal the normal situation—which is, metaphorically, feast or famine. A string of drought years can be followed by one or two very wet ones. In wet years much of the moisture received comes in the form of rather short but intense winter storms. A case in point is a monumental downpour recorded in January 1942 at Hoegee's Camp in the Front Range of the San Gabriels: more than 26 inches of rain fell in a 24-hour period. On another occasion in the San Gabriels, a rain gauge collected one inch in one minute. When dumped on steep slopes denuded of vegetation after a fire, such intense rainfall sends "debris flows"—torrents of water, rocks and soil with a consistency of wet aggregate concrete—down through the canyons.

Despite Nature's occasional temper tantrums, more than nine times out of ten your outings in Los Angeles County are likely to coincide with dry weather and temperatures in a moderate register—for at least part of the day. Few other areas around the country, and probably no other great city in the world, can offer such good odds.

**Reading the Rocks**

A good way to approach the subject of L.A. County's geology is to think about the *geomorphology*, or shape and structure, of the landscape. Of California's many geomorphic provinces, the County claims parts of three: the Los Angeles Basin, the Transverse Ranges, and the Mojave Desert. The bulk of the county's urban area dominates the Basin province, while the mostly undeveloped San Gabriel Mountains and semi-developed Santa Monica Mountains (the two containing the majority of the hikes written up in this guide) belong to the Transverse Ranges. Since only a few of

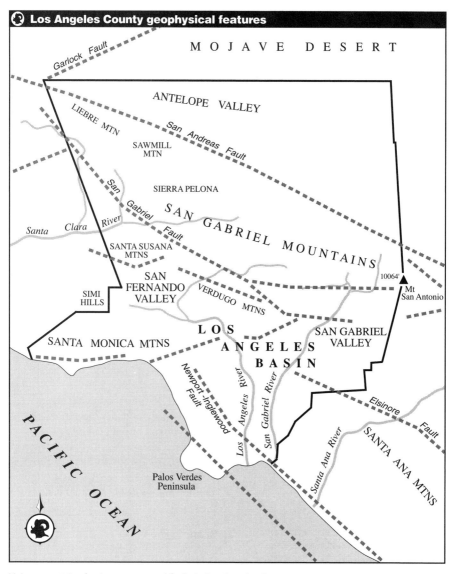

Major mountains, basins, steams, and faults in Los Angeles County

the trips in this guide border on, and none actually touch, the Mojave Desert, it will not be discussed in any detail here.

The Los Angeles Basin province extends from the base of the San Gabriel and Santa Monica Mountains in the north to the Santa Ana Mountains and San Joaquin Hills of Orange County on the south. It's a huge, deeply folded basin filled to a depth of up to 6 miles by some volcanic material and land-deposited sediments, but mostly by sediments of marine origin—sand and mud deposited on the ocean bottom from 80 million years ago to as recently as 1 million years ago.

Then, after uplift during the past 1–2 million years, the surface of the basin accumulated a layer of terrestrial sediment shed from the surrounding hills and mountains. The basin, in fact, would still be filling with sediment today were it not for the installation of flood-control barriers in the mountains, dams to catch debris at the mouths of the canyons, and more than 2000 miles of storm drains and concrete-lined flood channels that carry flood waters to the sea. (Amazingly, some of the sediment cleaned out from behind the flood-control dams is trucked back up into the mountains; there's no room for it down in the city!)

The Transverse Ranges province encompasses in Los Angeles County the Santa Monica and San Gabriel mountains, plus the mini-ranges of Liebre Mountain, Sawmill Mountain, and Sierra Pelona lying northwest of the San Gabriels. Outside L.A. County, the province takes in part of the coastal mountains of Santa Barbara and Ventura County, and the San Bernardino and Little San Bernardino mountains. As indicated by the name "Transverse," these east-west trending mountains stand crosswise to the usual northwest-southeast grain of California's other major mountain groups—Coast Ranges, Sierra Nevada, and Peninsular Ranges. This "kink" in the alignment of California's mountains is mirrored by a similar east-west jog in the San Andreas Fault, which defines the north edge of the San Gabriel Mountains.

The San Andreas Fault, of course, represents the boundary between two of the earth's major tectonic plates—the largely oceanic Pacific Plate and the largely continental North American Plate. For at least 10 million years, lands on the west side of the boundary have been sliding (often lurching) northwest relative to lands on the east side. Currently the average rate of movement is about 2 inches per year—enough, if it continues, to put Los Angeles abreast of San Francisco about 10 million years from now. A growing body of evidence now suggests that the movements along the San Andreas Fault do not simply involve one plate slipping past another; they also produce compression, which accelerates and possibly controls the process of mountain building along the central and southern California coast. In the area of the kink, centered on the San Gabriel Mountains, the compression forces are greatest. In this view, the San Gabriels are being squeezed horizontally about a tenth of an inch each year, and being thrust upward much more rapidly than that. At the same time, the Los Angeles Basin, which is underlain by folded and crumpled structures under its blanket of sediment, may be losing an average of a quarter acre per year due to compression.

The kink in the San Andreas Fault, and therefore in the alignment of the coastal mountains, might be explained by the fact that the part of the North American Plate over Nevada and Utah is stretching and spreading outward because it is thin and is closer to the earth's mantle there. The western Mojave Desert, which rides on the western edge of the North American Plate, may be jamming against the plate boundary, producing the kink.

Regardless of what has pushed them to their present heights, the mountains of the Transverse Range are relatively young as upthrust units—only a few million years old. This is not true of the ages of most of the rocks that compose them. The oldest rock found exposed in the Santa Monica Mountains—Santa Monica Slate—checks out at about 150 million years. Some rocks in the San Gabriels are representative of the oldest found on the Pacific Coast—over 600 million years of age.

The geologic history of the San Gabriels, which have been called the most complicated mountain range in North America, may never be fully deciphered. As one expert put it, "The San Gabes look like a flake kicked around on plate boundaries for hundreds of millions of years."

Caught in the tectonic frenzy of the moment, San Gabriel Mountains are surging upward as fast as any mountain range on earth, They are also disintegrating at a spectacular rate. Although they consist mainly of durable granitic rocks, much like those in the sturdy Sierra Nevada, the San Gabriel rocks have been through a tectonic meat grinder. Like mountains made of soft material, the tops of the San Gabriels are rounded. But the slopes are often appallingly steep and unstable. An average of 7 tons of material disappears from each acre of the front face each year, most of it coming to rest behind debris barriers and dams below. As you hike through the San Gabriel Mountains, and also the Santa Monicas (which to a lesser degree suffer erosion problems), the ultimate futility of dam-building, road-building, even trail-building in many places will become readily apparent. Like sand-castles waiting for the next ocean tide, the manmade improvements and even the natural vegetation clinging to mountain slopes wait for advancing tides of fire, flood, and earthquake to sweep them away.

### Native Gardens

As mentioned earlier, Los Angeles County's varied climate, topography, and geology have set the stage for a remarkable diversity of plants. There's a second reason too: Los Angeles County, and coastal Southern California for that matter, lies between two major groups of flora: a southern group represented by drought-tolerant plants characteristic of northern Mexico, and a northern group represented by moisture-loving plants typical of the Sierra Nevada and California's north coastal ranges. As the climate fluctuated, seesawing from cool and wet to warm and dry over the past million years or so, species from both groups invaded the present-day county borders. Once established, many of these species remained in protected niches even as the climate turned unfavorable for them. Some survived unchanged; others evolved into unique forms. Some are present today only in very specific habitats.

Several common, widely distributed trees—gray pine, limber pine, bigleaf maple, valley oak, and California buckeye—reach their southernmost limits on the Pacific coast in or near Los Angeles County. California walnut and bigcone Douglas-fir, the former a foothill-dwelling tree and the latter an inhabitant of the higher mountains, have more restricted ranges centered approximately on the L.A. Basin. The Joshua tree, the trademark of the Mojave Desert, reaches its westernmost limit near Interstate 5 in northern L.A. County, and is widely distributed in the Antelope Valley and along the northern base of the San Gabriels.

The bulk of Los Angeles County's undeveloped and naturally vegetated land can be grouped into several general classes, which botanists often call plant communities or plant associations. In a broader sense, these are biological communities, because they include animals as well as plants. Several of the major plant communities in the county are briefly described, in the order you would encounter them on a journey from the coast, up into the San Gabriel High Country, and then down to the desert.

The *sage-scrub* (or coastal sage-scrub) community lies mostly below 2000 feet elevation, on south-facing slopes in the Santa Monica Mountains, the Simi Hills, the Santa Susana Mountains, and on some of

Sacred Datura

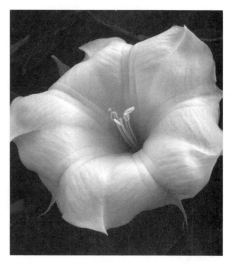

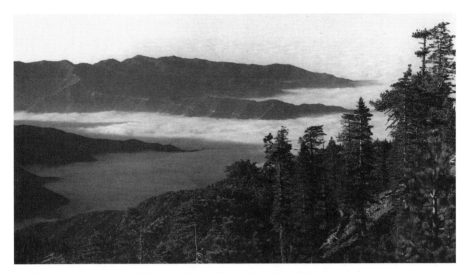

Coniferous forest (above) and chaparral (below) in the San Gabriel Mountains

the lower, hotter slopes of the San Gabriel Mountains. The dominant plants are small shrubs, typically California sagebrush, black sage, white sage, and California buckwheat. Two larger shrubs often present are laurel sumac and lemonade berry, which, like poison oak, are members of the sumac family. In some areas along the coast, prickly-pear cactus thrives within this community. Interspersed among the somewhat pliable and loosely distributed shrubs is a variety of grasses and wildflowers, green and colorful during the rainy season, but dry and withered during the summer and early fall drought. Much of the sage-scrub vegetation is "summer-deciduous"—dormant and dead-looking during the warmer half of the year, lush green and aromatic during the cool, wet half.

The *chaparral* community is commonly found between 1000 and 5000 feet elevation just about anywhere there's a slope that hasn't burned recently. Were it not for roads, firebreaks, and other interruptions, the chaparral would run in wide unbroken swaths along the flanks of most of the county's mountains. At low elevations, chaparral (which requires more moisture than sage-scrub) tends to stick to slopes protected from the full glare of the sun. At

higher elevations, which get more rainfall, chaparral takes over the south slopes, while oaks and conifers thrive on slopes receiving less sun. The dominant chaparral plants include chamise, scrub oak, manzanita, toyon, mountain mahogany, and various forms of ceanothus ("wild lilac"). Yuccas, known for their spectacular candle-shaped blooms, often frequent the chaparral zones. The chaparral plants are tough and intricately branched, evergreen shrubs with deep root systems that help the plants survive during the long, hot summers. Chaparral is sometimes referred to as "elfin forest"—a good description of a mature stand. Without benefit of a trail, travel through mature chaparral, which is often 15 feet high and incredibly dense all the way up from the ground, is almost impossible.

The *coniferous forest,* which has two phases in Los Angeles County, takes over roughly above 4000 feet elevation, at least in areas with sufficient rainfall. The "yellow-pine" phase includes conifers such as bigcone Douglas-fir, ponderosa pine, Jeffrey pine, sugar pine, incense cedar, and white fir, and forms tall, open forest. These species are often intermixed with live oaks, California bay (bay laurel), and scattered chaparral shrubs such as manzanita and mountain mahogany. Higher than about 8000 feet, in the "lodgepole-pine" phase, lodgepole pine, white fir, and limber pine are the indicator trees. These trees, somewhat shorter and more weather-beaten than those below, exist in small, sometimes dense stands, interspersed with such shrubs as chinquapin, snowbrush, and manzanita.

*Pinyon-juniper woodland* is found in narrow zones bordering the Antelope Valley and along the semi-arid Soledad Canyon area southwest of Palmdale, elevation roughly 3000–5000 feet. Here are found a couple of rather stunted conifers—the one-leafed pinyon pine and the California juniper. Usually these trees do not predominate, but are mixed with typical chaparral shrubs.

*Joshua tree woodland,* found in scattered locales along the north base of the San Gabriel Mountains, and more abundantly on rocky hills poking up from the Antelope Valley floor, is dominated by an outsized member of the yucca family—the Joshua tree. (L.A. County's best spot to view them is Saddleback Butte State Park east of Lancaster—not covered in this guidebook.)

Aside from this coast-to-desert cross-section of plant communities, there are others of more restricted range:

*Southern oak woodland,* widely distributed in coastal and inland valleys and on some of the mountains near Antelope Valley's western tip, consists of dense to open groves of live oak, valley oak (near the coast), black oak (near the desert), and California walnut trees. Scattered conifers such as Coulter pine, gray pine, and bigcone Douglas-fir intermix with the oaks in some areas.

*Riparian* (streamside) *woodland,* one of the rarest (in terms of the land it covers) communities, thrives at lower and mid-elevations where water is always present on or close to the surface. Massive live oaks, sycamores, alders, bigleaf maples and cottonwoods, and a screen of water-hugging willows are the hallmarks of riparian woodland. Not only is this kind of environment essential for the continued survival of many kinds of birds, animals, and fish, it is also very appealing to the senses. Riparian woodland is somewhat reminiscent of Eastern forests, with a palpable sense of dampness year round. Much of this habitat in Southern California has been destroyed or is threatened by continued urbanization and attendant development of water resources or flood-control measures.

Other communities found in snippets along the coast or far afield in the Mojave Desert are *rocky shore, coastal strand, coastal salt marsh, freshwater marsh, grassland, sagebrush scrub, creosote-bush scrub,* and *alkali sink.* In many places in the foothills and mountains of the county you will also find planted trees introduced from other parts of the world. Eucalyptus, pepper, and other exotic trees are often on the sites of many old ranches, while many roadsides, especially in the Angeles National Forest, have been planted with drought-resistant cypress trees and non-native pines. Some of the non-urbanized areas of the county are natural grasslands given over to agriculture and grazing. In areas characterized by heavy grazing, one finds grassy flats and bald slopes—sometimes called *potreros* (pastures)—supporting mostly non-native vegetation like wild oats, filaree, fennel, mustard, and thistle.

Early-to-mid spring is the best time to appreciate the cornucopia of Los Angeles County's plant life. Many of the showiest species—spring wildflowers, for example—brighten the sage-scrub and chaparral zones at that time, and other plants exhibit fresh new growth. Peak periods for wildflowers vary according to elevation, slope, and proximity to coastal fogs. Generally, April is the best month.

One of the county's best wildflower spots (not covered in the trip descriptions that follow) is the Antelope Valley California Poppy Reserve, a small state park west of Lancaster. Parched and uninspiring 10 or 11 months of the year, it comes alive (in years of average rainfall or better) with carpets of orange poppies around April. These desert-

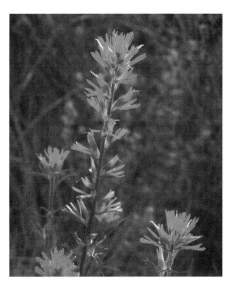

Indian Paintbrush

dwelling members of a species that is more at home in the valleys and hills of central California evidently invaded the Antelope Valley through low-elevation passes to the west.

## Creatures Great and Small

One's first sighting of a mountain lion, a bighorn sheep, an eagle, or any other seldom-seen form of wildlife is always a memorable experience. Because of the diversity and generally broad extent of its habitats, and the inaccessibility of many of its wilderness areas, Los Angeles County plays host to a healthy population of indigenous creatures. If you're willing to stretch your legs a bit and spend some time in areas favored by wild animals, you'll eventually be rewarded with some kind of close visual contact.

The most numerous large creature in the county is the mule deer, with a population of at least several thousand. Deer are abundant in areas of mixed forest and scattered chaparral up in the higher mountains, and also close to the coast in the Santa Monica Mountains. Deer like to have a protective screen of vegetation near them at all times, and a good supply of tasty leaves to munch

on, so you won't often see them in wide-open spaces.

The mountain lion, once hunted to near-extinction in California, has made a substantial comeback. In Los Angeles County perhaps two dozen lions roam the San Gabriel Mountains, and a few more have been spotted in the Santa Monica Mountains. They're secretive, but wide-ranging creatures, so you're much more likely to spot the tracks of this cat than meet one face to face. Still, several serious attacks and two fatalities involving mountain lions have occurred in California in the last two decades, so caution is warranted (learn more about this in the next section: Health, Safety, and Courtesy).

Bobcats, which pose no danger unless cornered and harassed, are encountered on occasion in L.A.'s wild spaces, scampering through the canyons of the Santa Monicas or zipping across the Angeles Crest Highway at night.

A number of black bears (some of them "problem bears" deported from Yosemite, and others apparently the result of gradual migration south from the Sierra Nevada) inhabit the deeper canyons of the San Gabriels. They can be a nuisance at the both the developed campgrounds and the trail campgrounds of Angeles National Forest.

Coyotes are universally abundant, adapting to just about any habitat (except the urban core) with ease. At the foot of the mountains, where the urban-wildland interface is often a matter of a backyard fence or the curb of a cul-de-sac, coyotes make regular forays into the suburbs to snatch small pets or obtain water and food left unattended.

The county's most interesting (and surprisingly abundant) large mammal is the bighorn sheep. Several hundred of these agile animals maintain a tough existence on the steep slopes and rocky crags of the San Gabriel Mountains. Unlike mule deer, the bighorn prefer lightly vegetated, rugged terrain, on which they are capable of escaping almost any predator. They also shun contact with humans, although it's not unusual to spot them quite near such popular High Country summits as Mount Williamson and Mount Baden-Powell. The sheep are superbly adapted to surviving on meager supplies of water and coarse vegetation, conditions that characterize the San Gabriel and Sheep Mountain wilderness areas, which were set aside partly for their benefit.

The county's mammals also include gray fox, raccoon, and various rabbits, squirrels, woodrats, and mice. Amphibians include tree frogs, salamanders, and pond turtles. Many streams supporting populations of rainbow trout exist in the San Gabriels. Some are artificially stocked to meet the demand of fishermen; others are natural fisheries where catch-and-release is the only method allowed. The tiny, unarmored three-spine stickleback, an endangered species, inhabits streams in Soledad and Bouquet canyons.

Among the commonly seen reptiles are rattlesnakes, discussed in the next section.

Bird life is varied in the county, not only because of the coast-to-desert range of habitats, but also because the county lies along the Pacific Flyway route of spring-fall migration and also serves some overwintering birds.

Los Angeles County is also an ancestral home of several other creatures symbolic of wild America. The California condor, a large vulture with a wingspan of up to 9 feet, was commonly seen over the San Gabriel and Santa Monica Mountains in the 19th Century. By the 1980s the condor population statewide had declined so precipitously that the remaining few condors were captured, taken to zoos, and bred in captivity with the eventual goal of returning their offspring to the wild. This last-ditch strategy worked. Now there are hundreds of California condors, some housed in zoos and many others released into the wild areas of Arizona, central and Southern California, and Baja California. Peregrine falcons are another comeback success story. These birds, which can achieve speeds of 200 miles per hour when diving for prey, have established nests on L.A. skyscrapers, as well as on secluded cliffs in Southern California's mountains.

Hunted and trapped with vigor until the late 19th Century, grizzly bears were once the terror of the San Gabriel Mountains. (Thankfully for hikers, they won't return.) Also gone are the pronghorn antelope that once wintered in the Antelope Valley. Unaccustomed to barriers in their natural open habitat, the pronghorn would not cross or jump over even the most trivial obstacles. Fences and railroads built across Mojave Desert migration routes sealed their fate—death by starvation.

## HEALTH, SAFETY, AND COURTESY

Good preparation is always important for any kind of recreational pursuit, and hiking Southern California's backcountry is no exception. Although most of our local environments are usually not hostile or dangerous to life and limb, there are some pitfalls to be aware of.

### Preparation and Equipment

An obvious safety requirement is being in good health. Some degree of physical conditioning is always desirable, even for the trips in this book designated as easy or moderate. The more challenging trips, rated moderately strenuous to very strenuous, require stamina and occasionally some technical expertise. Fast walking, running, bicycling, swimming, inline skating, aerobic dancing, or any similar exercise that develops both the leg muscles and the aerobic capacity of the whole body are recommended as preparatory exercise.

For long trips over rough, cross-country terrain (there are several of these in this book) there is no really adequate way to prepare other than practicing the activity itself. Start with easy- or moderate-length cross-country trips first to accustom the leg muscles to the peculiar stresses involved in walking over uneven terrain and scram-

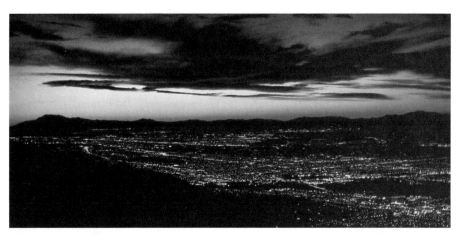

Los Angeles city lights from Mount Lowe

bling over boulders, and to acquire a good sense of balance. Sturdy hiking boots are recommended for such travel.

Several of the hiking trips in this book reach elevations of 7000 feet or more—altitudes at which sea-level folks may notice a big difference in their rate of breathing and their energy. A few hours or a day spent at altitude before exercising will help almost anyone acclimate, but that's often impractical for short day trips. Still, you might consider spending a night at Buckhorn Campground (6450′) or Crystal Lake Campground (5800′) before taking a hike along the Angeles Crest, or at Manker Flats Campground (6000′) before tackling Old Baldy. Altitude sickness strikes some victims at elevations as low as 8000 feet. If you become dizzy or nauseous, or suffer from congested lungs or a severe headache, the antidote may be as simple as descending one or two thousand feet.

Your choice of equipment and supplies on the longer hikes in this book can be critically important. The essentials you should carry with you at all times in the backcountry are the things that would allow you to survive, in a reasonably comfortable manner, one or two unscheduled nights out. It's important to note that no one ever plans these nights! No one plans to get lost, injured, stuck, or pinned down by the weather. Always do a "what if" analysis for a worst-case scenario, and plan accordingly. These essential items are your safety net; keep them with you on dayhikes, and take them with you in a small day pack if you leave your backpack and camping equipment behind at a campsite.

Chief among the essential items is *warm clothing*. Inland Los Angeles County is characterized by wide swings in day and night temperatures. In mountain valleys, for example, a midday temperature in the 70s or 80s can be followed by a subfreezing night. Layer your clothing: it is better to take along two or more middleweight outer garments than rely on a single heavy or bulky jacket to keep you comfortable at all times. Add to this a cap, gloves, and a waterproof or water-resistant shell (a large trash bag will do in a pinch) and you'll be quite prepared for all but the most severe weather experienced in Southern California.

In hot, sunny weather, sun-shielding clothing is another "essential." This would normally include a sun hat and a light-colored, long-sleeve top.

*Water* and *food* are next in importance. Most streams and even some springs in the mountains have been shown to contain unacceptably high levels of bacteria or other contaminants. Even though some of the remote watersheds are probably pristine, it's wise to treat by filtering or chemical methods any water obtained outside of developed camp or picnic sites. Unless the day is very warm or your trip is a long one, it's usually easiest to carry (preferably in sturdy plastic bottles) all the water you'll need. Don't underestimate your water needs: during a full day's hike in 80° temperatures you may require as much as a gallon of water. Food is needed to stave off hunger and keep energy stores up, but it is not as essential as water in a survival situation.

Down the list further, but still "essential," are a *map* and *compass* (or a GPS unit and the knowledge of its use); *flashlight; fire-starting devices* (examples: waterproof matches or lighter, and candle); and *first-aid kit.*

Items not always essential, but potentially very useful and convenient, are sunglasses, pocket knife, whistle (or other signaling device), sunscreen, and toilet paper. A cell phone may be of use in an emergency, but be aware that it may fail to work for one reason or another, or you could easily be out of range of an antenna relay in just about any remote location.

The essential items mentioned above should be carried by every member of a hiking party, because individuals or splinter groups may end up separating from the party for one reason or another. If you plan to hike solo in the backcountry, being well-equipped is very important. If you hike alone, be sure to check in with a park ranger or leave your itinerary with a responsible person. In that way, if you do get stuck, help will probably come to the right place—eventually.

## Special Hazards

Other than getting lost or pinned down by a sudden storm, the four most common hazards found in the L.A. County backcountry are steep, unstable terrain; icy terrain; rattlesnakes; and poison oak.

Exploring some parts of the San Gabriel Mountains—even by way of the trails—involves travel over structurally weak rock on steep slopes. The erosive effects of flowing water, of wedging by roots and by ice, and of brush fires tend to pulverize such rock even further. Slips on such terrain usually lead to sliding down a hillside some distance. If you explore cross-country, always be on the lookout for dangerous run-outs, such as cliffs, below you. The side-walls of many canyons in the San Gabriels may look like nice places to practice rock-climbing moves, but this misconception has contributed to many deaths over the years.

Statistically, mishaps associated with snow and ice have caused the greatest number of fatalities in the San Gabriel Mountains. This is not because the San Gabriels are somehow inherently more dangerous than other ranges. Rather, it is because inexperienced lowlanders, never picturing their backyard mountains as true wilderness areas, are attracted here by the novelty of snow and the easy access by way of snow-plowed highways. Icy chutes and slopes capable of avalanching can easily trap such visitors unaware. Winter travel in the more gentle areas of the high country can be accomplished on snowshoes or skis; but the steeper slopes require technical skills and equipment such as ice axe and crampons, just as in any other high mountain range.

Rattlesnakes are fairly common in most parts of Los Angeles County below about 7000 feet. Seldom seen in either cold or very hot weather, they favor temperatures in the 75–90° range—mostly spring through fall in the lower areas, and summer in the higher mountains. Most rattlesnakes are as interested in avoiding contact with you as you are with them. The more hazardous areas include rocky canyon bottoms with running streams. Watch carefully where you put your feet, and especially your hands, during the warmer months. In brushy or rocky areas where sight distance is short, try to make your presence known from afar. Tread with heavy footfalls, or use a stick to bang against rocks or bushes. Rattlesnakes will pick up the vibrations through their skin and will usually buzz (unmistakably) before you get too close for comfort.

Poison oak grows profusely along many of the county's canyons below 5000 feet. It is often found on the banks of streamcourses in the form of a bush or vine, where it prefers semi-shady habitats. Quite often, it's seen beside or encroaching on well-used trails. Learn to recognize its distinctive three-leafed structure, and avoid touching it with skin or clothing. Since poison oak loses its leaves during the winter months (and sometimes during summer and fall drought), but still retains some of the toxic oil in its stems, it can be extra hazardous at that time because it is harder to identify and avoid. Mid-weight pants, like blue jeans, and a long-sleeve shirt will serve as a fair barrier against the toxic oil of the poison oak plant. Do, of course, remove these clothes as soon as the hike is over, and make sure they are washed carefully afterward.

Here are a few more tips:

Ticks can sometimes be a scourge of overgrown trails in the sage-scrub and chaparral country, particularly during the first warm spells of the year, when they climb to the tips of shrub branches and lie in wait for warm-blooded hosts. Ticks are especially abundant along trails used by cattle, deer, or coyotes. If you can't avoid brushing against vegetation along the trail, be sure to check yourself for ticks frequently. Upon finding a host, a tick will usually crawl upward in search of a protected spot, where it will try to attach itself. If you can be aware of the slightest irritations on your body, you'll usually intercept ticks long before they attempt to bite.

For decades, encounters with mountain lions (cougars) were almost never reported in Southern California. This began to change in the 1990s, due, in part certainly, to an increase in cougar population, a decrease in cougar habitat (especially in areas where suburban and rural housing development is increasing), and abnormal geographic displacement of deer, a prime source of food for cougars.

Several incidents involving cougars stalking or menacing campers, hikers, and mountain bikers have occurred throughout Southern California in the last 20 years. In the worst such incident, a woman was attacked and killed by a cougar while hiking near Cuyamaca Peak in San Diego County. The following precautions are urged for all persons entering cougar country, which may include virtually every non-urban Los Angeles County locale:

- Hike with one or more companions.
- Keep children close at hand.
- Never run from a cougar. This may trigger an instinct to attack.
- Make yourself "large," face the animal, maintain eye contact with it, shout, blow a whistle, and do not act fearful. Do anything to convince the animal that you are not its prey.

Despite the recent interest in and the increased use of hiking trails in Los Angeles County, there is paradoxically less money (especially in Angeles National Forest) for building and maintaining them. Much of that work is left to volunteer crews nowadays. In the chaparral areas, trails can become overgrown quickly, so that travel along them can become an exercise in bushwhacking. Traveling certain trail-less canyon bottoms and ridgelines also involves some bushwhacking. Blue jeans (despite their reputation as being worthless in cold, wet conditions) are very good at protecting your legs when you're dodging or pushing through dry chaparral.

## Camping and Permits

Overnight camping in roadside campgrounds is not always a restful experience. Off-season camping (late fall through early spring) offers relief from crowds, but not from chilly nighttime weather. Campgrounds in Angeles National Forest are less well supervised than those in the

Santa Monica Mountains, and therefore sometimes attract a noisy crowd. In my experience, facilities with a "campground host" promise a better clientele, and a better night's sleep.

The nice advantage of a developed campground is that you can always have a campfire there—unless the facility itself is closed. On the national forest trails, campfires are allowed most of the year in the stoves provided at trail camps or on ground cleared to bare mineral soil to a 5-foot radius (campfire builders must also carry a shovel to bury the embers). Fire permits, valid for the length of a fire season, must be obtained from the Forest Service for the use of any campfire or flame device (camp stoves, gas lanterns) on the trail from May 15 to the first soaking rains of the following fall or winter. Often during that period, a "very high fire danger" is declared and Stage I restrictions go into affect which prohibit open wood fires, but allow the operation of gas stoves in the above-mentioned cleared areas. "Extreme fire danger" conditions may either close parts of National Forest areas to all entry, or result in Stage II restrictions for campers—no fire use of any kind outside of developed recreation sites.

Be aware that any jurisdiction—national forest, state, county, city, or private—may declare fire closures in which all access is prohibited during critical fire conditions. Call first if you're in doubt.

Angeles National Forest allows "remote," primitive-style camping: under this policy, you are not restricted to staying at a developed campground or designated trail camp. For sanitation reasons, you are required to locate your primitive camp at least 200 feet from the nearest source of water. And, of course, you must observe the fire regulations stated earlier. Contact the Forest Service to confirm these rules if you intend to do any remote camping.

Most federally managed wilderness areas around the state require special wilderness permits for entry. At present, however, permits are not required for San Gabriel Wilderness, nor for Sheep Mountain Wilderness *except* at the East Fork Station gateway, where self-registering permits are offered. Cucamonga Wilderness in San Bernardino County (included in one hike in this book) does require a wilderness permit.

**Other Regulations**

This book contains much trail information of interest to mountain bikers. Mountain-biking regulations, however, vary according to jurisdiction. Currently, bikes are allowed on all Angeles National Forest roads and trails except the Pacific Crest Trail and trails within wilderness areas. Elsewhere, bikes are usually permitted on fire roads, but not on "single-track" trails. Mountain bikers should yield the right-of-way to both hikers and equestrians.

Deer hunting season in Angeles National Forest occurs during mid-autumn. Although conflicts between hunters and hikers are rare, you may want to confine your explorations at that time to the state, county, and city parks, where hunting is prohibited.

Once allowed over a wide area of the mountains, target shooting is now legally restricted to a small number of private shooting ranges and designated shooting areas in Angeles National Forest. Some illegal shooting continues to take place in canyons just off some of the mountain highways. Try to report this kind of activity to the sheriff or a ranger. Shooting in the lawful pursuit of game is easy to distinguish from automatic-weapon fire in undesignated areas.

**For Your Protection**

There is always some risk in leaving a vehicle in an unattended area. Automobile vandalism, burglary, and theft are small but distinct possibilities. Report all theft and vandalism of personal property to the county sheriff, and report vandalism of public property to the appropriate park or forest agency.

Obviously it is unwise to leave valuable property in an automobile. To prevent theft of the car, you can disable your car's ignition system or use a locking device on the steering wheel. Many of the routes in this book are written up as one-way, point-to-point trips requiring either a car shuttle (leaving cars at both ends) or an arrangement by which someone drops you off and later picks you up. Choose the latter method if you're concerned about security.

### Trail Courtesy

Whenever you travel in the natural areas of the county, you take on a burden of responsibility—keeping the backcountry as you found it. Aside from common-sense prohibitions against littering, vandalism, and illegal fires, there are some less obvious guidelines every hiker should be aware of. We'll mention a few:

Never cut trail switchbacks. This practice breaks down the trail tread and hastens erosion. Improve designated trails by removing branches, rocks, or other debris if you can. Springtime growth can quite rapidly obscure pathways in the chaparral country, and funding for trail maintenance is often scarce—so try to do your part by joining a volunteer trail crew or by performing your own small maintenance tasks while walking the trails.

Report any damage to trails or other facilities to the appropriate ranger office.

When backpacking, be a "no trace" camper. Leave your campsite as you found it—or leave it in an even more natural condition.

Collecting specimens of minerals, plants, animals, and historical objects without special permit is prohibited in state and county parks. This means common things, too, such as pine cones, wildflowers, and lizards. These should be left for all visitors to enjoy. Some limited collecting of items like pine cones may be allowed on the national forest lands—check first.

We've covered most of the general regulations associated with the use of the public lands in Los Angeles County. But you, as a visitor, are responsible for knowing any additional rules as well. The capsulized summary for each hike described in this book includes a reference to the agency responsible for the area you'll be visiting. Addresses and phone numbers for those agencies appear in Appendix 4.

### Where and When to Go

Clearly, two of the most detrimental aspects of living in most parts of Los Angeles are air pollution and traffic congestion. Air pollution affects, to a greater or lesser

The Gabrielino Trail above Oakwilde

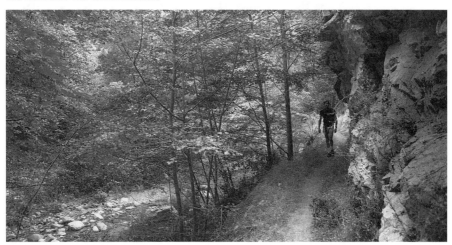

degree, all of the trips in this book, and traffic congestion affects (at least at certain times) how quickly you can escape the city and be on your merry way down the trail. In this section we'll look into some of the strategies you can use to sidestep these difficulties and also take advantage of optimum conditions of weather and visibility.

Beating the traffic is not too difficult once you're out of the urban core. On weekdays, the flow of automobiles is mostly inward toward congested parts of the city during the morning, and outward during the afternoon and evening. Driving out of town early on weekend mornings is a breeze, but getting back into town later in the afternoon can be a bit problematical.

Nearly all the trails of Los Angeles County are refreshingly underutilized on weekdays. Sometimes you can walk for hours without seeing another traveler. Fair-weather weekends bring large numbers of people to a relatively small number of popular trailheads, while other trailheads have plenty of room for parking. Chantry Flat and Sunset Ridge (Millard Canyon), both easily accessible from San Gabriel Valley communities, have outside gates that can and do close to incoming traffic whenever the parking situation gets intolerable. The moral of all this is: hike on weekdays when you can, or on weekends as long as you get an early start.

There's a strong belief, even among most Southern Californians, that summer equals the hiking season. This prejudice probably comes from the fact that so many Southland residents have emigrated from other areas where this may be true. Actually, summer is the worst season to visit most of the wild lands of Los Angeles County. Summer and early fall is a time of drought, when much of the chaparral and scrub vegetation blanketing the mountain slopes turns drab and crispy, and the land bakes under a near-vertical sun. Summer hikes can be rewarding, however, if the trip is not long, and you get an early-morning start.

Summer—early summer especially—is fine for areas above 6000 feet or 7000 feet. Some of the highest elevations in the San Gabriel Mountains don't experience much of a "summer" at all, the snows of winter disappearing in July or not long before the first subfreezing nights of September or October. Summer is also a perfectly good time to visit the beaches, and the lower slopes and canyons of the Santa Monica

Oak woodland, Solstice Canyon

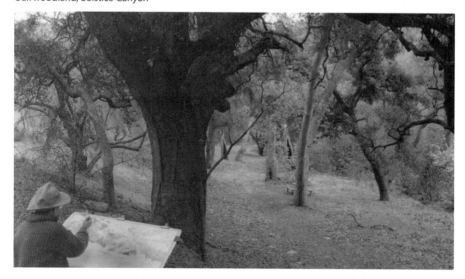

Mountains that benefit from the coastal breezes.

Late fall brings autumn color to the oak woodlands and wet canyons of the county. The leaves of the valley oak, black oak, and walnut turn a crispy yellow in the valleys and on the hillsides. Bigleaf maples, cottonwoods, willows and sycamores contribute similar hues to canyon bottoms spotted with red-leafed poison oak vines. This is a time when the marine layer over the coastline and basin often lies low (at least in the morning) while the air above can be extraordinarily clean and dry.

Instead of suffering through days-long episodes of bad weather in winter, we Southern Californians usually experience a string of sunny days interspersed with short, rainy spells. Some storms are followed by very clear weather along with cold winds from the north. This is when you should "seize the moment": hop in the car, and head for a trail in the nearby foothills or mountains leading to some prominent high point. The views will often stretch from snow-covered peaks to the island-dotted Pacific Ocean.

Spring comes on gradually, each week a little warmer (with a heat wave or two tossed in) and a little hazier. The marine layer is thicker now, but superb views are still possible from mile-high summits in the San Gabriels such as Mount Lowe and Strawberry Peak. Sunrises can be dramatic up there, with much of the surrounding lowland enveloped in a bank of low clouds. Annual wildflowers seem to pop up everywhere, wild lilacs paint the hillsides white and blue, and the scents of sage and nectar float on the air. When the marine layer is very deep, fogs bearing light drizzle may envelop the canyons of the Santa Monicas and San Gabriels, like the mists of Sherwood Forest. The High Country is often snowbound through May, although it may be possible to approach some of the passes and high points by way of southern routes.

In any season, the infamous Los Angeles smog can seriously affect your enjoyment of wild areas. At worst, the eye-smarting, lung-irritating air can turn an otherwise pristine watershed into one that looks like a hellish abyss. Strict emissions controls implemented over the past three decades have resulted in dramatic improvements in the air quality; still, the Los Angeles region is noted for having the poorest air quality in the nation. So for now and in the future, a good strategy is simply to try to evade the smog by judicious choices of where and when to go.

Often, that's not very hard. Prevailing ocean breezes keep the western Santa Monica Mountains fairly clean most of the year. The High Country and northern slopes of the San Gabriels are more affected by marine air moving up the Santa Clara River valley than by dirty air blown in from the city. For example, Charlton-Chilao Recreation Area, just 10 air-line miles from the edge of the L.A. Basin, gets an average of only about 40 slightly smoggy days a year.

Air pollution often and seriously affects such L.A.-Basin-bordering areas as Griffith Park, the Verdugo Mountains, the Santa Susana Mountains, the Puente Hills, and the Front Range of the San Gabriels. But there are clear spells as well. Much of the smog originating in the L.A. Basin is photochemically produced (sunlight reacting on automobile exhaust gases), so morning air tends to be cleaner than afternoon air. Weekends are a little cleaner than weekdays, because traffic volumes are somewhat reduced.

When the weather is stable, and a strong temperature inversion (warmer air overlying cooler air) exists, the smog-bearing marine layer stays close to the ground until about midday. By afternoon local sea breezes are transporting it east to Riverside and San Bernardino counties, and up the Front Range canyons and slopes.

Less commonly, regional winds kick the smog north or northeast into the Antelope Valley, west along the Malibu coast to Oxnard and Ventura, or south as far as San

Diego. Sometimes smog covers the whole county as a gauzy curtain, but more often it lies quite close to the ground in a localized area, leaving upwind areas with clear, blue skies.

An awareness of wind and weather patterns can help you decide where to find the cleanest air. Failing that, you can always set forth with a "plan B" as well as "plan A." While doing field work for this book, I usually kept sets of maps for at least two widely separate areas of the county in my car. Plan B was successfully invoked several times.

## Using This Book

Whether you wish to use this book as a reference tool or as a guide to be read cover to cover, you should take a few minutes to read this section. Herein I explain the meaning of the capsulized information that appears before each trip description, and also describe the way in which trips are grouped together geographically.

One way to expedite the process of finding a suitable trip, especially if you're unfamiliar with hiking opportunities in Los Angeles County, is to turn to Appendix 1, "Best Hikes." This is a cross-reference of the most highly recommended hikes described in this book.

Each of the 200 hiking trips belongs to one of 29 geographical areas, which are organized as chapters in this book. Each chapter has its own introductory text and map. The chapters are grouped according to "regions" within Los Angeles County. Chapters 1 and 2 cover the county's coastline areas. Chapters 3–11 cover the "basin and foothill" areas, which include the L.A. Basin and the small mountain ranges bordering it. Chapters 12–16 encompass the majority of the Santa Monica Mountains. Chapters 17–27 cover the Angeles National

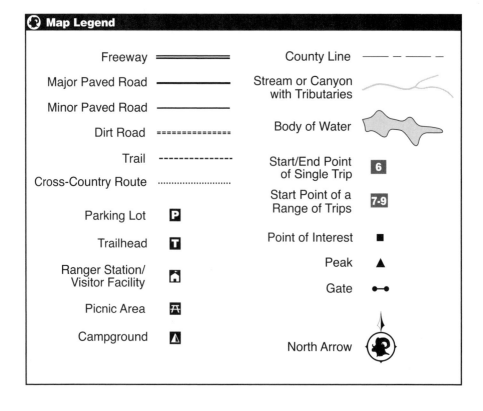

Forest, which is nearly synonymous with the San Gabriel Mountains. Chapter 28 and 29 cover a small number of hikes on Santa Catalina Island, which technically belongs to Los Angeles County.

Since the easternmost Santa Monicas (Griffith Park and the Hollywood Hills) lie cheek-by-jowl next to the urban basin, I've grouped these areas with the basin and foothills region. The Santa Monica Mountains region of this book includes a few hikes that spill over into Ventura County, so as to preserve the integrity of coverage of the Santa Monica Mountains National Recreation Area. Also, the Angeles National Forest region picks up two hikes along the L.A.-Ventura county line (partly in Los Padres National Forest) and three hikes just beyond the L.A.-San Bernardino county line.

The index map of Los Angeles County and vicinity (on pages vi and vii) shows the coverage of each chapter map, and the Contents shows the page numbers for each region, chapter, and trip.

The introductory text for each area includes any general information about the area's history, geology, plants, and wildlife not included in the trip descriptions. Important information about possible restrictions or special requirements (wilderness permits, for example) appears here, too, and you should review this material before starting on a hike in a particular chapter. In particular, you should be aware that nearly all trips on Angeles National Forest land require that you post a "National Forest Adventure Pass" on your parked car. The rules are constantly in a state of flux—but basically, visitors must purchase an adventure pass (parking permit) for the privilege of parking their cars along roadsides, in picnic grounds, or at trailheads in any national forest in Southern California. The permit, which costs $5 daily or $30 yearly, can be purchased at any national forest office or ranger station, and at virtually every Southern California outdoor equipment and sports vendor.

Each chapter also contains a sketch map of the locations and routes of all hikes in the area covered by that chapter. The numbers in the squares on those maps correspond to trip numbers in the text. These boxed numbers refer to the start/end points of out-and-back and loop trips. The point-to-point trips have two boxed numbers, indicating separate start and end points. For some hikes, the corresponding chapter map alone is complete enough and fully adequate for navigation; for other hikes, more detailed topographical or other maps are recommended. A legend for the maps appears on page 18.

## Capsulized Information

The following is an explanation of capsulized information appearing at the beginning of each trip description. If you're simply browsing through this book, these summaries alone can be used as a tool to eliminate from consideration hikes that are either too difficult, or perhaps too trivial, for your abilities.

### DISTANCE

An estimate of total distance is given. Out-and-back trips show the sum of the distances of the out and back segments. After the trail distance, I've noted whether the trip, as described, is a loop, an out-and-back route, or a point-to-point trip, requiring a car shuttle. There is some flexibility, of course, in the way in which a hiker can actually follow the trip.

### HIKING TIME

This figure is for the average hiker, and includes only the time spent in motion. It does not include time spent for rest stops, lunch, etc. Fast walkers can complete the routes in perhaps 30 percent less time, and slower hikers may take 50 percent longer. We assume the hiker is traveling with a light day pack. Hikers carrying heavy packs could easily take twice as long, especially if they are traveling under adverse weather conditions. Remember, too, that the progress made by a group as a whole is limited by the pace of the slowest member or members.

## ELEVATION GAIN/LOSS

These are an estimate of the sum of all the vertical gain segments and the sum of all the vertical loss segments along the total length of the route (includes both ways for out-and-back trips). This is often considerably more than the net difference in elevation between the high and low points of the hike.

## DIFFICULTY

This overall rating takes into account the length of the trip and the nature of the terrain. The following are general definitions of the five categories:

**Easy:** Suitable for every member of the family.

**Moderate:** Suitable for all physically fit people.

**Moderately Strenuous:** Long length, substantial elevation gain, and/or difficult terrain. Suitable for experienced hikers only.

**Strenuous:** Full day's hike (or overnight backpack) over a long and often difficult route. Suitable only for experienced hikers in excellent physical condition.

**Very Strenuous:** Long and rugged route in extremely remote area. Usually requires two days. Suitable only for experienced hikers/climbers in top physical condition.

Each higher level represents more or less a doubling of the difficulty. On average, moderate trips are twice as hard as easy trips, moderately strenuous trips are twice as hard as moderate trips, and so on.

## TRAIL USE

**Suitable for Backpacking:** Many of the trips in this book are not. Some parks and trails are closed at night, others allow night hiking but prohibit camping. Sometimes, over-night camping is permitted at some spot off the route yet nearby.

**Suitable for Mountain Biking:** The trip, as described, is open to mountain biking, and is reasonably safe for that activity. Since regulations governing the use of mountain bikes on trails may change, it is a good idea to check with the agency having jurisdiction over the area.

**Dogs Allowed:** This indicates that dogs are allowed on the trail, generally on a leash no longer than 6 feet.

**Good for Kids:** These trips are especially recommended for inquisitive children. They were chosen on the basis of their safety and ease of travel, and their potential for entertaining the whole family.

## BEST TIMES

This is the seasonal range estimated as best for each trail. Nearly all of the short trips in this book are suitable year round. Some of the longer trips in the warmer, interior areas are simply too hot during the summer season. Hikes at high altitude can become inaccessible during the winter because of road closures, or they may be dangerous because of snow and ice. Generally, however, the range of months indicates when the hike is most rewarding.

## AGENCY

These code letters refer to the agency, or office, that has jurisdiction or management over the area being hiked (for example, ANF/LARD means Angeles National Forest, Los Angeles River District). You can contact the agency for more information. Contact data is listed in Appendix 4.

## OPTIONAL/RECOMMENDED/REQUIRED MAP(S)

The topographic maps listed under this heading are U.S. Geological Survey 7.5-minute series topographic maps. Usually, they are the most complete and accurate maps of the physical features (if not always the cultural features and trails) of the area you'll be traveling in. They are especially useful in the remote mountain areas, which have experienced few or no changes in topography. Persons familiar with the terrain in a particular trip area may be able to do without a "recommended" map, as long as some other map is substituted. However, a "required" topographic map (noted for some of the most remote trips in the book) is one that is essential for successful navigation. Topographic maps are typically stocked by backpacking, outdoor sports, and map shops. Topographic maps on CD format and topographic-map images downloadable from the Internet are becoming popular alternatives to purchasing hard-copy topographic maps. In many parks and open-space areas close to the populated areas of the county, excellent hiking maps are now being provided to visitors at entrances and trailheads for free or at minimal cost.

## NOTES

Only one of these terrain designations appears in the "Notes" section for a given trip, indicating the general character of the terrain encountered. Light footwear (running or walking shoes) is appropriate for easy terrain, while sturdy hiking boots are recommended for more difficult terrain.

**Easy Terrain:** roads, trails, and easy cross-country hiking

**Moderate Terrain:** cross-country boulder hopping and easy scrambling

**Difficult Terrain:** nontechnical climbing required (Warning: These trips should be attempted only by suitably equipped, experienced hikers adept at traveling over steep or rocky terrain requiring the use of the hands as well as the feet.)

Nontechnical climbing includes everything up to and including Class 3 on the rock climber's scale. While ropes and climbing hardware are not required, a hiker should have a good sense of balance, and enough experience to recognize danger-ous moves and situations. The safety and stability of heavy hiking boots are especially recommended for this kind of trip. Hazards may include loose or slippery rocks and rattlesnakes (don't put your hands in places you can't see clearly).

"Bushwhacking" indicates cross-country travel through dense brush is required. I have noted this when trips require a substantial amount of off-trail "bushwhacking." Wear long pants and be especially alert for rattlesnakes.

Only one of these two designations appears in the "Notes" section: "Marked Trails/ Obvious Routes" or "Navigation Required." (Warning: Trips for which navigation skills are required should be attempted only by hikers skilled in navigation techniques and map and compass or GPS use.)

Unambiguous cross-country routes up a canyon, for example, are noted as having "Marked Trails/Obvious Routes." The hiker, of course, should never be without a map in any remote area, even if there are marked trails or the route seems obvious.

## DIRECTIONS

Whenever driving directions are given for trips in the rural or remote areas of Los Angeles County, certain reference points along numbered highways may be keyed to the roadside mile markers posted at frequent intervals. County highways often have small paddle-shaped signs with mileage figures on them. State highways have reflective paddles stenciled with numbers like "29.54." The mileage signs may appear at half mile intervals, one mile intervals, or at irregular intervals. When the driving directions stipulate a turn at, say, mile 39.7, this does not mean there is necessarily a marker at that exact spot. Rather it would typically indicate a spot 0.3 mile from a mile post labeled 40.0. In general, highway mileage increases northward for north-south highways, and increases eastward for east-west highways.

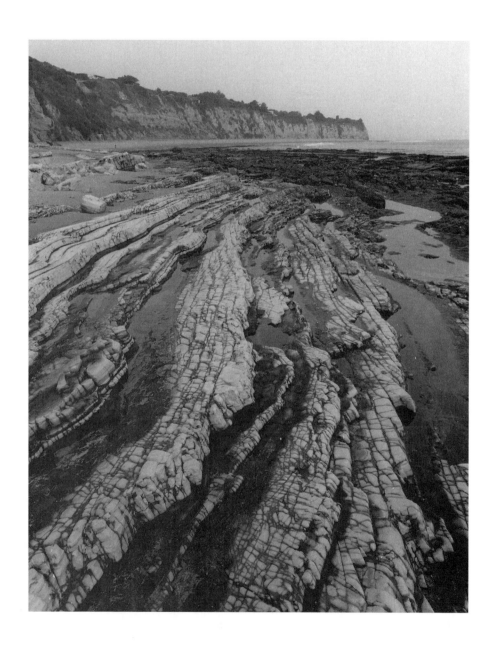

# chapter 1

# Coastline:
# Malibu Coast

**F**abled Malibu stretches 25 miles from the edge of the Los Angeles Basin at Santa Monica up-coast toward the Ventura County line. This odd, ribbon-like community—the home of many of L.A.'s rich and famous—doggedly follows the course of the narrow, curvy Pacific Coast Highway, itself confined to a precariously unstable coastal terrace at the foot of the Santa Monica Mountains. Parts of Malibu consist of unbroken rows of townhouses perilously jammed between the highway and the surf. Just back of the coastal strip, stilted houses have gained airy footholds on precipitous slopes overlooking the coast. Periodic wildfires sweeping over the mountains and the erosive battering of the ocean waves have done little to discourage urban-style growth. But a rising anti-growth sentiment among residents may well accomplish what nature has failed to do.

If you like strolling on crowded public beaches, or ogling fancy houses, the Malibu coastline has plenty of both. Quieter stretches of coastline, removed from the sight of houses and the roar of traffic, are a little harder to find, but are well worth seeking out. These include (in the middle section of Malibu) Malibu Lagoon State Beach, which has a salt-water lagoon favored by migrating birds, a surfing beach, and a pier, as well as Malibu Bluffs Park.

If you're an avid hiker, though, you'll head a little farther west to a stretch of coastline wrapping around the flat-topped headlands of Point Dume. This southward-pointing promontory, jutting into the Pacific Ocean some 20 miles west of Santa Monica, is a widely visible landmark. Just east of the point itself, an unbroken cliff wall shelters a secluded beach from the sights and sounds of the civilized world. On this beach, you can forget about whatever else may lie just over the cliff rim; your world is simply one of crashing surf, tangy salt spray, pearly sand, and fascinating tidepools.

Dume Cove at low tide

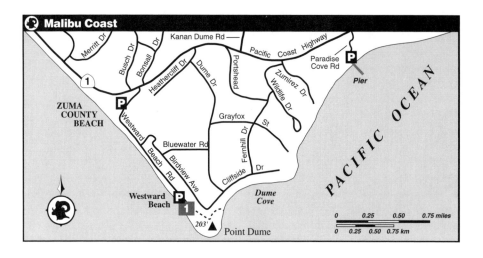

## trip 1  Point Dume to Paradise Cove

| | |
|---|---|
| **Distance** | 4.2 miles round trip, Out-and-back |
| **Hiking Time** | 3 hours (round trip) |
| **Elevation Gain/Loss** | 400'/400' |
| **Difficulty** | Moderate |
| **Trail Use** | Good for kids |
| **Best Times** | All year (passable during low tide) |
| **Agency** | NPS |
| **Optional Map** | USGS 7.5-min *Point Dume* |
| **Notes** | Marked trails/obvious routes, moderate terrain |

**DIRECTIONS** From Santa Monica drive west (up the coast) on Pacific Coast Highway about 25 miles to Westward Beach Road. Turn south and follow Westward Beach Road to its end, where there is a spacious parking lot.

A pleasant walk anytime the tide is low, this trip is doubly rewarding when the tide dips as low as -2 feet. The rocky coastline below the cliffs of Point Dume harbors a mind-boggling array of marine plant and animal life, much of it underwater most of the time. That includes, based on what I've seen myself: limpets, periwinkles, chitons, tube snails, sandcastle worms, sculpins, mussels, shore and hermit crabs, green and aggregate anemones, three kinds of barnacles, and two kinds of sea stars. Extreme low tides occur during the afternoon two or three times each month from October

through March. Consult tide tables to find out exactly when.

From the parking lot at Westward Beach you have two choices. The shorter, much easier route profiled here (and the only practical alternative during all but extremely low tides) is the trail slanting left up the cliff. On top you'll come to an area popular for sighting gray whales during their southward migration in winter. You'll also discover a state historic monument. Point Dume was christened by the British naval commander George Vancouver, who sailed by in 1793. As you stand on Point Dume's apex, note the

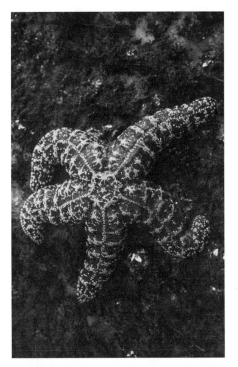

Sea star in tide pool, Point Dume coast

The alternate route is appropriate for expert climbers only (and definitely not appropriate for small children). During the lowest or low tides, you can edge around the point itself, making your way by hand-and-toe climbing in a couple of spots over huge, angular shards of volcanic rock along the base of the cliffs. The tidepools here and also to the east along Dume Cove's shoreline harbor some of the best displays of intertidal marine life in Southern California. This visual feast will remain for others to enjoy if you refrain from taking or disturbing in any way the organisms that live there. Be aware that exploring the lower intertidal zones can be hazardous. Be very cautious when traveling over slippery rocks, and always be aware of the incoming swells. Don't let a rogue wave catch you by surprise.

The going is easy once you're on Dume Cove's ribbon of sand. You may see signs posted here that warn against nude bathing and sunning. This was once a popular nude beach, much to the chagrin of some of those living in the cliffside mansions overlooking the area.

When you reach the northeast end of Dume Cove, swing left around a lesser point and continue another mile over a somewhat wider beach. You can travel as far as Paradise Cove, site of an elegant beach-side restaurant and private pier, 2.1 miles from your starting point.

You can return the way you came.

marked contrast between the lighter sedimentary rock exposed on the cliff faces both east and west, and the darker volcanic rock just below. Like the armored bow of an icebreaker, this unusually tough mass of volcanic rock has thus far resisted the onslaught of the ocean swells. After you descend from the high point, some metal stairs will take you down to crescent-shaped Dume Cove.

# chapter 2

# Coastline:
# Palos Verdes Peninsula

Forged by local uplift of the sea floor roughly 2 million years ago, Palos Verdes lay surrounded by the ocean for hundreds of thousands of years. Today the vast sheet of alluvium filling the L.A. Basin connects Palos Verdes to the mainland—yet in a figurative sense Palos Verdes has never really lost its identity as an island.

When the South Bay cities of Torrance and Long Beach are cloaked by fog or brown haze, Palos Verdes often stands head and shoulders above the murk. Sometimes you can stand on top enjoying views of far-away Santa Catalina Island and Old Baldy, but fail to make out L.A. Harbor only a few miles away.

Palos Verdes is a very distinct economic and cultural island as well. Rimmed by oil refineries, gritty industrial neighborhoods, and wall-to-wall people, the peninsula itself is dominated almost exclusively by opulent ranch-style homes and sprawling, lavishly landscaped estates. The contrast is startling.

Fortunately, Palos Verdes offers miles of near-pristine coastline and a big patch of hillside open space for any explorer on foot to enjoy. You can start with easy Trip 1 below for an overview of the area, and later graduate to one of the tougher scrambles (Trips 2-4) along the base of the coastal cliffs.

Top of the peninsula view at Palos Verdes

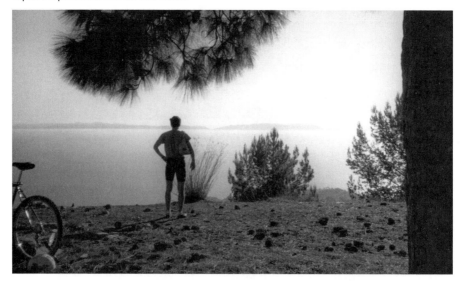

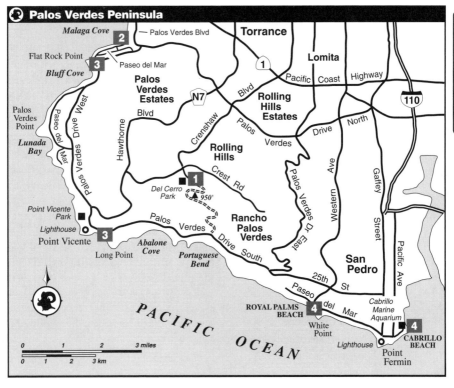

**Palos Verdes Peninsula**

---

**trip 1**  **Top of the Peninsula**

|  |  |
|---|---|
| **Distance** | 1.6 miles round trip |
| **Hiking Time** | 1 hour (round trip) |
| **Elevation Gain/Loss** | 350'/350' |
| **Difficulty** | Easy |
| **Trail Use** | Dogs allowed, good for kids |
| **Best Times** | All year |
| **Agency** | CORPV |
| **Optional Maps** | USGS 7.5-min *Torrance, San Pedro* |
| **Notes** | Marked trails/obvious routes, easy terrain |

**DIRECTIONS** Drive south on Crenshaw Boulevard, one of L.A.'s longest and busiest thoroughfares, all the way to its southern end. Park either at the dead-end of the road or at nearby Del Cerro Park.

At Del Cerro Park on the top of the Palos Verdes peninsula, you need only climb a small, grassy hill to take in one of L.A.'s truly great ocean views. With a little bit more ambition, you can hoof it less than a mile to an even more panoramic view spot.

Ideally, you could be here when a chilly north wind (which usually follows the passage of major winter storms) cleanses the Southland of polluted air. But don't neglect the early spring. During March and April the sages, native wildflowers and weedy grasses magically transform the normally drab-colored hillsides into tapestries of velvet green. Even with hazy skies, however, the view seems ethereal.

At Crenshaw's dead end, step around the steel gate and follow the dirt fire road beyond. This road traces Crenshaw's proposed extension down to Palos Verdes Drive South at Portuguese Bend, a project that will likely never be realized.

Soon you're in a rare patch of open space surrounded by, but largely removed from, the curving avenues and palatial estates of Rancho Palos Verdes. Since the mid-1950s, when more than 100 houses were destroyed or seriously damaged by landslides in the Portuguese Bend area, most of the steep area above the Bend has remained off-limits to development.

At 0.5 mile, stay right as lesser trails branch left. Continue a curving descent until you reach a flat area about 0.3 mile farther. Leave the road there and make a beeline for the top of a 950-foot knoll, dotted with planted pines, on the left. Atop this serene little overlook you'll enjoy a 150-degree view of the ocean, with Santa Catalina Island sprawling at center stage in the south. If the air is very clear, try to spot San Nicolas Island, some 70 miles away to the southwest.

The knoll you're standing on is a remnant of one of the 13 marine terraces that have made the Palos Verdes hills a textbook example familiar to geology students. The 13 terraces, rising like rounded and broken stairs from sea level to 1300 feet, are the result of wave erosion modified by uplift and fluctuating sea levels during the past 2 million years. From this spot (despite the effects of decades of grading and construction on some of the adjacent ridges) you will probably recognize at least seven of the terraces in the topography around you.

## trip 2 Malaga Cove to Bluff Cove

see map on p. 27

| | |
|---|---|
| **Distance** | 2.0 miles, Loop |
| **Hiking Time** | 1½ hours |
| **Elevation Gain/Loss** | 200'/200' |
| **Difficulty** | Moderate |
| **Trail Use** | Good for kids |
| **Best Times** | All year (only at low tide) |
| **Agency** | PVESP |
| **Optional Map** | USGS 7.5-min *Redondo Beach* |
| **Notes** | Marked trails/obvious routes, moderate terrain |

**DIRECTIONS** From Palos Verdes Drive West in Palos Verdes Estates, turn north on Via Corta. After 0.5 mile, make a right on Via Arroyo. One more right turn, on Paseo del Mar, takes you to a parking area in front of the Malaga Cove Intermediate School.

If dancing across wave-rounded boulders is your cup of tea, you'll enjoy this moderately difficult rock-hop along the northernmost edge of the Palos Verdes peninsula. With near-vertical cliffs on one side and foamy surf on the other, you'll truly feel that you're treading the edge of the continent. Shoes or boots with good ankle support are recommended to deal with the uneven terrain.

Find the top of the paved pathway at the far end of Paseo del Mar and walk down to the beach at Malaga Cove. Turn left along the shoreline and make your way over the obstacle course of wave-pounded rocks. After a short mile you arrive at Flat Rock Point, a popular area for tidepooling when the tide is low. Wide, curving Bluff Cove lies just ahead. From there, take the pathway on the left going back up the cliff to Paseo del Mar. You can then return to your car by strolling the four blocks of Paseo del Mar leading back to the school. Lining both sides of this street are some of Palos Verdes' most attractively landscaped mansions—very nice to admire even if you can't own one.

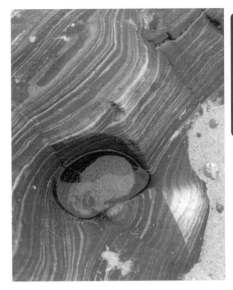

Wave-sculpted bedrock, Palos Verdes West Shore

## trip 3  **Bluff Cove to Point Vicente**

see map on p. 27

| | |
|---|---|
| **Distance** | 5.7 miles, Point-to-point |
| **Hiking Time** | 4 hours |
| **Elevation Gain/Loss** | 200'/200' |
| **Difficulty** | Moderately strenuous |
| **Best Times** | All year (low tide recommended) |
| **Agency** | PVESP |
| **Optional Map** | USGS 7.5-min *Redondo Beach* |
| **Notes** | Marked trails/obvious routes, moderate terrain |

**DIRECTIONS** *North End:* From Palos Verdes Drive West in Palos Verdes Estates, turn north on Via Corta. After 0.5 mile, make a right on Via Arroyo. After one block, turn left on Paseo del Mar. Go 0.5 mile to the spot where a pathway (Flat Rock Point Trail) descends to the shoreline at Bluff Cove. *South End:* From eastbound Palos Verdes Drive South, 0.8 mile south of Hawthorne Boulevard, take the exit to the Point Vicente Fishing Access parking lot.

This long trek down Palos Verdes' wild west side visits crescent-shaped Lunada Bay plus a half dozen mini-coves, and traverses the wave-torn base of the sea cliffs below Point Vicente. Time your hike so that low tide occurs when you're below the lighthouse at Point Vicente, which is one of the tighter spots along the coastline. Set up a car shuttle in advance—unless you plan to add 4.5 miles to your trip by walking back on Palos Verdes Drive West. If you're out during the late morning or noon hour on a sunny day, you may want to reverse the route from that described here in order to avoid facing the sun the whole way. Shoes or boots with good ankle support are recommended to deal with the uneven terrain, but do realize that exposure to salt water may shorten their life.

On the Flat Rock Point Trail, you descend quickly to Bluff Cove. Onward to Lunada Bay, the going is quite easy—you'll be on pebbles, and sometimes a thin ribbon of sand, as long as you stay close to the base of the cliffs. Often there are occasions where you can walk out farther to tidepools that are well exposed during -1 foot tides or lower. These moderately rich pools contain green anemones, crabs, and especially purple sea urchins—but probably not too many of the more interesting creatures such as sea stars.

At around 2 miles, short of Palos Verdes Point (aka Rocky Point) you'll come upon the dismembered remains of the freighter *Dominator*, which ran aground in 1961. Rusting pieces of the ship now litter a stretch of coastline nearly a half mile long.

Once around the point, the beautiful, semicircular Lunada Bay lies before you. The beige-tinted sedimentary cliffs encircling the bay are of Monterey shale, a thinly bedded and easily eroded formation that composes about 90 percent of the exposed rock on the Palos Verdes peninsula. The formation consists of former sea floor rich in diatoms, the skeletons of microscopic single-celled plants that float about in the ocean. A steep trail leads up the cliff at Lunada Bay to connect with Paseo del Mar. The first two of the half dozen indentations pocking the coastline beyond Lunada Bay also have steep paths going up to Paseo del Mar. Keep this in mind if you want to "bail out" and avoid the more rugged and rocky shoreline ahead.

Rock hopping becomes *de rigeur* in the last mile before Point Vicente. Some hand and foot work will get you over the piles of broken rocks just below the whale-watching overlook and lighthouse. A short way ahead you'll come to a steep path slanting up the cliff to the Point Vicente Fishing Access parking lot at the end of the traverse.

Before or after your hike, consider visiting nearby Point Vicente Park. Open daily, the park features an interpretive center, which includes a nice relief map of the peninsula and offers great views of the winter-migrating gray whales from the brink of the sea cliffs.

The Point Vicente lighthouse

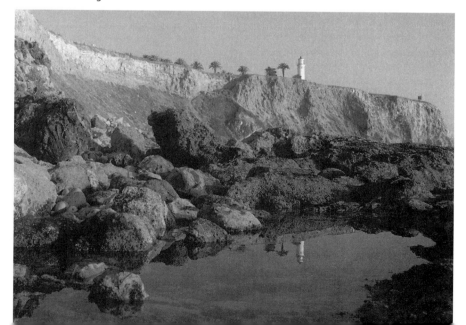

## trip 4 White Point to Cabrillo Beach

see map on p. 27

**COASTLINE**

| | |
|---|---|
| **Distance** | 3.0 miles, Point-to-point |
| **Hiking Time** | 2 hours |
| **Elevation Gain/Loss** | 100'/100' |
| **Difficulty** | Moderate |
| **Best Times** | All year (low tide recommended) |
| **Agency** | RPB |
| **Optional Map** | USGS 7.5-min *San Pedro* |
| **Notes** | Marked trails/obvious routes, moderate terrain |

**DIRECTIONS** *West End:* Start at Royal Palms Beach, where Western Avenue intersects with Paseo del Mar in San Pedro. *East End:* Finish at the Cabrillo Marine Aquarium, near the south end of Pacific Avenue in San Pedro.

Pressed hard and fast against the densely populated community of San Pedro, the rocky ribbon of coastline between White Point and Cabrillo Beach looks out over a 20-mile, watery gap separating Santa Catalina Island from the mainland. On clear winter days the island seems to float like a dusky shadow over the sparkling surf.

From Royal Palms Beach, walk east past White Point, making your way over tilted slabs of sedimentary rock and small boulders. Here, and on the bluffs above are the skimpy remains of early-century resorts and spas that capitulated to the 1933 Long Beach earthquake and decades of pounding surf. The checkered history of this stretch of coastline is interpreted in a display at the Cabrillo Marine Aquarium, which lies at the end of this hike.

At about 1.5 miles, before the shoreline terrace you're following narrows to practically nothing at Point Fermin, you'll spot some metal steps going up the bluff. This is your safe ticket to getting past Point Fermin. (If the tide is extremely low and the surf is relatively calm—conditions that are most likely to occur on only a few afternoons during the fall—expert scramblers

can try to edge around the point itself and reach the sand of Cabrillo Beach beyond.) Point Fermin's cliff faces, though not the highest on the peninsula, present the wildest scene on the peninsula. When I scooted over them during a -1 foot tide, dozens of sleek, black cormorants perched on tiny niches above observed my every move.

At the top of the metal stairs, a path leads to the west end of Point Fermin Park, a grassy strip popular among joggers and strollers. Keep heading east along the edge of the cliffs, passing the antique Point Fermin Lighthouse, built in 1874 with materials shipped around Cape Horn. Farther east a big landslide blocks your way, so you turn inland a little to reach Shepard Street. Follow this street east, to Pacific Avenue, and continue straight ahead on Bluff Place down to Cabrillo Beach. Here you can enjoy the only true beach for miles in either direction, and pay a visit to the aquarium, which features some excellent marine and historical exhibits. If you want to stretch your legs further, try walking out to sea atop the San Pedro breakwater, one of several artificial barriers protecting the Los Angeles/Long Beach harbor complex from ocean swells.

# chapter 3

# Basin and Foothills:
# Thousand Oaks & Moorpark

Interior Ventura County is dominated by long, parallel ridges associated with the Transverse Ranges, Shallow, often wide valleys lie between those ridges. Housing developments have spread far and wide over some of the valleys and hillsides here, but much open land remains.

Historical uses such as agriculture, cattle grazing, and oil production are fading in Ventura County, whereas habitat preservation and recreational opportunities are in greater demand. That is why key parcels of this spacious landscape are bit by bit being transferred into public ownership. One goal is to create a "Rim-of-the-Valley" natural area—a connected patchwork of open spaces stretching around the San Fernando Valley from Ventura County to Glendale.

While the two parks described in this chapter are not within Los Angeles County itself, they are located nearby and are easily accessible to San Fernando Valley residents. They were included in this guidebook for that reason.

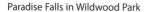

Paradise Falls in Wildwood Park

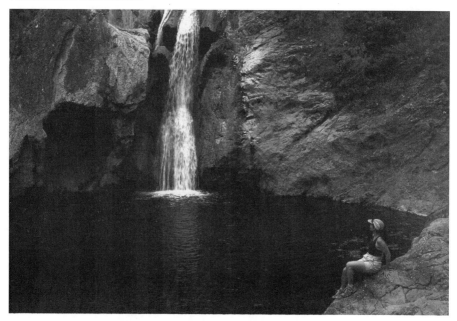

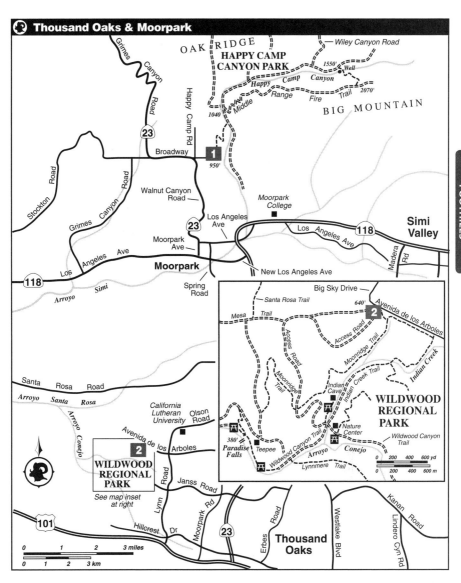

## Thousand Oaks & Moorpark

OAK RIDGE

HAPPY CAMP CANYON PARK

Wiley Canyon Road

Grimes Canyon Road

1550' Well

Happy Camp Canyon

Range Fire Trail

2070'

1040 Middle

BIG MOUNTAIN

Happy Camp Rd

23

Broadway

950'

1

Walnut Canyon Road

Moorpark College

Stockton Road

Grimes Canyon Road

Los Angeles Ave

23

Los Angeles Ave

118

Simi Valley

Moorpark Ave

Madera Rd

Moorpark

118

Los Angeles Ave

Simi

Arroyo

New Los Angeles Ave

Spring Road

Big Sky Drive

Santa Rosa Trail

640'

Avenida de los Arboles

Mesa Trail

Access Road

2

Access Road

Moonridge Trail

Indian Creek

Santa Rosa Road

Arroyo Santa Rosa

Arroyo Conejo

California Lutheran University

Olson Road

Moonridge Trail

Indian Cave

Indian Creek Trail

WILDWOOD REGIONAL PARK

Avenida de los Arboles

2

WILDWOOD REGIONAL PARK

See map inset at right

Lynn Road

Janss Road

380'

Paradise Falls

Teepee

Wildwood Canyon Trail

Nature Center

Arroyo Conejo

Wildwood Canyon Trail

Lynnmere Trail

0   200   400   600 yd

0   200   400   600 m

101

Hillcrest Dr

Moorpark Rd

23

Erbes Road

Thousand Oaks

Westlake Blvd

Kanan Road

Lindero Cyn Rd

0   1   2   3 miles

0   1   2   3 km

## trip 1  Happy Camp Canyon

| | |
|---|---|
| **Distance** | 9.4 miles round trip, Out-and-back |
| **Hiking Time** | 5 hours (round trip) |
| **Elevation Gain/Loss** | 700'/700' |
| **Difficulty** | Moderately strenuous |
| **Trail Use** | Suitable for mountain biking |
| **Best Times** | October through June |
| **Agency** | SMMC |
| **Optional Map** | USGS 7.5-min *Simi* |
| **Notes** | Marked trails/obvious routes, easy terrain |

see map on p. 33

**DIRECTIONS**  Follow the 118 Freeway west from Simi Valley or the 23 Freeway north from Thousand Oaks to the New Los Angeles Avenue exit. Go west 1 mile to Moorpark Avenue (signed Highway 23), turn right, and proceed 2.6 miles to where Highway 23 makes a sharp bend to the left. Keep going straight here, but then make an immediate right turn on Broadway. Proceed a short way to the east end of Broadway, where there's a spacious dirt parking lot and trailhead.

Happy Camp Canyon nuzzles in a crease between the long, rounded ridge called Big Mountain, just north of Simi Valley, and Oak Ridge, a taller parallel ridge to the north. These ridges and plenty more, like the Santa Monica Mountains, are caterpillar-like parallel segments of the Transverse Ranges, which stretch from Santa Barbara County in the west to San Bernardino County to the east.

Oil-bearing shales predominate in this region, evidenced by various oil wells and dirt roads built to access them scattered across the surrounding hillsides. On your ramble through the lower and middle parts of the canyon, keep an eye out for bright red stones, sometimes exhibiting a glassy texture, some right under you feet and others visible in outcrops. These rocks were formed by the slow combustion of organic material trapped in layers of shale.

Happy Camp Canyon itself remains quite pristine. Several groups of Chumash Indians called this place home in past centuries; later it became a part of an immense cattle ranch founded by a pioneer Simi Valley family. Purchased as a future state park in the late 1960s, it was later traded to Ventura County for use a regional park. Today, save for a few dirt roads and a smattering of artifacts from the days of cattle ranching, the 3000-acre canyon park serves as prime

Live Oaks in Happy Camp Canyon

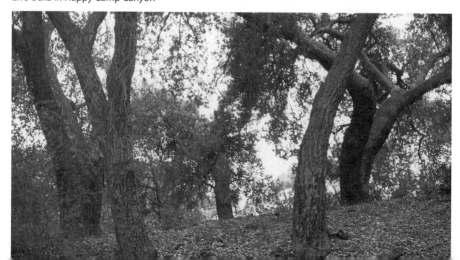

natural habitat for native plants and animals, and a restful retreat for hikers seeking to escape from the sights and sounds of city and suburban life.

From the trailhead, follow the path heading north and east along gentle, grassy slopes down onto the wide floor of Happy Camp Canyon. As you look down on a golf course at the canyon's mouth, note the terraced aspect of the landscape on both sides. These are fluvial (streamside) terraces—sedimentary deposits from earlier flows of Happy Camp Canyon's creek.

At 1.0 mile you join a dirt road in the bottom of the canyon, and 0.2 mile later you pass through a gate marking the start of the "wilderness" section of Happy Camp Canyon Park. Ignoring dirt roads on the right and left, keep straight (north) into the main canyon.

By 2.0 miles, the canyon floor has become narrow, you've turned decidedly east, and you are strolling through beautiful coast live-oak woods (plus native sycamore and walnut trees), which continue intermittently up the canyon in the next 3 miles. A little stream flows in the bottom of the canyon during, and for some weeks or months after, the winter rains. You're climbing at a gentle rate of about 200 feet of elevation gain per mile. You pass the ascending Wiley Canyon Road on the left at 4.1 miles, and at 4.7 miles you reach the site of an old well and pump. Large oak trees nearby provide enough shade for a convenient lunch stop. Savor the splendid isolation of this secluded retreat before you head back the same way.

An alternative to the out-and-back trip described above is available if you are energetic, especially if the air is clear enough to enjoy distant views: Continue following the graded dirt road about 300 yards past the well. The road ends, but a bulldozed track, eroded and very steep at first, curls 0.7 mile up the south slope of Happy Camp Canyon then joins Middle Range Fire Trail on the crest of Big Mountain. Use that ridge-running fire trail to return to lower Happy Camp Canyon at a point just above the gate marking the wilderness area boundary. This looping alternative route (beginning and ending at the trailhead) measures 10.5 miles, with elevation gains and losses of 1300 feet.

**trip 2  Paradise Falls**

|  |  |
|---|---|
| **Distance** | 3 miles, Loop |
| **Hiking Time** | 2 hours |
| **Elevation Gain/Loss** | 400'/400' |
| **Difficulty** | Moderate |
| **Trail Use** | Dogs allowed, good for kids |
| **Best Times** | All year |
| **Agency** | CRPD |
| **Optional Map** | USGS 7.5-min *Newbury Park* |
| **Notes** | Marked trails/obvious routes, easy terrain |

see map on p. 33

**DIRECTIONS**  Exit the Ventura Freeway (Highway 101) at Lynn Road in Thousand Oaks and follow Lynn Road north 2.5 miles to Avenida de los Arboles. Turn left and follow Avenida de los Arboles 1 mile west. At this point traffic goes sharply right on Big Sky Drive; you make a U-turn and park on the right at Wildwood Park's principal trailhead, open 8 a.m. to 5 p.m. Nearby curbside parking is also available.

**W**ildwood Park in Thousand Oaks is Ventura County's most scenic suburban park. The scenery here has been imprinted in the minds of many in the over-50 age group: the area was once a outdoor set for old Hollywood movies, as well as for television's *The*

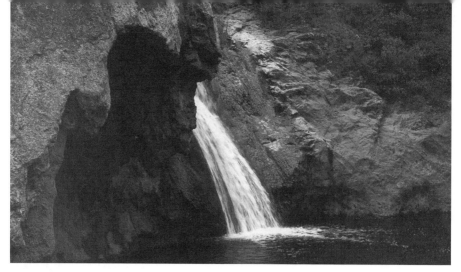

Paradise Falls

*Rifleman, Gunsmoke,* and *Wagon Train.* The short but steep hike—down and then up—described here takes you to Wildwood Park's scenic gem: the Arroyo Conejo gorge and Paradise Falls.

Three trails radiate from Avenida de los Arboles Trailhead. Two are wide and relatively unscenic dirt roads. The third (the one you want), the narrow and scenic Moonridge Trail, descends sharply from the east side of the parking area. This is the left side of the parking area as you drive in. Immediately after you start on it you come to a T-intersection amid oak woods. Turn right, remaining on Moonridge Trail. The trail descends a sunny slope covered with aromatic sage-scrub vegetation and dappled with succulent live-forever plants that sprout white, comical-looking flower stalks. There's a brief passage across a shady ravine using wooden steps and a plank bridge. At 0.5 mile, you cross over a dirt road and continue on the narrow Moonridge Trail.

Ahead, the trail curls around a deep ravine without gaining or losing a lot of elevation, edging into the crumbly sedimentary rock. This passage is exciting enough for hikers, and could be worrisome for parents with small kids. At 0.9 mile you join another dirt road and use it to descend toward a large wooden teepee structure on a knoll just below. Make a right at the teepee, further descending into the Arroyo Conejo gorge. As you descend, watch for the narrow side trail on the left that will take you straight down to Paradise Falls—a beautiful, 30-foot-high cascade that makes its presence known by sound before sight. The high water table in the canyon bottom ensures a nearly year-round flow of water.

After you've admired the falls, continue by climbing back up the slope in the direction you came, and by taking the fenced, cliff-hanging trail around the left (east) side of the falls. Beyond that fenced stretch, the narrow trail descends a little and sidles up alongside the creek, where large coast live oaks spread their shade. Soon, you'll find yourself continuing on a path of dirt-road width. Stay with that path until you reach a major crossroads. The small Wildwood Nature Center is just around the bend to the right, a short spur path to the walk-through Indian Cave lies on the left, and your return route up along Indian Canyon is straight ahead.

On the Indian Creek Trail, you pay your debt to gravity by ascending nearly 300 feet in about 0.7 mile. The beautifully tangled array of live oak and sycamore limbs along this trail keeps your mind off the climb. At one point, you can look down into a deep ravine where an inaccessible mini-waterfall and pool lie practically hidden. When you finally reach Avenida de los Arboles, turn left and return a short distance to the trailhead parking lot.

# chapter 4

# Basin and Foothills:
# Simi Hills

Up until the 1970s the pastoral grazing lands of the Simi Hills were remote from the city. Today, spill-over growth along the Ventura Freeway from the San Fernando Valley to Thousand Oaks has made substantial inroads. More grading and construction threatens to further usurp the habitat of the valley oak (the stately, spreading tree for which the city of Thousand Oaks is named), and snuff out an important wildlife corridor between the coastal Santa Monica Mountains and the remaining wild lands of the interior.

On the brighter side, nearly 4500 acres of Simi Hills ranchland—nearly the entire upper watershed of Cheeseboro and Palo Camado canyons—have been purchased by the National Park Service over the past 25 years for inclusion in the Santa Monica Mountains National Recreation Area. This has assured protection for most of the area's valley-oak savanna habitat, established a permanently protected link in the north-south wildlife migration corridor, and created a recreational resource for hundreds of thousands of people who have settled in the immediate area. In 2003, a big parcel of land on the west rim of the San Fernando Valley—the Ahmanson Ranch—was purchased with the help of state bond money and additional grants. The acquisition of this parcel, now titled the Upper Las Virgenes Canyon Open Space Preserve, ensures that an uninterrupted block of natural landscape can remain in between the San Fernando Valley and the city of Thousand Oaks.

Turtle Rock, Sage Ranch

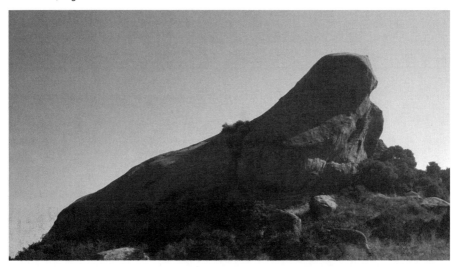

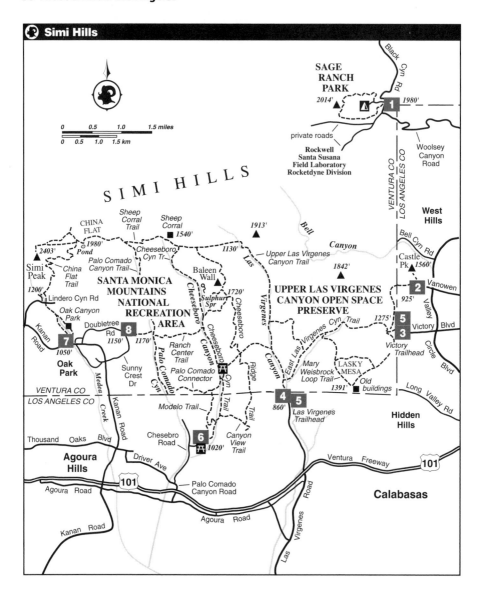

## trip 1  Sage Ranch

| | |
|---|---|
| **Distance** | 2.1 miles, Loop |
| **Hiking Time** | 1 hour |
| **Elevation Gain/Loss** | 400'/400' |
| **Difficulty** | Easy |
| **Trail Use** | Suitable for mountain biking, dogs allowed, good for kids |
| **Best Times** | October through June |
| **Agency** | SMMC |
| **Optional Map** | USGS 7.5-min *Calabasas* |
| **Notes** | Marked trails/obvious routes, easy terrain |

see map on p. 38

**DIRECTIONS** Sage Ranch's entrance and spacious parking lot is accessible by way of Woosley Canyon Road (the former Rocketdyne Road) from Chatsworth in the San Fernando Valley, or (more awkwardly) by way of the excessively narrow and squiggly Black Canyon Road from Simi Valley.

The 635-acre Sage Ranch owes its name not to the predominant sage-scrub vegetation growing there, but rather to the former owner of the ranch, one Orrin Sage, Sr. Mr. Sage grazed cattle here for a time and planted orange and avocado orchards on a portion of the property in 1981. Purchased by the state in 1990, this pocket-sized patch of publicly owned open space has become a model park for recreational activities such as hiking, birdwatching, and nature study. A 10-site campground within the park is available by reservation to organized groups only.

Tilted sandstone outcrops and boulders punctuate the landscape hereabouts, the result of uplift of Cretaceous marine sedimentary rock. This rock originated from layers of sandy muck deposited near the ocean shore some 70 million years ago. Framed by these sometimes dramatic outcrops, the hiker's view on a clear day extends broadly toward Simi Valley and the Santa Susana Mountains in the north, San Fernando Valley in the east, and the Santa Monica Mountains in the south. The closer-at-hand view to the south and west includes some worn-out-looking former Rocketdyne aerospace test facilities and buildings.

The single loop trail (with minor spurs) going around the property follows graded and ungraded roads, passing near dramatic rock formations known as Turtle Rock and Sandstone Ridge, and skirting a maintained grove of orange trees.

You can see Sage Ranch at its very best in early spring, a time when wildflower fragrances, mixed with the scent of orange blossoms, suffuse the air.

**BASIN AND FOOTHILLS**

## trip 2 Castle Peak

see map on p. 38

| | |
|---|---|
| **Distance** | 1.4 miles round trip, Out-and-back |
| **Hiking Time** | 1 hour (round trip) |
| **Elevation Gain/Loss** | 650'/650' |
| **Difficulty** | Moderate |
| **Trail Use** | Dogs allowed |
| **Best Times** | All year |
| **Agency** | LACRPD |
| **Optional Map** | USGS 7.5-min *Calabasas* |
| **Notes** | Marked trails/obvious routes, moderate terrain |

**DIRECTIONS** Park at El Escorpion Park, at the west end of Vanowen Street (a major San Fernando Valley thoroughfare), just west of Valley Circle Boulevard.

Topped by craggy blocks of white conglomerate rock, Castle Peak affords what is probably the most expansive view of San Fernando Valley's west side. From the top, a sea of ground-hugging subdivisions is seen lapping at the foot of the mountain and stretching toward a vaporous horizon. In the middle distance, a bevy of skyscrapers at Warner Center rises up starkly, symbolizing the valley's evolution toward a presumably more vertical type of metropolitan environment in the future.

To the Chumash Indians living in the Simi Hills centuries ago, Castle Peak was known as *Huan*, a gigantic monument used to keep track of repetitive celestial and earthly cycles. Every year during the winter solstice, Huan's pointed afternoon shadow swept across a Chumash village located near the mouth of Bell Canyon. Even today, there's a sense of timeless drama on Huan's summit as you watch (on a crystal-clear December or January afternoon especially) the shadows of the Simi Hills stretch across the urban plain.

Although Castle Peak's summit can be reached from all sides, the shortest and most direct route is from El Escorpion Park just below the southeast slope. Follow an old dirt road going west into a broad, valley-oak-dotted canyon. Soon you will spot, on the right, a steeply inclined path heading straight up toward Castle Peak's craggy summit. Some scrambling gets you to the highest outcrop.

Hawks and ravens patrol the air spaces above—and often below—you as you survey the landscape. If you wish, you can follow the trailless ridgeline east to Peak 1639 for a better view of the rolling Simi Hills to the west.

## trip 3  Lasky Mesa

see map on p. 38

| | |
|---|---|
| **Distance** | 3.4 miles, Loop |
| **Hiking Time** | 1½ hours |
| **Elevation Gain/Loss** | 500'/500' |
| **Difficulty** | Moderate |
| **Trail Use** | Suitable for mountain biking, dogs allowed, good for kids |
| **Best Times** | October through May |
| **Agency** | SMMC |
| **Optional Map** | USGS 7.5-min *Calabasas* |
| **Notes** | Marked trails/obvious routes, easy terrain |

**DIRECTIONS** Take Victory Boulevard (a major San Fernando Valley thoroughfare) all the way to its westernmost end, 0.8 mile west of Valley Circle Boulevard. The Victory Trailhead at the roadend is open during daylight hours.

**BASIN AND FOOTHILLS**

Lasky Mesa, an elevated, treeless plain in the southeast corner of the Upper Las Virgenes Canyon Open Space Preserve, offers sweeping vistas in any direction you care to look. That view is most impressively "open" on sparkling clear winter days—yet nothing beats being here in early spring in a year of average or better rainfall. That's when the whole area can acquire an almost impossibly vivid emerald-green sheen.

The route described here keeps you entirely on old dirt roads, which today are essentially maintained as wide, multi-use trails. Starting from the west side of the Victory Trailhead, you descend 0.1 mile to a trail junction, when you make a sharp left, briefly reversing your path (your return route lies on the right). You then wind uphill through valley oaks that are clinging to the grassy slopes.

Before long the climb moderates and spacious Lasky Mesa lies ahead. Meadowlarks and redwing blackbirds sing, accompanied by the droning hum of distant traffic on Highway 101, unseen from this vantage point. At 1.0 mile, stay left where a segment of the Mary Weisbrock Loop Trail intersects on the right.

At 1.3 miles you swing by some old ranch buildings that were used in the movie and television industries. Starting in 1914, motion-picture pioneer Jesse Lasky utilized the surrounding landscape for wide-screen settings Lasky described as "big scenes." Movies such as *Gone With the Wind* and *The Charge of the Light Brigade* were partially filmed here, as was the television series *Petticoat Junction*.

Bypass the ranch buildings and swing to the right (north), remaining on the Mary Weisbrock Loop Trail. Continue north, ignoring other old ranch roads, signed against entry, which lead into an off-limits habitat restoration zone to the west. At 1.8 miles, keep straight where the north segment of the loop trail comes in from the right.

Now you begin a delightful descent down off the mesa, past fine specimens of coast live oak, and later through willow trees. Turn right at the next trail junction (2.2 miles) and head east, uphill, on the East Las Virgenes Canyon Trail, which will take you back toward your starting point.

# trip 4 Upper Las Virgenes Canyon

| | |
|---|---|
| **Distance** | 5.4 miles round trip, Out-and-back |
| **Hiking Time** | 2½ hours (round trip) |
| **Elevation Gain/Loss** | 400'/400' |
| **Difficulty** | Moderate |
| **Trail Use** | Suitable for mountain biking, dogs allowed, good for kids |
| **Best Times** | October through June |
| **Agency** | SMMC |
| **Optional Map** | USGS 7.5-min *Calabasas* |
| **Notes** | Marked trails/obvious routes, easy terrain |

see map on p. 38

**DIRECTIONS** Exit Highway 101 at Las Virgenes Road, and go 1.4 miles north to the end of the road. The Las Virgenes Trailhead at the roadend is open during daylight hours.

Upper Las Virgenes Canyon is one of those places where you can make the sight and sound of a huge metropolitan area simply disappear after a short drive from a major freeway and only a few minutes' walk. The area even seems removed from the flight paths of major aircraft.

The out-and-back jaunt into the upper canyon is a great one for kids, too. What creatures might they discover? Cottontail rabbits, for sure. A frog perhaps, or (as I did) a scorpion. If the kids get tired, you can turn back anytime. Expect to encounter two or three foot-wetting and possibly muddy stream crossings in the early part of the hike.

From the trailhead, simply head north on the main trail (an old dirt road), which imperceptibly gains elevation in the canyon's initially wide flood plain. In a couple of places ahead, narrow side trails higher on the canyon slope exist, but they may be too heavily overgrown by vegetation to follow. All along the way, enjoy the toasty, pungent fragrances of wild grape vines and riparian vegetation baking in the sun. There are enough oaks, sycamores, and willows around to keep much of the trail decently shaded, even during the middle of the day.

After about 2.5 miles the ascent into the upper canyon quickens, and you go sharply up and sharply down twice. Afterward, you bend right and transit a gorgeous gallery of overarching coast live oak limbs. The trail then executes a hairpin turn and starts to climb out of the canyon at a point below Peak 1913. You've come 2.7 miles from the start, and this is good place to turn back—for this casual hike at least. If your goal is to connect to the extensive trail systems lacing through Cheeseboro and Palo Comado canyons to the west, then by all means press on.

## trip 5  Victory to Las Virgenes

see map on p. 38

| | |
|---|---|
| **Distance** | 2.8 miles, Point-to-point |
| **Hiking Time** | 1½ hours |
| **Elevation Gain/Loss** | 50'/450' |
| **Difficulty** | Moderate |
| **Trail Use** | Suitable for mountain biking, dogs allowed, good for kids |
| **Best Times** | All year |
| **Agency** | SMMC |
| **Optional Map** | USGS 7.5-min *Calabasas* |
| **Notes** | Marked trails/obvious routes, easy terrain |

**DIRECTIONS** *East End:* Take Victory Boulevard (a major San Fernando Valley thoroughfare) all the way to its westernmost end, 0.8 mile west of Valley Circle Boulevard. The Victory Trailhead at the roadend is open during daylight hours. *West End:* Exit Highway 101 at Las Virgenes Road, and go 1.4 miles north to the end of the road. the Las Virgenes Trailhead at the roadend is open during daylight hours.

**BASIN AND FOOTHILLS**

This one-way traverse across the Upper Las Virgenes Canyon Open Space Preserve—easy for just about anyone when traveled in the east-to-west, downhill direction as suggested here—can be pleasantly accomplished anytime the weather is not excessively hot. You start in a saddle at the head of the upper east branch of Las Virgenes Canyon (the site of the Victory Trailhead) and finish at the north terminus of Las Virgenes Road (Las Virgenes Trailhead). For an afternoon hike, consider reversing the direction so as to avoid having sun glare in your eyes the entire way. The driving distance from one trailhead to the other measures 8 miles by way of Victory Boulevard, Valley Circle Boulevard, Highway 101, and Las Virgenes Road.

From the Victory Trailhead, descend 0.1 mile to a trail junction and veer right. You're on the East Las Virgenes Canyon Trail, which twists and turns a bit as it swoops into a shallow, tributary of Las Virgenes Canyon. You're also on the signed Juan Bautista de Anza National Historical Trail, which rather closely traces the famed overland route of the 1775–76 Spanish expedition. On that expedition, some 30 families traveled from southern Arizona into California. Most settled in the San Francisco Bay Area.

On your gradually descending route, stay on the East Las Virgenes Canyon Trail

as two other trails intersect on the left and the right. Enjoy the spacious vistas of wide-open grassland, highlighted here and there by valley and live oaks, willows, and sycamores. The scene is most impressive when the sun angle is low, as in early morning or late afternoon.

After traveling for a total of 2.5 miles you arrive at the "confluence" of Las Virgenes Canyon's east and main branches. Turn left there on the Upper Las Virgenes Canyon Trail and complete the remaining short distance over to the Las Virgenes Trailhead.

*Valley oak below Lasky Mesa*

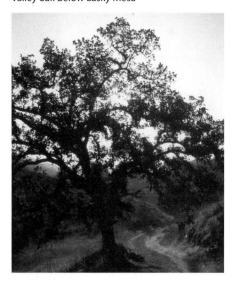

# trip 6  Cheeseboro Canyon

see map on p. 38

| | |
|---|---|
| **Distance** | 6.5 miles, Loop |
| **Hiking Time** | 3 hours |
| **Elevation Gain/Loss** | 850'/850' |
| **Difficulty** | Moderate |
| **Trail Use** | Dogs allowed |
| **Best Times** | November through May |
| **Agency** | NPS |
| **Optional Map** | USGS 7.5-min *Calabasas* |
| **Notes** | Marked trails/obvious routes, easy terrain |

**DIRECTIONS**  Take the Chesebro[sic] Road exit from the Ventura Freeway, go north about 200 yards, and then turn right on the signed Chesebro Road. Drive 0.7 mile north to Cheeseboro Canyon's entrance and trailhead on the right.

Instantly a hit when it first opened to the public in the late 1980s, Cheeseboro Canyon now draws a host of hikers, mountain bikers, equestrians, and even some wheelchair explorers to its network of old roads and newer trails. Friendly rangers patrol the roads and trails on horseback, eager to tell anyone willing to lend an ear about the park's natural features and wildlife (deer and coyotes, especially).

For a good overview of the entire area, follow the 6.5-mile route described here, which goes up the canyon floor and back along the east ridge. Two optional, worthwhile side trips could add more miles—if you're up to it. If you're traveling on a mountain bike, be aware that they are allowed only on the wide trails designated for such use, not for the entire trip described here.

Starting from the trailhead, the wide Cheeseboro Canyon Trail goes east and then bends north up the wide, nearly flat canyon floor, while the Modelo Trail slants left and curves up along the canyon's rounded west wall. At 1.6 miles, near the Palo Comado Connector trail joining from the west, you come upon a pleasant trailside picnic area. Stay on the main, wide trail going north along the Cheeseboro Canyon bottom, passing statuesque valley oaks, which are deciduous, and gnarled coast live oaks, which retain their leaves year round.

After 2.5 miles, turn right on the steep, narrow Baleen Wall Trail—no mountain bikes allowed on the ascending stretch ahead—and begin climbing the grass- and sage-covered east canyon wall. (From this junction you could make an out-and-back side trip: By keeping straight on the main trail, you would pass some sulfurous-smelling seeps and later emerge in an open valley dotted with sandstone boulders. An old sheep corral made of wire lies in the upper reaches of Cheeseboro Canyon, 2 miles from the Baleen Wall turnoff.)

After some huffing and puffing up the Baleen Wall Trail, you come to a powerline access road roughly following the east ridgeline. (Here you could begin a second side trip by going north along the road 0.5 mile to the lip of the Baleen Wall, a whitish sedimentary outcrop, for an impressive view of the upper canyon.)

To continue on the main route, walk south on the powerline access road, the Cheeseboro Ridge Trail, past a large water tank and down to a trail junction. Turn right and continue descending toward the picnic area you passed earlier. From there, retrace your steps down the Cheeseboro Canyon Trail back to the trailhead.

# trip 7  Oak Canyon Park

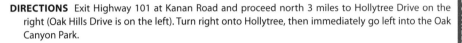

| | |
|---|---|
| **Distance** | 1.0 mile, Loop |
| **Hiking Time** | ½ hour |
| **Elevation Gain/Loss** | 100'/100' |
| **Difficulty** | Easy |
| **Trail Use** | Good for kids |
| **Best Times** | All year |
| **Agency** | RSRPD |
| **Optional Map** | USGS 7.5-min *Thousand Oaks* |
| **Notes** | Marked trails/obvious routes, easy terrain |

see map on p. 38

**DIRECTIONS** Exit Highway 101 at Kanan Road and proceed north 3 miles to Hollytree Drive on the right (Oak Hills Drive is on the left). Turn right onto Hollytree, then immediately go left into the Oak Canyon Park.

Oak Canyon Community Park, just north of Agoura Hills in the Ventura County suburb of Oak Park, is a model for suburban growth that doesn't have to bulldoze everything in sight. The 60-acre park, surrounded on three sides by new housing developments, straddles Medea Creek, which arises on the south slope of Simi Peak and flows year round.

From an information board near the parking lot you may obtain a leaflet that will guide you counterclockwise around a loop with numbered posts. You can either go that way, starting with a stretch on concrete and asphalt, or else go the opposite way by heading straight down to the creek from the park's spacious lawn. The creekside stretch is perfect for small kids, who will doubtless enjoy the magical atmosphere of overhanging oak limbs, the whisper of trickling water, and (of course) mud.

For further exploration and a good view of the immediate area, you can venture onto the chaparral-clad slopes rising to the west. Beyond Oak Canyon Park itself, pathways continue along Medea Creek through the suburbs—south toward Thousand Oaks Boulevard, and north to Lindero Canyon Road. At the latter, the China Flat Trail begins an ascent toward China Flat and Simi Peak (see Trip 8).

# trip 8  China Flat Loop

see map on p. 38

| | |
|---|---|
| **Distance** | 9.8 miles, Loop |
| **Hiking Time** | 5½ hours |
| **Elevation Gain/Loss** | 2300'/2300' |
| **Difficulty** | Moderately strenuous |
| **Trail Use** | Dogs allowed |
| **Best Times** | November through May |
| **Agency** | NPS |
| **Optional Maps** | USGS 7.5-min *Calabasas, Thousand Oaks* |
| **Notes** | Navigation required, easy to moderate terrain |

**DIRECTIONS**  Exit Highway 101 at Kanan Road and drive north 2.2 miles to Sunnycrest Drive. Turn right and continue 0.8 mile to a trail entrance on the right signed public recreation trail. At this point, the street's name changes to Doubletree Road. Abundant curbside parking is available.

This rambling loop route includes a little of everything: a long ascent up pristine Palo Camado Canyon, a visit to a reflecting pool (well, an old stock pond) at China Flat, broad views of the surrounding suburbs from Simi Peak, a passage through Oak Canyon Park, and a concluding stretch on suburban streets. Although the route as described here is customized for hikers, mountain bikers can at least appreciate the stretch through Palo Camado Canyon and into China Flat. The trek to the summit of Simi Peak and the descent on the China Flat Trail are generally not suitable and sometimes unsafe for riding on any sort of wheels.

From the trailhead, travel east through grassland for 0.5 mile over a rise and downhill into broad Palo Camado Canyon. Turn left on the dirt road going left, up the canyon, and enjoy a pleasant stroll amid stately sycamores and gnarled live oaks. Unlike Cheeseboro Canyon to the east, Palo Camado is pleasantly free from the visual annoyance of powerlines. Wildlife is plentiful hereabouts but often circumspect. Deer, bobcats, coyotes, rabbits, owls, and various birds of prey can be spotted here, especially in the early morning.

At around 1.5 miles, the canyon divides. Keeping to the right of the right tributary,

Pond at China Flat

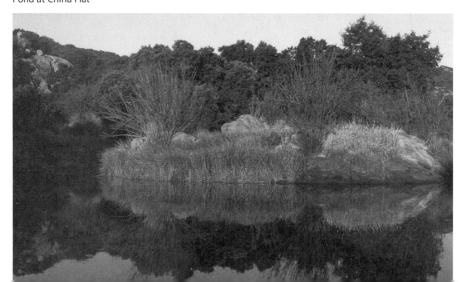

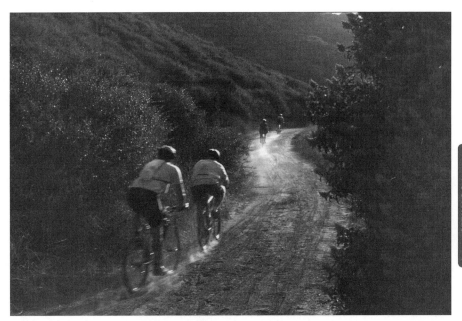

Cycling upper Palo Comado Canyon

the dirt road begins a vigorous and some-times crooked ascent. Looking behind you, you gaze upon a lovely tapestry of canyon-bottom woods and slopes adorned with dense patches of chaparral and sandstone outcrops.

After assuming a more gentle gradient at 2.6 miles, you pass over a summit at 3.3 miles and proceed another 0.2 mile down-hill to the edge of oak-dotted China Flat. On your left lies an old stock pond forming a small reflecting pool when it brims with water during and after the rainy season.

Continue west through China Flat, stay-ing left at the next junction. Beyond the oaks to your left (south), the China Flat Trail climbs a ridge and goes down the far side. This is your way back to suburbia, but for now don't miss the side trip to Simi Peak, which is 1.0 mile away by trail. Keep going west by veering right on a pathway going up a gradual incline. This pathway eventually curls up Simi Peak's north slope, becoming very steep and rocky in the last 200 yards. South and west from the jagged summit, your gaze takes in the broad sweep

of the Santa Monica Mountains and scat-tered patches of cityscape embedded in the rolling landscape below.

After visiting the peak, return to China Flat and turn right on the China Flat Trail. You duck under a canopy of oaks, climb for a few minutes, pass over a saddle, and finally descend 1.5 miles on a disused and sometimes eroded dirt road to the edge of a housing development. You emerge either at King James Court, or just around the corner on Lindero Canyon Road. Cross Lin-dero Canyon Road and proceed on one or another pathway heading southeast down along the oak-lined Medea Creek drainage. Soon you find yourself on Oak Canyon Park's nature trail (see Trip 7), where you can either follow a bike path on the left, or stick to a wide dirt path along trickling Medea Creek itself. You emerge near the park's entrance, where you can find water and restrooms.

Now only 1.3 miles remain—entirely on sidewalks. Use Hollytree Drive and Double-tree Road to get back to your starting point by the shortest route.

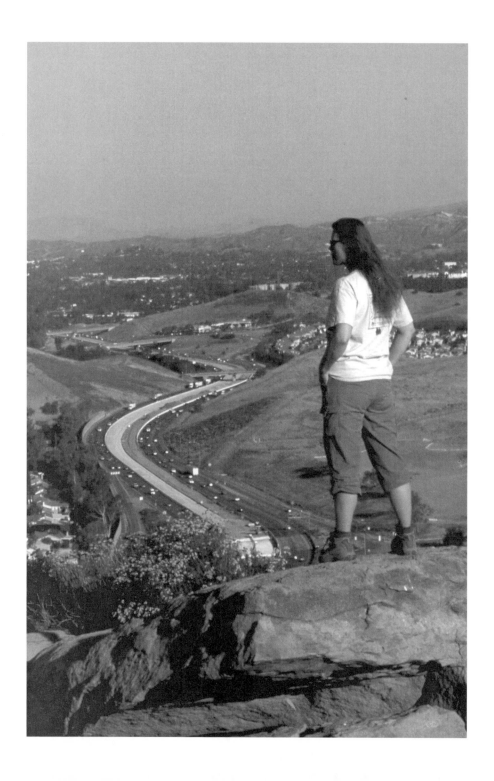

# chapter 5

# Basin and Foothills:
# Santa Susana Mountains

**B**arren and austere when viewed by midday light, but soft and pillowy under the sun's slanting rays, the Santa Susana Mountains, rising from the northeast corner of the San Fernando Valley, have long been recognized as an important reservoir of open space. Conservation organizations have spearheaded the effort to acquire from private interests bits and pieces of what will hopefully become a broad tapestry of protected land for wildlife habitat and low-impact recreation.

Overlooking the valley from the east end of the range is 672-acre O'Melveny Park, the second biggest (after Griffith Park) city park in Los Angeles. Noted for its picture-perfect picnic grounds with white fences and towering eucalyptus trees, the park also challenges hikers with several miles of steep, backcountry fire roads and primitive trails.

Behind, or north of, O'Melveny Park, on slopes facing the Santa Clarita Valley, lie some 6000 acres of attractively wooded ridges and canyons that are a part of the Santa Clarita Woodlands State Park and various parks and preserves acquired or managed by the Santa Monica Mountains Conservancy. Four trips in this chapter explore this surprisingly beautiful patch of open space.

Farther west, hikers can enjoy a network of riding and hiking paths in suburban Porter Ranch, ascend the south slope of Oat Mountain, probe the narrow confines of Devil Canyon, trace an old stagecoach trail that preceded the 20th-Century roads through Santa Susana Pass, and climb view-rich Rocky Peak. Worth mentioning (but not included as a "trip" in this chapter) is Stony Point in Chatsworth, a spectacular but graffiti-scarred pile of sandstone boulders popular among rock-climbing enthusiasts and scramblers of all ages.

The 12 trips of this chapter give a taste of what is currently available for hikers in the Santa Susanas. The presently existing parks and open spaces in this area are but a part of a visionary "Rim-of-the-Valley" natural area that will include, it is hoped, a trail stretching 100 miles around the north rim of the San Fernando Valley—from Ventura County to Glendale.

On the Hummingbird Trail overlooking the 118 Freeway

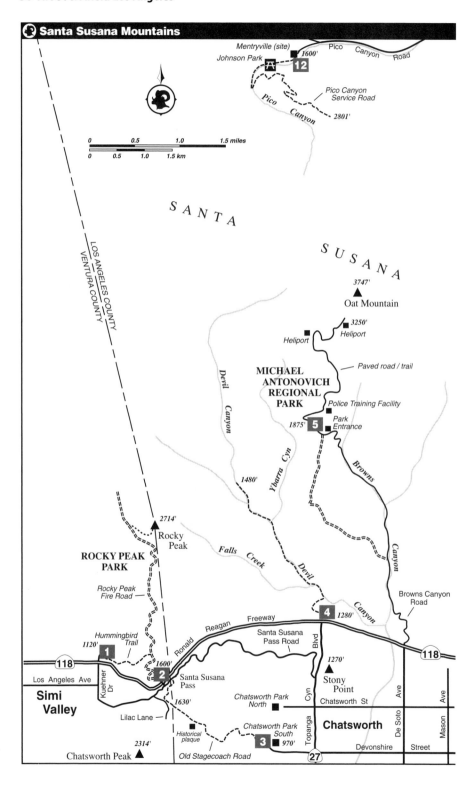

**Santa Susana Mountains**

Mentryville (site)
Pico Canyon Road
Johnson Park
*1600'* 12
Pico Canyon Service Road
Pico Canyon
*2801'*

0        0.5        1.0        1.5 miles
0     0.5     1.0     1.5 km

S A N T A

S U S A N A

*3747'*
Oat Mountain

*3250'*
Heliport
Heliport

MICHAEL
ANTONOVICH
REGIONAL
PARK

Paved road / trail

Police Training Facility

*1875'* 5
Park
Entrance

LOS ANGELES COUNTY
VENTURA COUNTY

Devil Canyon

Ybarra Cyn

*1480'*

Browns Canyon

*2714'*
Rocky Peak

ROCKY PEAK
PARK

Falls Creek

Devil

Rocky Peak
Fire Road

Browns Canyon
Road

4 *1280'*

Canyon

Ronald Reagan Freeway

Santa Susana
Pass Road

Hummingbird
Trail
*1120'*

Blvd

*1270'*
Stony
Point

118

1

*1600'*

118

Los Angeles Ave

Kuehner Dr

2

Santa Susana
Pass

Chatsworth Park
North

Chatsworth St

De Soto Ave

Mason Ave

Simi
Valley

*1630'*

Lilac Lane

Chatsworth Park
South

3 *970'*

Topanga Cyn

Chatsworth

*2314'*
Chatsworth Peak ▲

Historical
plaque

Old Stagecoach Road

Devonshire Street

27

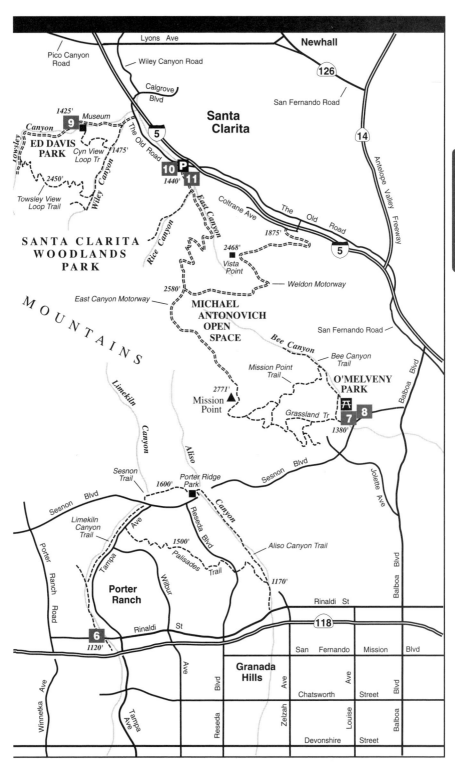

# trip 1 Hummingbird Trail

see map on p. 50

| | |
|---|---|
| **Distance** | 4.5 miles round trip, Out-and-back |
| **Hiking Time** | 3 hours (round trip) |
| **Elevation Gain/Loss** | 1150'/1150' |
| **Difficulty** | Moderately strenuous |
| **Trail Use** | Dogs allowed, good for kids |
| **Best Times** | October through May |
| **Agency** | SMMC |
| **Optional Map** | USGS 7.5-min *Santa Susana* |
| **Notes** | Marked trails/obvious routes, easy to moderate terrain |

**DIRECTIONS** Exit the 118 Freeway at Kuehner Drive in Simi Valley. Drive north 0.1 mile and park off pavement on the right side of Kuehner. This is the site of a future trailhead for the Hummingbird Trail. Do not park at the north end of Kuehner, where curbside parking is prohibited.

The Hummingbird Trail starts at the extreme northeast corner of Simi Valley (both the valley and the city of same name) and deviously ascends boulder-studded slopes to the crest of a long ridge leading north to Rocky Peak. This out-and-back jaunt is perfect for early-morning exercise, when the trail lies mostly in shadow. Hikers and runners use it, as well as some intrepid mountain bikers who may risk life and limb on a couple of the steeper, more slippery pitches.

Signs along Kuehner Drive, just north of the 118 Freeway direct hikers north alongside the road shoulder for about 200 yards to a path veering right, just shy of where Kuehner ends at the entryway to a gated community. Follow this sketchy path down to the bottom of a ravine, called Hummingbird Creek, where the well-defined trail starts. (These directions will likely change when a housing project at the foot of the trail, stalled as of 2009, is completed and the trail is rerouted around it.)

After veering south to reach a point close to the freeway embankment, the trail switches back and starts to dart upward, trending east via many zigs and zags, sometimes over barren rock. This continues more or less unabated until about 2 miles into the hike, where the trail straightens, heads straightforwardly east, and finally reaches the Rocky Peak Fire Road at a point 0.8 mile north of the fire road's origination point alongside the 118 Freeway at Santa Susana Pass.

Along the way up and the way back down you're seldom out of earshot of traffic on the neighboring freeway. Yet there are consistently panoramic views to enjoy whenever you want to take a break. If you have a camera it's fun to pose your hiking companion atop any number of rounded boulders alongside the trail, with a background, perhaps, of the geometric patterns of subdivisions on the flat Simi Valley floor.

# trip 2  Rocky Peak

| | |
|---|---|
| **Distance** | 5.6 miles round trip, Out-and-back |
| **Hiking Time** | 3 hours (round trip) |
| **Elevation Gain/Loss** | 1200'/1200' |
| **Difficulty** | Moderately strenuous |
| **Trail Use** | Suitable for mountain biking, dogs allowed |
| **Best Times** | October through May |
| **Agency** | SMMC |
| **Optional Map** | USGS 7.5-min *Santa Susana* |
| **Notes** | Marked trails/obvious routes, easy to moderate terrain |

see map on p. 50

**DIRECTIONS**  From the San Fernando Valley, take 118 Freeway west and exit at the Santa Susana Pass/ Rocky Peak offramp. Park in the dirt lot on the right. Those approaching eastbound from Simi Valley and Ventura County will find there is no eastbound offramp here; instead, access to the trailhead is by way of Santa Susana Pass Road.

In 1990 the Santa Monica Mountains Conservancy entered negotiations with entertainer Bob Hope to purchase Rocky Peak Park—a 4369-acre parcel of land overlooking the Simi and San Fernando valleys. Today, the entire spread—long locked up in private ownership and more recently threatened by creeping suburbia— welcomes hikers and bikers who can start their trip, conveniently enough, at the end of a freeway offramp.

A look at a topographic map of the area reveals a loopy pattern of closely spaced contour lines, indicative of terrain topped by immense boulder piles. The sandstone that underlies this area dates from the Cretaceous period more than 65 million years ago. Relatively recent uplift, weathering, and erosion has carved this rock into impressively huge and intricate structures at the surface.

Rocky Peak vista

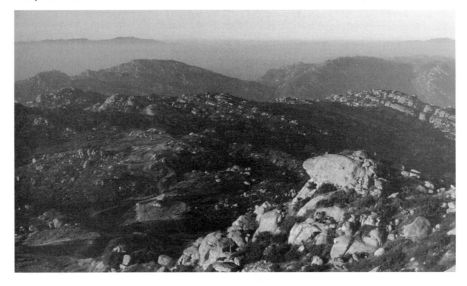

**BASIN AND FOOTHILLS**

Your ascent from the trailhead begins immediately on the Rocky Peak Fire Road. At 0.8 mile, note the junction of the Hummingbird Trail (see Trip 1) on the left. Keep climbing. At about 1.5 miles, your relentless ascent is temporarily reversed by a brief drop into a little flat where, on the right, you can find shade and rest under a lone live-oak tree.

After passing larger and more impressively convoluted outcrops of sandstone, the fire road tops out on a prominent ridgeline (2.4 miles). There an older, disused road joins on the right, leading circuitously toward Rocky Peak—only a little higher but well worth a side trip of 0.4 mile for the sake of a fabulous view. This old road peters out quickly, but hikers (not mountain bikers) can follow an informal path ahead. As the path becomes indistinct, you face a somewhat scratchy scramble over a false summit, down and back up to the highest pile of boulders.

The Rocky Peak summit defines a waypoint on the boundary between Los Angeles County and Ventura County. The view from the top at best encompasses large parts of these two counties, plus the Pacific Ocean—partly obscured by the undulating Santa Monica Mountains.

## trip 3  Old Stagecoach Road

see map on p. 50

| | |
|---|---|
| **Distance** | 2.6 miles round trip, Out-and-back |
| **Hiking Time** | 1½ hours (round trip) |
| **Elevation Gain/Loss** | 650'/650' |
| **Difficulty** | Moderate |
| **Trail Use** | Good for kids |
| **Best Times** | All year |
| **Agency** | SSPSHP |
| **Optional Maps** | USGS 7.5-min *Oat Mountain, Santa Susana* |
| **Notes** | Navigation required, easy terrain |

**DIRECTIONS** Drive to the west end of Devonshire Street, 0.5 mile west of Topanga Canyon Boulevard, in Chatsworth. Park at Chatsworth Park South, which is open 8 a.m. to sunset daily.

Clear-air vistas of the San Fernando Valley and surrounding mountain ranges are as spectacular as they come when seen from the Old Stagecoach Road above Chatsworth. The boulder-stacked hillsides rising from the valley seem strongly reminiscent of the golden backdrops seen in old Western movies and television shows, because they really did play a background role in many of those productions.

The area traversed by the Old Stagecoach Road has recently been incorporated into the new 670-acre Santa Susana Pass State Historic Park. The pass has been (and continues to be) a key link in a major coastal transportation corridor connecting northern and southern California. The Spanish Army Captain Gaspar de Portola passed this way in 1769, blazing a trail from San Diego to Monterey Bay. The route later became a part of the El Camino Real (King's Highway), which linked the Spanish system of presidios, pueblos, and missions along California's coast and coastal-inland valleys. Today, railroad tracks and the Simi Valley Freeway traverse the Santa Susana Pass slightly north of where an earlier, devilishly steep road called the Devil's Slide, was built to accommodate stagecoaches. Surprisingly, this long-abandoned stage route can be traced today on foot.

Because the state historic park is new and a plan for development of marked trails is in the works, the directions here may differ somewhat from what you will find when you visit.

At Chatsworth Park South, pick up the path indicating the Old Stagecoach Road on the left. After reaching the west boundary of Chatsworth Park (0.4 mile) you start climbing into the bouldered hills, where a maze of roads and old vehicle tracks may complicate route-finding. Head generally southwest and uphill to a low ridge distinguished by a row of bushy olive trees (0.6 mile). From there, turn right (northwest) up the ridge and aim toward a large, white, rectangular plaque embedded in sandstone on the hillside about 0.4 mile away. You're now on a well-preserved section of the Devil's Slide, a key link in the 1860–90 coastal stage road linking Los Angeles and San Francisco. As you walk up the hard sandstone bed, notice the carefully hewn drainage chutes on both sides. With a little detective work you may also find a couple of old cisterns, used to capture rainwater for relay teams of horses that pulled wagons up the formidable grade.

The tiled historical plaque, installed in 1939, remains in good shape. Beyond the plaque, you can follow the stagecoach road bed another 0.3 mile to the Devil's Slide summit (1630′), where you cross the L.A.–Ventura county line and reach a trailhead sign on Lilac Lane in an area of scattered residences. North, behind a hill, is today's Santa Susana Pass, threaded by the Simi Valley Freeway and the older Santa Susana Pass Road. Some 600 feet below you is the 1.4-mile-long Santa Susana railroad tunnel, whose east entrance can be seen back near Chatsworth Park South.

## trip 4  Devil Canyon

|  |  |
|---|---|
| **Distance** | 4.6 miles round trip, Out-and-back |
| **Hiking Time** | 2½ hours (round trip) |
| **Elevation Gain/Loss** | 450′/450′ |
| **Difficulty** | Moderate |
| **Trail Use** | Suitable for mountain biking, dogs allowed, good for kids |
| **Best Times** | October through June |
| **Agency** | SMMC |
| **Optional Map** | USGS 7.5-min *Oat Mountain* |
| **Notes** | Marked trails/obvious routes, easy terrain |

see map on p. 50

**DIRECTIONS**  Exit the 118 Freeway at Topanga Canyon Boulevard in Chatsworth. Turn north and immediately go west on Poema Place. On the hillside to the right, just below a newly constructed condominium complex, is a small dirt lot, which (perhaps temporarily) serves as a trailhead for the Devil Canyon Trail.

A surprisingly cool and pleasant retreat just back of the hot, dry northwest corner of the San Fernando Valley, Devil Canyon sports abundant growths of live oak and willow and a small, intermittent stream. Fire and flood have long since removed almost all traces of an old auto road in the canyon; in its place hikers and mountain bikers have beaten down a narrow trail. Come here in the early spring to enjoy the blooming ceanothus on the hillsides, or in winter (wear an old pair of shoes) if you don't mind tramping through lots of good, clean mud.

From the dirt lot, note the path and accompanying wooden fence a short distance up the hill. This new, rerouted (as of 2008) segment of trail passes alongside and behind a just-built condominium complex, and descends into Devil Canyon beyond.

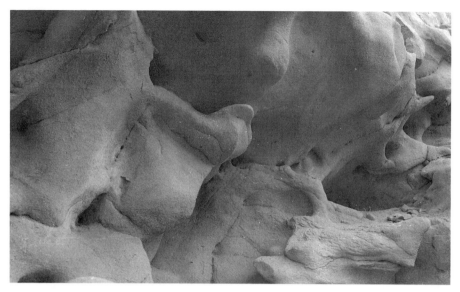

Devil Canyon wall

The at-first uninspiring scenery improves greatly as you swing around a couple of sharp bends and lose sight of wall-to-wall condos on the bluff above. Scattered riparian vegetation accompanies you most of the way as you work your way up along the canyon bottom.

You can go as far as a pipe gate (2.3 miles), pausing along the way to admire the wind- and water-carved sandstone bedrock along both sides of the canyon. This sandstone, a part of the same formation exposed at Stony Point and Santa Susana Pass, originated from sediments laid down in a marine environment roughly 80 million years ago. Shallow caves can be found in Devil Canyon's tributaries—especially Falls Creek—if you don't mind a little bushwhacking.

## trip 5  Oat Mountain

see map on p. 50

| | |
|---|---|
| **Distance** | 4.6 miles round trip, Out-and-back |
| **Hiking Time** | 2½ hours (round trip) |
| **Elevation Gain/Loss** | 1400′/1400′ |
| **Difficulty** | Moderately strenuous |
| **Trail Use** | Suitable for mountain biking, dogs allowed |
| **Best Times** | October through May |
| **Agency** | SMMC |
| **Optional Map** | USGS 7.5-min *Oat Mountain* |
| **Notes** | Marked trails/obvious routes, easy terrain |

**DIRECTIONS**  Exit the 118 Freeway at De Soto Avenue in Chatsworth. The northern extension of De Soto is called Browns Canyon Road. Follow this narrow, twisty road around some outlying houses, up along the Browns Canyon stream, and finally up a steep hill to the main Antonovich Park entrance. There's a lower parking lot on the left, but continue about 0.4 mile farther to an large upper lot just shy of where the road is blocked to public traffic.

A rambling patch of newly acquired open space that goes by the long-winded name of Michael D. Antonovich Regional Park at Joughin Ranch spreads over a south-facing slope, culminating in a 3747-foot summit called Oat Mountain. On this trip, you drive about halfway up the mountain (as measured from the San Fernando Valley floor) and travel on foot most of the remaining distance to Oat Mountain, which technically lies on private property. On a clear day, the ever more spacious view gets ever more stupendous; on a hazy or smoggy day you won't like either the impaired view or the dirty air moving in and out of your lungs.

After parking in the upper lot—as far as you can drive on Browns Canyon Road—trudge on, uphill and sometimes steeply so, continuing on the same road. By 0.5 mile into the hike, you're passing the various buildings of a Los Angeles Police Department training facility, and the sharp increase in elevation gain so far has yielded a significantly wider panorama of the vast, flat, and densely populated San Fernando Valley below. Above the training facility, the close-at-hand landscape assumes a more impressive character, with wild grasses—mostly wild oats, after which the peak above was named—bending in a supple fashion in the zephyrs of springtime, or chafing in the dry breezes of the other seasons.

At 1.0 mile you traverse a cattle grate and temporarily enter a parcel where cattle graze contentedly. Soon, after crossing a second grate, you're back in Antonovich parkland, where the ascent quickens. The valley view to the south now assumes a pseudo-aerial character, and the green or golden (depending on the season) slopes seem to roll sensuously upward, downward, and sideways.

At 2.0 miles, alongside a heliport (a large flat spot for fire-fighting helicopters to land), you start to get a view to the north, which consists of miles of ridges sparsely dotted with valley oaks, and an occasional rocker pump struggling to extract the very last drop of crude oil remaining in the permeable strata far below.

Keep going a bit farther to a second heliport, this one on the right, which offers perhaps the most comprehensive vista so far. After contemplating the scene and taking a deep pull from your water bottle, it's time to return. Use the same route—a possibly knee-jarring experience at times.

Oat Mountain

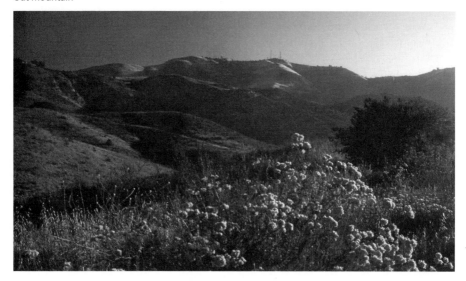

see map on p. 50

# trip 6  Porter Ranch Loop

|                     |                                          |
|---------------------|------------------------------------------|
| **Distance**        | 8.0 miles, Loop                          |
| **Hiking Time**     | 4 hours                                  |
| **Elevation Gain/Loss** | 1000'/1000'                          |
| **Difficulty**      | Moderately strenuous                     |
| **Trail Use**       | Suitable for mountain biking, dogs allowed |
| **Best Times**      | October through May                      |
| **Agency**          | LACRPD                                   |
| **Optional Map**    | USGS 7.5-min *Oat Mountain*              |
| **Notes**           | Marked trails/obvious routes, easy terrain |

**DIRECTIONS** Exit the 118 Freeway at Tampa Avenue in the Northridge area. Go north for one block, turn left on Rinaldi Street, go about one block, and find a place to park where Rinaldi crosses Limekiln Canyon Park.

The open spaces and trails lacing well-to-do Porter Ranch could serve as a nice model for community development anywhere in the Southland. Of course, it could be also be argued that the world would be better off without the square miles of new housing developments here and elsewhere along the rim of the San Fernando Valley. But at least local residents—and the public at large—have the opportunity to wander the remaining vestiges of two riparian canyons and a cliff-rimmed hillside blanketed with aromatic sage.

Suitable for horses and mountain bikes as well as hikers, this trip is best taken on a cool day. A look at this chapter's map (or any street map of the area) reveals ways to abbreviate the trip if you don't want to go the full 8 miles.

From Rinadi Street, pick up the equestrian trail going north through the landscaped linear park along Limekiln Canyon's trickling creek. After crossing the creek twice on bridges you come to a split (0.7 mile) where one branch of the trail bends easily left and follows a ravine toward a subdivision. Take the main branch (right), which goes up toward the shoulder of Tampa Avenue. You pass under a concrete bridge (a gated entrance road serving houses west of Limekiln Canyon); pass a junction with the Palisades Trail (your return route); cross Sesnon Boulevard; and finally join the Sesnon Trail, 1.8 miles from the start.

Follow the Sesnon Trail east over a hump to Ormskirk Avenue. Turn south, walk through Porter Ridge Park, and go left on Sesnon Boulevard to where it dead ends on the edge of steep-sided Aliso Canyon. Walk around the pipe gate on the left and down into Aliso Canyon.

After following the canyon bottom for 1.3 miles (to 4.0 miles from the start) you turn right on the Palisades Trail, which doubles back up a ravine, climbs a slope, passes some houses, and reaches Reseda Boulevard. Cross Reseda, continue uphill on the west sidewalk for about 0.3 mile, and then veer off on the wide trail, bordered by a wooden fence, descending left along a sage-covered slope.

Soon you start contouring along the base of some craggy, sedimentary bluffs—the so-called palisades. You're well above the valley floor here, so the view takes in thousands of rooftops in the foreground and the purple Santa Monica Mountains rising above the valley haze in the south.

At 6.5 miles the Palisades Trail goes over a saddle and then it drops down to Tampa Avenue. Pick up the Limekiln Canyon Trail on the far side and return to your car, retracing your earlier steps.

## trip 7  Bee Canyon

| | |
|---|---|
| **Distance** | 2.0 miles round trip, Out-and-back |
| **Hiking Time** | 1½ hours (round trip) |
| **Elevation Gain/Loss** | 250'/250' |
| **Difficulty** | Moderate |
| **Trail Use** | Dogs allowed, good for kids |
| **Best Times** | All year |
| **Agency** | LACRPD |
| **Optional Map** | USGS 7.5-min *Oat Mountain* |
| **Notes** | Marked trails/obvious routes, easy to moderate terrain |

see map on p. 50

**DIRECTIONS** Exit the 118 Freeway at Balboa Boulevard in Granada Hills. Drive north 2 miles to Sesnon Boulevard. Go left (west) and continue 0.6 mile to the parking lot for O'Melveny Park on the right.

O'Melveny Park's Bee Canyon is a terrific place for exploring with little ones. Presided over by sky-scraping cliffs and shaded by a veritable jungle of young willow saplings, this is natural L.A.'s answer to Disneyland's Adventureland. During most of the year water seeps, or flows, down the canyon's silty bottom, so you'd better wear old shoes if you intend to probe the canyon's upper, nearly trailless reaches.

From the park's entrance, follow the paved trail uphill though the tree-shaded picnic grounds. After the path turns to dirt simply follow the path of least resistance into the hills, straight up the V-shaped gorge ahead, which is Bee Canyon. On the left (southwest) side of the canyon, live oak and California walnut trees stand as battered but proud survivors of fire and flood. On the right, barren sedimentary cliffs soar 500 feet. Movements along the Santa Susana thrust fault, which cuts east-west across the Santa Susanas, have helped produce this towering feature. In the wetter times of year water seeps out of cracks in the layered rock above and dribbles down several of the steep gullies. (Note: the cliffs are unstable and are not suitable for climbing.)

At 0.5 mile beyond the picnic area, the main trail bends left to climb the canyon's south wall. A less-traveled trail continues ahead through willow thickets, becoming more and more obscure the farther you venture. Soon you're scrambling over eroded banks and tree roots, and squishing through mud puddles. By the time the going gets really rough, you'll be at or near the north boundary of the park—a good turnaround point.

**BASIN AND FOOTHILLS**

## trip 8 Mission Point

| | |
|---|---|
| **Distance** | 4.7 miles, Loop |
| **Hiking Time** | 3 hours |
| **Elevation Gain/Loss** | 1450'/1450' |
| **Difficulty** | Moderately strenuous |
| **Trail Use** | Suitable for mountain biking, dogs allowed |
| **Best Times** | November through May |
| **Agency** | LACRPD |
| **Optional Map** | USGS 7.5-min *Oat Mountain* |
| **Notes** | Marked trails/obvious routes, easy terrain |

see map on p. 50

**DIRECTIONS** Exit the 118 Freeway at Balboa Boulevard in Granada Hills. Drive north 2 miles to Sesnon Boulevard. Go left (west) and continue 0.6 mile to the parking lot for O'Melveny Park on the right.

Two centuries ago the treeless bump called Mission Point overlooked an arid valley dotted with Indian villages. One century ago, the same vantage point would have revealed an early housing boom amid the citrus groves on the valley floor. Today (whenever the smog chances to clear away) the 150-degree view of the San Fernando Valley takes in a seemingly endless grid of rectilinear streets and avenues, plus all the visible infrastructure of a city-within-a-city of more than 1.5 million people.

Start your hike on the Grassland Trail, west of the park office. The trail darts up a narrow, almost barren ridge dividing two parallel ravines. California walnut trees dot the bottoms of these ravines. Chances are good you'll spot a deer or a coyote, or a roadrunner flitting across your path.

Keep straight where a nature trail joins on the left. After plenty of huffing and puffing due to the elevation gain, you'll reach a wide fire road. Turn right and continue climbing, on looping curves, toward Mission Point. (You can shave off some distance, if not effort, by following a footpath going straight up the mountain along the easement of an underground gas pipeline.) Nearing the summit you'll pass a knoll topped by a cluster of live-oak trees. This tiny oak copse makes a fine picnic spot with a good view to boot.

A small stone monument atop Mission Point's shadeless summit (2 miles into the hike) memorializes physician Mario De Campos, a lover of the local mountains. Down in the valley 3 miles southeast, you'll spot the newer Los Angeles Reservoir as well as the dry bed of its predecessor, the Van Norman Reservoir, whose dam very nearly failed during the 1971 Sylmar earthquake. To the west, carved into the dry south slopes of the Santa Susanas, are old oil wells and a tangle of cliff-hanging roads built to serve them.

For a look at the much more agreeable and verdant north slopes of the Santa Susanas, walk farther north about 0.3 mile to where the road begins its descent into the Santa Clarita Woodlands area. There you can get a glimpse of canyon country dotted with live oak, valley oak, walnut, and bigcone Douglas-fir trees. Why the big difference in vegetation? Simply the slope aspect, whereby the south-facing slopes bake in year-round sun, while the north-facing slopes experience far more shade and far less evaporation of moisture.

On your return to the O'Melveny Park entrance, descend below Mission Point using the road you followed uphill. This time, take the Mission Point Trail to the left, which will take you down, sometimes steeply, into Bee Canyon. Once you reach the canyon floor, turn downstream and hike the remaining short distance out to the picnic area and your starting point.

# trip 9 Towsley Canyon/Wiley Canyon Loop

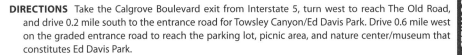
see map on p. 50

| | |
|---|---|
| **Distance** | 4.8 miles, Loop |
| **Hiking Time** | 3 hours |
| **Elevation Gain/Loss** | 1400'/1400' |
| **Difficulty** | Moderately strenuous |
| **Trail Use** | Suitable for mountain biking, dogs allowed |
| **Best Times** | October through June |
| **Agency** | SMMC |
| **Optional Map** | USGS 7.5-min *Oat Mountain* |
| **Notes** | Marked trails/obvious routes, easy terrain |

**DIRECTIONS** Take the Calgrove Boulevard exit from Interstate 5, turn west to reach The Old Road, and drive 0.2 mile south to the entrance road for Towsley Canyon/Ed Davis Park. Drive 0.6 mile west on the graded entrance road to reach the parking lot, picnic area, and nature center/museum that constitutes Ed Davis Park.

The Santa Clarita Woodlands Park, north of the arid San Fernando Valley and just east of Santa Clarita's dry hills and valleys, encompasses a surprising assortment of strange geologic features and several amazingly lush canyons and north-facing hillsides. For 120 years, Chevron Corporation (formerly Standard Oil of California) owned this land, using it for oil production and limited grazing. In 1995, over 3000 acres of this land was transferred to the Santa Monica Mountains Conservancy. With subsequent additions of open space, the protected area now includes about 6000 acres. Here, as elsewhere on the metropolitan fringe of Los Angeles, it is hard to believe such near-pristine and sublime landscapes can exist so close to a population of millions.

The loop through Towsley and Wiley canyons described here, partly on old roads and partly on "single-track" trail, visits narrow canyon bottoms and sunny ridges, all

Sandstone outcrop, Towsley Canyon

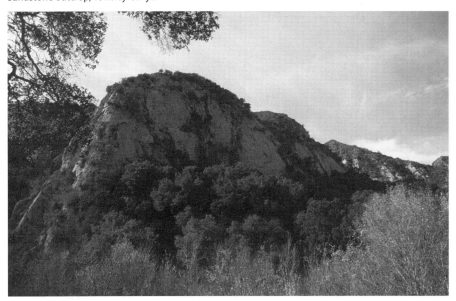

the while exposing you to an ever-changing array of habitats: riparian woodland, oak and walnut woodlands, coastal sage scrub, chaparral, and grassland.

From Ed Davis Park start walking west on the graded service road going up the wide floodplain of Towsley Canyon. Notice the foamy beige water flowing in the canyon's creek, the faint sulfurous smell, and gobs of tar in places. Well before any oil was extracted for commercial purposes here, the Tataviam Indians of the area used naturally occurring asphalt for medicinal applications and to seal their basketry.

The scenery improves dramatically as you reach, at 0.9 mile, the portals of The Narrows, a slotlike cleft worn through layers of sandstone and conglomerate tilted nearly vertical. The Santa Susana Mountains were built through geologic uplift along thrust faults—a process dramatically demonstrated during the catastrophically damaging 1994 Northridge quake, an event that actually caused the Santa Susanas to rise a foot or more. With all the compression going on, both underground and at the surface, it is not surprising to see a variety of folds (synclines and anticlines) in the rocks exposed here and elsewhere in the Santa Clarita Woodlands.

After a brief passage through The Narrows, you encounter a split in the road. Stay left. After another 200 yards, stay left again, and begin climbing the canyon slope to the left on what is called the Towsley View Loop Trail. It quickly evolves into a narrow, or single-track, trail (easy to negotiate on foot, tougher on a mountain bike) that steadily ascends on switchbacks through sage scrub and later through some gorgeous, almost pure stands of California walnut. Higher still the tree canopy thins, with scattered oaks and pungent bay laurel clinging to the hillsides. There you catch sight of the hills and valleys of Santa Clarita to the north and east, which are increasingly being overrun with cookie-cutter subdivisions.

After reaching a high point of 2450 feet, the trail begins to pitch downward, executing a circuitous and sometimes steep descent down drier slopes into the shady depths of Wiley Canyon. Joining a dirt road there (3.4 miles), you turn left and head north, making your easy way down-canyon. At 4.1 miles, look carefully for your next turn, on the Canyon View Loop Trail which ascends to the left. A final, crooked 0.7-mile traverse on this trail takes you over a summit and back down to Ed Davis Park, your starting point.

## trip 10  Rice Canyon

| | |
|---|---|
| **Distance** | 2.5 miles round trip, Out-and-back |
| **Hiking Time** | 1½ hours (round trip) |
| **Elevation Gain/Loss** | 350'/350' |
| **Difficulty** | Easy |
| **Trail Use** | Dogs allowed, good for kids |
| **Best Times** | All year |
| **Agency** | SMMC |
| **Optional Map** | USGS 7.5-min *Oat Mountain* |
| **Notes** | Marked trails/obvious routes, easy terrain |

see map on p. 50

**DIRECTIONS** Take the Calgrove Boulevard exit from Interstate 5, turn west to reach The Old Road, and drive 0.8 mile south to the trailhead on the right. This is just before The Old Road goes under Interstate 5.

A pleasant little retreat in almost any season, Rice Canyon hides amid the foothills of the Santa Susana Mountains, just outside the busy suburban community of Santa Clarita. Even on the sunniest days, you can find dark pools of shade here, and much cooler temperatures.

From the trailhead, you start with an uninteresting 0.3-mile hike south on an old ranch road to an old water trough and other evidence of former cattle ranching. Look on the right side of the road for the narrow trail going into Rice Canyon, where it is noted that mountain bikes are not allowed. This nearly 1-mile-long trail is enchanting for kids and adults alike—a veritable fairyland complete with a limpid brook and a shade-giving assortment of sycamore, willow, and cottonwood trees, plus four kinds of oak: scrub oak, coast live oak, canyon live oak, and valley oak.

In the upper part of Rice Canyon, the trail begins to rise sharply along the slope to the right. After climbing sharply for a few minutes, you get a nice view south of steep slopes plunging sheer from the crest of the Santa Susana Mountains. Here and there, higher in elevation, you'll spot bigcone Douglas-fir trees, a relative of Douglas-firs more commonly found much farther north in California and up the Pacific coast.

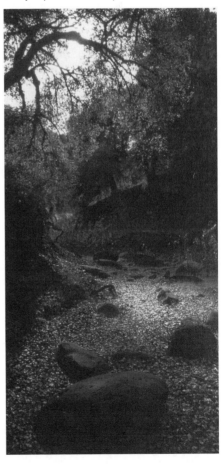
Shady depths of Rice Canyon

see map on p. 50

**trip 11** **East Canyon Loop**

| | |
|---|---|
| **Distance** | 6.5 miles, Loop |
| **Hiking Time** | 3½ hours |
| **Elevation Gain/Loss** | 1300'/1300' |
| **Difficulty** | Moderately strenuous |
| **Trail Use** | Suitable for mountain biking, dogs allowed |
| **Best Times** | October through May |
| **Agency** | SMMC |
| **Optional Map** | USGS 7.5-min *Oat Mountain* |
| **Notes** | Marked trails/obvious routes, easy terrain |

**DIRECTIONS** Take the Calgrove Boulevard exit from Interstate 5, turn west to reach The Old Road, and drive 0.8 mile south to the trailhead on the right. This is just before The Old Road goes under Interstate 5.

Verdant East Canyon tucks into steep, north-facing slopes just below the crest of the Santa Susana Mountains. The canyon receives an average of about 20 inches of rainfall annually—just enough, in an environment sheltered from sun's south-slanting rays, to support an island-like array of scraggly bigcone Douglas-fir trees. This evergreen species tends to thrive higher up in the nearby San Gabriel Mountains, but in this area some specimens can be found at elevations as low as 2000 feet.

Except for some steep pitches here and there, the looping route into East Canyon

described here is perfect for mountain biking. You'll see plenty of cyclists on the route, which consists of a combination of paved and dirt roads.

From the trailhead, head southeast (on foot or bike) on The Old Road, first under the traffic lanes of Interstate 5 and then parallel to freeway. The road's name suggests that this is the defunct U.S. Highway 99 over Newhall Pass which has since been replaced by the modern Interstate 5. Stay on The Old Road's shoulder so as to keep away from the light automotive traffic that still exists here. After a probably tedious

Early-morning marine layer over San Fernando Valley

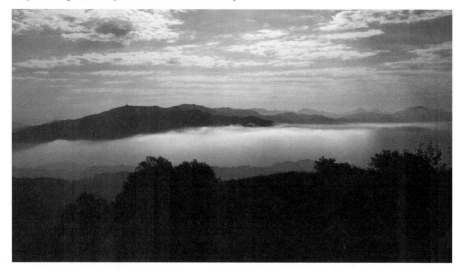

(on foot, at least) 1.5 miles, you reach Weldon Canyon Road, which crosses over Interstate 5 on a narrow overpass. Make a right at Coltrane Avenue on the far side of that overpass and continue 0.1 mile to Weldon Motorway (a fire road) on the left. The fire road's initial ascent is excruciating, but the uphill grade soon moderates.

The scenery turns gorgeous as you climb, especially during the early morning on many a day, when the entire San Fernando Valley lies unseen beneath a marine-layer blanket of clouds. To the east, the rounded summits of the San Gabriel Mountains rise into a sapphire sky, sometimes flecked with cirrus clouds. Near at hand, note the coast live oaks and a small number of bigcone Douglas-firs dotting the slopes.

At 2.2 miles, there's a private road on the left; stay right and proceed along a narrow ridge with dramatic dropoffs on both sides.

Some California walnut trees can be seen here. At 2.9 miles (elevation 2468') there's a rest stop with a shade ramada overlooking the East Canyon drainage to the north and east.

Continue following the same narrow ridge—essentially the south rim of East Canyon—until you reach a junction of fire roads at 4.3 miles. A left turn here could take you to Mission Point and O'Melveny Park (Trip 8). You go right, however, and begin the long and sometimes steep descent into East Canyon. Note more fine specimens of bigcone Douglas-firs along the way, their wandlike limbs reaching wide.

By 5.7 miles, you arrive alongside East Canyon's trickling stream, and enter a strip of gorgeous riparian/oak-woodland. Your starting point along The Old Road lies a short mile ahead.

BASIN AND FOOTHILLS

## trip 12  Pico Canyon

| | |
|---|---|
| **Distance** | 6.0 miles round trip, Out-and-back |
| **Hiking Time** | 3 hours (round trip) |
| **Elevation Gain/Loss** | 1250'/1250' |
| **Difficulty** | Moderately strenuous |
| **Trail Use** | Suitable for mountain biking, dogs allowed |
| **Best Times** | October through May |
| **Agency** | SMMC |
| **Optional Maps** | USGS 7.5-min *Newhall, Oat Mountain* |
| **Notes** | Marked trails/obvious routes, easy terrain |

see map on p. 50

**DIRECTIONS** Exit Interstate 5 at Pico Canyon Road in Santa Clarita, and drive west 2.5 miles to the gated park entrance (open daily, sunrise to sunset). Continue 0.4 mile farther to the large parking lot/trailhead at the historic site of Mentryville.

Pico Canyon cuts deeply into the northern Santa Susana Mountains, a few miles south of the Six Flags Magic Mountain amusement park. The canyon is considered to be the birthplace of the oil industry in California (ignoring the small-scale use of oil tar as a caulking agent by early Native Americans and missionaries). All of the wells in the canyon are capped today, and the surrounding property has become a part of the publicly accessible Santa Clarita Woodlands Park.

Historic Mentryville is today a gentrified ghost town. A number of structures in this former oil boom town remain intact: an 1890s barn and chicken coop, the 1898 home of oil driller Charles Alexander Mentry, and the Felton schoolhouse built in 1885 to serve more than 100 families residing in the canyon at that time.

From Mentryville, either by foot or by mountain bike, you may travel up the canyon as little as 1 mile to the rest stop known as Johnson Park, or as many as 3 miles to a canyon-rim perch offering a panoramic view of the entire Santa Clarita region. The former option is fine for an easy stroll anytime; the latter option involves significant effort and elevation gain, whether you go by foot or bike.

As you proceed uphill into Pico Canyon from Mentryville, you'll be right alongside the canyon's sluggishly flowing creek. Enjoy the green ribbon of riparian vegetation and trees—mostly live oaks, valley oaks, and arroyo willows. Natural tar still seeps into the stream, and it isn't unusual to catch a pungent whiff of it on the passing breeze.

At Johnson Park, a former oil-company picnic site with picnic benches and restrooms, don't mistake the wooden oil derrick you'll see there for a historic artifact; it's in fact an accurate replica of an early 20th Century oil rig.

At 1.3 miles up the canyon from Mentryville, two historical plaques indicate the site of the Pico Canyon Oil Field Well Number 4, which was not only California's first commercially successful oil well, but also the longest continuously operating oil well in the world (1876 to 1990) at the time of its closure. Its yield of 150 barrels of oil per day was modest compared to modern oil wells.

On ahead a short distance, the Pico Canyon service road, graded dirt at this point, bends sharply left and rises very steeply onto the brushy slope of the canyon, where the view expands to include the looping coaster tracks at Magic Mountain. After many twists and turns, 3.0 miles into the hike, the road ends at a flat spot some 1200 feet higher than your starting point. Look for a rusty old sign indicating a defunct Union Oil well. Intrepid hikers have forged a sketchy path along the ridgeline connecting this point to the Towsley Canyon unit of the Santa Clarita Woodlands Park, which lies southeast of here. Your easy option, to be sure, is to return via the same route.

Oil derrick replica at Johnson Park

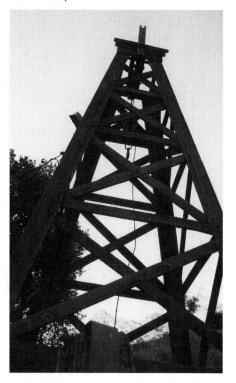

# chapter 6

# Basin and Foothills: Desert Gateway

**M**illions of years of geologic tumult can be read in the frozen stone exposed to casual view as you drive the Antelope Valley Freeway (Highway 14) between Interstate 5 and the Mojave Desert city of Palmdale. The area is chock full of fault-sliced sedimentary rock formations, twisted and turned into a variety of forms. On a geologic time scale, of course, the rocks are anything but solid and unmoving. The collapse of a freeway ramp over Interstate 5 near the Antelope Valley Freeway during the 1971 Sylmar earthquake, and again during the 1994 Northridge quake were pointed reminders of that.

Some of most magnificent rock formations in this "desert gateway" area of northern Los Angeles County can be found in Vasquez Rocks Natural Area. The Pacific Crest Trail passes through this smallish park, wending its way from the Mexican border to the Canadian border. In June 1993 a "golden spike" ceremony was held not far away in Soledad Canyon to commemorate the completion of the final link of trail tread in that 2640-mile-long pathway.

The desert gateway area is also notable as a significant "wind gap" between the coastal valleys of Ventura and Los Angeles counties, and the interior desert. Often on spring and summer afternoons the canyon serves as a conduit for cool, hazy marine air flowing east toward the southwestern Mojave Desert. Less common are the hot, dry Santa Ana winds of fall and early winter that scream through the area in the opposite direction.

Also included in this chapter is Placerita Canyon Park, which nestles comfortably at the foot of one of the more verdant slopes of the San Gabriel Mountains. The park's wild backcountry sector is complemented by a very civilized nature center—the envy of many a national park—housing exhibits on local history, pre-history, geology, plants, and wildlife.

Placerita Canyon's fascinating history is highlighted by the discovery of gold there in 1842. That event, which touched off California's first (and relatively trivial) gold rush, predated by six years John Marshall's famous discovery of gold at Sutter's Mill in northern California. When you first arrive at Placerita, you may want to check out the wheelchair-accessible Heritage Trail, which leads to the "Oak of the Golden Dream," the exact site (according to legend) where gold was discovered by a herdsman pulling up wild onions for his after-siesta meal.

In the bucolic early 1900s, Placerita settlers grew vegetables and fruit, raised animals, and tapped some small reserves of a very high-grade "white" oil. Right out of the ground, the fuel was suitable for home heating and lighting purposes—and even for powering a Model T Ford.

By the 1950s, Placerita Canyon had become one of the more popular generic Western site locations used by Hollywood's movie makers and early television producers. The canyon was eventually acquired as parkland.

Completing the short list of hikes presented in this chapter is a stroll up Whitney Canyon, right off the Antelope Valley Freeway in Santa Clarita. All locales in this chapter can be reached in a half hour or less from most parts of the San Fernando Valley.

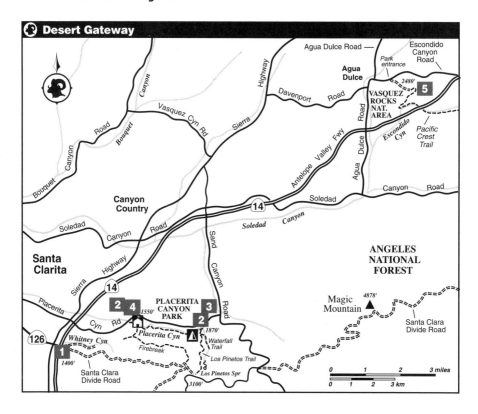

## trip 1  Whitney Canyon

|  |  |
|---|---|
| **Distance** | 2.0 miles round trip, Out-and-back |
| **Hiking Time** | 1 hour (round trip) |
| **Elevation Gain/Loss** | 100'/100' |
| **Difficulty** | Easy |
| **Trail Use** | Suitable for mountain biking, dogs allowed, good for kids |
| **Best Times** | All year |
| **Agency** | SMMC |
| **Optional Maps** | USGS 7.5-min *Oat Mountain, San Fernando* |
| **Notes** | Marked trails/obvious routes, easy terrain |

**DIRECTIONS** Follow the Antelope Valley Freeway (Highway 14) north from Interstate 5. Take the first exit, San Fernando Road (Highway 126), turn east, and enter a large Park and Ride lot. This doubles as a "free" trailhead for Whitney Canyon and for the Santa Clara Divide Road, which is a major western access into Angeles National Forest. You can also park in a lot beyond a gate to the north for a small day-use fee.

The dry and desolate landscape you behold at the trailhead hides a pleasant thing or two not far up Whitney Canyon. Using an old dirt road, head east up the canyon, which remains broad and unin- teresting for the first half mile. You'll pass under some massive high-voltage power- lines, and then the scenery improves. The canyon bottom narrows, and massive live oaks and sycamores arch overhead, creating inviting pools of shade, even on hot summer days. The excessively gnarled appearance of the trees suggests that they are the survivors of multiple wildfires over decades and centuries of time.

Past a second set of large powerlines, and just beyond an old wall of light-colored masonry on the right, a small tributary canyon opens on the right (south) side, just shy of where the old road peters out. Poke into this little ravine, and you will soon come upon a cattail-choked freshwater marsh. A covey of quail might explode from this oasis as you approach it. In back of the marsh look for an artesian sulfur spring—a clear pool of water with sulfurous bubbles coming up.

## trip 2 Placerita Canyon

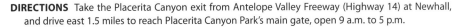

| | |
|---|---|
| **Distance** | 3.6 miles round trip, Out-and-back |
| **Hiking Time** | 2 hours (round trip) |
| **Elevation Gain/Loss** | 400'/400' |
| **Difficulty** | Moderate |
| **Trail Use** | Dogs allowed, good for kids |
| **Best Times** | All year |
| **Agency** | PCP |
| **Optional Map** | USGS 7.5-min *Mint Canyon* |
| **Notes** | Marked trails/obvious routes, easy terrain |

see map on p. 68

**DIRECTIONS** Take the Placerita Canyon exit from Antelope Valley Freeway (Highway 14) at Newhall, and drive east 1.5 miles to reach Placerita Canyon Park's main gate, open 9 a.m. to 5 p.m.

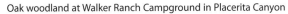

Placerita Canyon's melodious creek flows decently about half the year (winter and spring), caressing the ears with white noise that echoes from the canyon walls. During the fall, when the creek is bone-dry, you make your own noise instead by crunching through the crispy leaf litter of the sycamores.

Starting at Placerita Canyon Park's nature center, cross a bridge and pick up the trail heading east up the canyon's live-oak-shaded flood plain. Down by the grassy banks you'll see wild blackberry vines, lots of willows, and occasionally sycamore, cottonwood and alder trees.

After a while, the canyon narrows and becomes a rocky gorge. Soaring walls tell the story of thousands of years of natural erosion, as well as the destructive effects of hydraulic mining, which involved aiming

Oak woodland at Walker Ranch Campground in Placerita Canyon

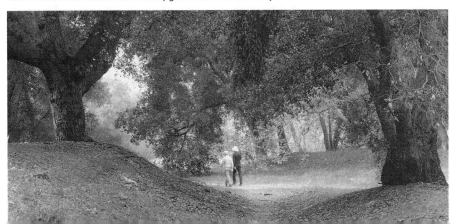

high-pressure water hoses at hillsides to loosen and wash away ores. Used extensively in northern California during the later Gold Rush, "hydraulicking" was finally banned in 1884 after catastrophic damages to waterways and farms downstream. At Placerita Canyon, several hundred thousand dollars worth of gold was ultimately recovered, but at considerable cost and effort.

At about 1 mile you reach a split. The right fork climbs a little onto the chaparral-clad slopes to the south, while the left branch connects with a trail going up to a parking area on Placerita Canyon Road and then goes upstream along the willow-choked canyon bottom. Follow either branch, but try taking the other on the return leg of the hike.

Using either route you eventually reach the scant remains of some early 20th-Century cottages hand-built by settler Frank Walker, his wife, and some of his 12 children. The area is now the site of the large campground catering to organized groups (drinking water available here). Amid a parklike setting of live oaks and gentle slopes, you'll discover a sturdy chimney and a cement foundation. Back by the nature center stands another cabin built by Walker, but modified later for use in the television series *Hopalong Cassidy*.

## trip 3  Los Pinetos Waterfall

see map on p. 68

|  |  |
|---|---|
| **Distance** | 1.6 miles round trip, Out-and-back |
| **Hiking Time** | 1 hour (round trip) |
| **Elevation Gain/Loss** | 350'/350' |
| **Difficulty** | Moderate |
| **Trail Use** | Dogs allowed |
| **Best Times** | All year |
| **Agency** | PCP |
| **Optional Maps** | USGS 7.5-min *Mint Canyon, San Fernando* |
| **Notes** | Marked trails/obvious routes, easy terrain |

**DIRECTIONS**  Take the Placerita Canyon exit from Antelope Valley Freeway (Highway 14) at Newhall, and drive east 3.5 miles to reach Placerita Canyon Park's Walker Ranch Trailhead (at mile 5.4 on Placerita Canyon Road).

**N**ourished by springs, Los Pinetos Canyon harbors at least a tiny trickle of water virtually the year round. About midway up this short tributary of Placerita Canyon is a sublime little grotto, cool and dark except when the sun passes almost straight overhead. If you come here after gully-washing rains, you'll find a true waterfall; otherwise you can just listen to water dribbling down the chute and enjoy the serenity of this private place just 3 miles—and a world away—from the edge of the L.A. metropolis.

Walk down to the Walker Ranch group campground and turn south on the Waterfall Trail into Los Pinetos Canyon. Don't confuse this trail with the signed Los Pinetos Trail going up the slope west of the canyon bottom. The Waterfall Trail momentarily climbs the canyon's steep west wall, then drops onto the canyon's sunny flood plain. Presently you bear right into a narrow ravine (Los Pinetos Canyon), avoiding a wider tributary bending left (east).

Continue, now on an ill-defined path, past and sometimes over water-polished, metamorphic rock. Live oaks and bigcone Douglas-firs cling to the slopes above, and a few bigleaf maples grace the canyon bottom. The bigcone Douglas-fir, a Southern

California variant of the Douglas-fir of the Pacific Northwest, is abundant in the San Gabriel Mountains from elevations of about 2000 feet (as here) up to about 6000 feet. The bigleaf maple, also common in the Pacific Northwest, has gained a foothold in the San Gabriels as well, especially in moist canyons and ravines.

About 0.2 mile after the first fork in the canyon, there's a second fork. Go right and continue 50 yards to the base of the waterfall—the end of the line in this branch of the canyon.

### trip 4  Manzanita Peak to Los Pinetos Canyon

see map on p. 68

|  |  |
|---|---|
| **Distance** | 7.0 miles, Loop |
| **Hiking Time** | 4 hours |
| **Elevation Gain/Loss** | 1800'/1800' |
| **Difficulty** | Moderately strenuous |
| **Trail Use** | Suitable for backpacking, dogs allowed |
| **Best Times** | October through June |
| **Agencies** | PCP and ANF/SCMRD |
| **Recommended Maps** | USGS 7.5-min *Mint Canyon, San Fernando* |
| **Notes** | Navigation required, easy terrain |

**DIRECTIONS**  Take the Placerita Canyon exit from Antelope Valley Freeway (Highway 14) at Newhall, and drive east 1.5 miles to reach Placerita Canyon Park's main gate, open 9 a.m. to 5 p.m.

The grand tour of Placerita Canyon country takes you swiftly up a steep trail and fire break to the top of a ridge spur of the San Gabriels, and then easily back downward via the Los Pinetos and Placerita Canyon trails. Start the hike early (the park gate opens at 9 a.m.) so you avoid broiling in the midday sun while ascending. If you

Bigleaf maple leaves in Los Pinetos Canyon

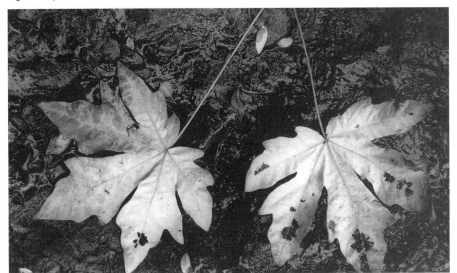

want to make this an overnight trip, you have the option of making camp on Angeles National Forest lands, subject to fire regulations. Contact the Santa Clara/Mojave Rivers Ranger District (see Appendix 4) for more information about that.

Start by picking up the Hillside Trail just behind the restroom building near the west end of the picnic area in Placerita Canyon Park. Climb past oaks and chaparral to a point just short of the camouflage-painted water tank. There you'll find an unmarked but well-worn trail heading straight up the ridge. After 0.5 mile on this you come to a side trail on the right leading 100 yards to the top of a rounded knoll dubbed Manzanita Mountain. Not much manzanita grows hereabouts, due to repeated wildfires. From this point on, you're on Angeles Forest lands until you reach the lower part of the Los Pinetos Trail.

Just past the side trail you come to a wide, sandy fire break. Turn left and tackle the first of several extremely steep pitches you'll encounter on the undulating fire break during the next 1.8 miles. At 2.6 miles you join Whitney Canyon Road, at the high point in elevation along the route. From there, it's downhill the rest of the way.

Turn left (east) and head for Wilson Canyon Saddle, a popular destination for equestrians and mountain bikers who come up from the San Fernando Valley via Wilson Canyon Road from Olive View Drive in Sylmar. Scramble up either of the two bumps on the ridgeline just east of here for a stupendous view (weather permitting) of the metropolis below. It's quiet here whenever the marine layer gets thick enough to smother the ridgeline in fog. At other times, when sound refracts upward through the inversion layer, the muffled roar of tens of thousands of cars on the network of freeways below comes through loud and clear.

Picking up the Los Pinetos Trail on the north side of the saddle, you begin a pleasant descent through splendid live-oak woodlands, and you lose all sight and sound of the city. Here and there you'll find nice specimens of the California walnut (black walnut) tree, a small deciduous tree with colorful foliage in the fall. The range of this trademark Southern California tree is limited to the margins of the L.A. Basin and the mountainous interiors of Ventura and Santa Barbara counties. Much of its habitat in Los Angeles County has been usurped by urbanization.

Down past a couple of switchbacks you come to Los Pinetos Spring, on the right, where non-potable water is stored for firefighting. Continue your descent on the trail ahead, winding amid thick growths of chaparral—ceanothus, scrub oak, chamise, sugar bush, mountain mahogany, manzanita, and sage—along the slope west of Los Pinetos Canyon. At 5.2 miles you reach Walker Ranch campground (water available here). From there, head west down the well-trodden trail through Placerita Canyon back to the starting point.

## trip 5 Vasquez Rocks Natural Area

| | |
|---|---|
| **Distance** | 2.0 miles round trip, Out-and-back |
| **Hiking Time** | 1 hour (round trip) |
| **Elevation Gain/Loss** | 150'/150' |
| **Difficulty** | Easy |
| **Trail Use** | Dogs allowed, Good for kids |
| **Best Times** | All year |
| **Agency** | VRNA |
| **Optional Map** | USGS 7.5-min *Agua Dulce* |
| **Notes** | Marked trails/obvious routes, easy terrain |

see map on p. 68

**DIRECTIONS** Exit the Antelope Valley Freeway at Agua Dulce Road. Drive north about 1.5 miles to where the road turns east and becomes Escondido Canyon Road. Look for the Vasquez Rocks Natural Area entrance on the right, and drive in on a dirt road, past the ranger office, to the picnic area 0.5 mile southeast.

**BASIN AND FOOTHILLS**

A perennial location for filming Old West movies and sci-fi extravaganzas, the distinctive Vasquez Rocks may be familiar to you from episodes of *The Lone Ranger, Bonanza, Star Trek, 24,* and movies such as *Blazing Saddles* and *Austin Powers.* Somehow these tilted slabs look impossibly high and steep when you first see them. But that illusion is dispelled when you try to climb them—none rise more than about 150 feet into the air, and there's almost always an easy way up. The best of the rocks are included in the 932-acre Vasquez Rocks Natural Area, named after Tiburcio Vasquez, a notorious 19th-Century bandito who reputedly used the park's cliffs and caves to hide from vigilantes and sheriffs' posses.

Geologically speaking, the rocks are west-dipping outcrops of sandstone and fanglomerate layers belonging to the Vasquez Formation. Here and in the surrounding area, the Vasquez Formation and the overlying Mint Canyon Formation constitute a 20,000-foot-thick sequence of sediments laid down 8–15 million years ago. The sandstone developed from fine-grained deposits laid down along gentle streams and shallow

Vasquez Rocks outcrop

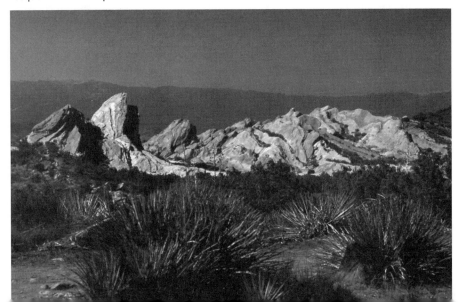

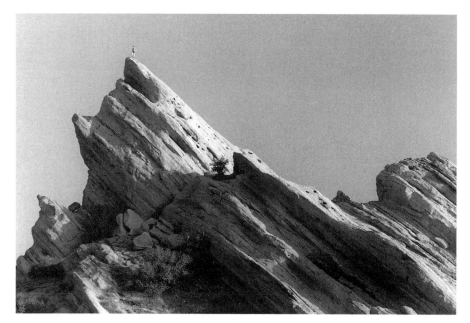

Vasquez Rocks

ponds. The fanglomerate (resembling conglomerate rock) developed from layers of coarse, broken rock deposited on what were probably alluvial fans at the base of steep mountains. More recently, faulting uplifted these layers, inclining them roughly 45 degrees to the horizontal. Erosion put on the final touches, producing the sheer east-facing exposures you'll see throughout the park.

The park includes a large picnic area, a couple of well-trampled nature trails, and a segment of the Pacific Crest Trail. That scenic stretch of the PCT is described here.

Start walking from the pepper tree at the far (southeast) end of the picnic area. Find the signed PCT route, which follows an old dirt road along a ridge trending south and southwest. After 0.5 mile, the PCT dives downward off the ridge, reaches the bottom of Escondido Creek, and turns sharply left to follow the canyon uphill (east). A 2007 fire singed the sycamores and incinerated everything else here, but the plentiful supply of water underground will ensure a rapid recovery of the riparian vegetation.

Make your way upstream into a lush riparian zone filled with willows and cottonwoods, right underneath the stony gaze of some spectacular overhanging cliffs of sandstone and conglomerate rock. High above on one jutting edge above, you might spot a lone, battered juniper.

Go as far as the point where the PCT drops right in the creekbed, bound for a nearby tunnel that takes the trail under the freeway. This a good spot to turn around and retrace your steps, enjoying a new perspective of the same great scenery.

# chapter 7

# Basin and Foothills:
# Glendale & Verdugo Mountains

Like a ship caught fast on a sandbar, the Verdugo Mountains protrude above what would otherwise be an unbroken sheet of alluvial deposits slanting down from the foot of the San Gabriel Mountains toward the San Fernando Valley. The narrow, sloping La Crescenta valley divides the Verdugos from the San Gabriels to the east, while the pancake-flat San Fernando Valley stretches nearly 20 miles to the west.

The Verdugos are, in fact, geologic cousins of the San Gabriels; they're only about half as high, but similar in origin and form. Both are youthful, fault-block ranges of unconsolidated crystalline (granitic and metamorphic) rocks, pushed skyward by vertical movements along faults at their bases.

The Verdugo Mountains stand as a remarkable island of undeveloped land—a haven for wildlife such as deer and coyotes—completely encircled by an urbanized domain. A number of trailheads in and around the city of Glendale provide public access by foot or mountain bike to the mountain slopes. The network of pathways includes wide, smooth fire roads built many decades ago to accommodate fire trucks and to service hilltop antenna installations, plus a number of narrow hiking trails constructed since the 1980s. These routes are your ticket to hours of healthy exercise and enjoyable views whenever the air turns clean and transparent.

In addition to hikes in the Verdugo Mountains, this chapter also includes Deukmejian Wilderness Park at the north extremity of the city of Glendale, and Haines Canyon just above the community of Tujunga, both of which lie at the foot of the San Gabriel Mountains.

Stream in Dunsmore Canyon, Deukmejian Wilderness Park

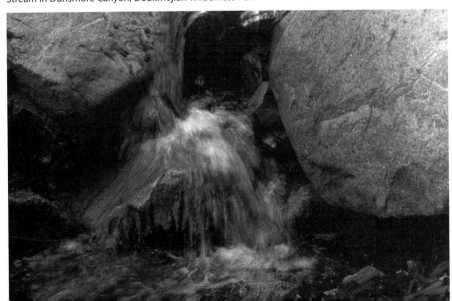

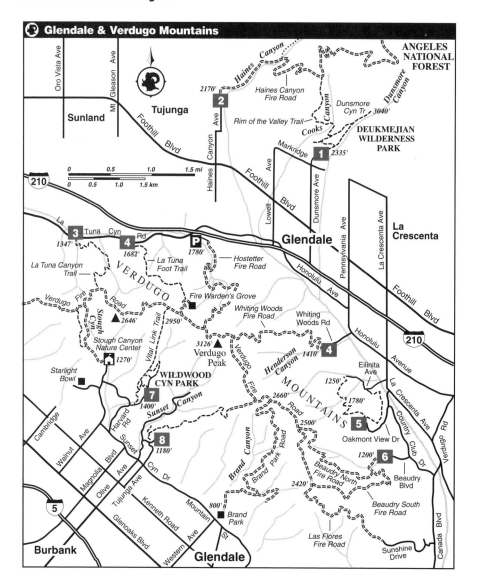

**Glendale & Verdugo Mountains**

# trip 1  Deukmejian Wilderness Park

see map on p. 76

| | |
|---|---|
| **Distance** | 2.4 miles, Loop |
| **Hiking Time** | 1½ hours |
| **Elevation Gain/Loss** | 900'/900' |
| **Difficulty** | Moderate |
| **Trail Use** | Suitable for mountain biking, dogs allowed, good for kids |
| **Best Times** | All year |
| **Agency** | GPR |
| **Optional Maps** | USGS 7.5-min *Sunland, Burbank, Condor Peak* |
| **Notes** | Marked trails/obvious routes, easy terrain |

**DIRECTIONS**  From Foothill Boulevard in Glendale, follow Dunsmore Avenue north for 1 mile to the Deukmejian Wilderness Park entrance. Park at the old stone barn, where the hike begins.

Not many small cities can boast of three mountain ranges within its border, but Glendale does. Stretching east and north from the San Fernando Valley, the city takes in substantial parts of the San Rafael Hills and the Verdugo Mountains, plus a small slice of the San Gabriel Mountains at the city's northern extremity. At this northernmost spot in Glendale, overlooking the foothill communities of La Crescenta and Tujunga, lies Deukmejian Wilderness Park, named after former California governor George Deukmejian. The park's 700 acres are drained by two ravines with steep gradients: Cooks Canyon and Dunsmore Canyon. During the mid-20th Century, the area alongside Dunsmore Canyon stream was used by the Le Mesnager family as a vineyard. An old stone barn at the trailhead is reminiscent of that time.

From the parking area find and follow the Dunsmore Canyon Trail (a fire road), which wastes no time in a relentless and shadeless ascent that matches the gradient of the Dunsmore Canyon stream alongside it. After nearly one mile of distance and 700

feet of ascent, the road ends. Duck under the cover of the streamside alders and enjoy the sound of the happy little stream tumbling over and around boulders of various sizes. Major floods occasionally rearrange the streambed rocks, creating mini-cascades that are probably temporary. The crystalline purity of the water at this spot is remarkable. Also, the 3000-foot elevation here ensures that on many days you can be well above the smog level.

Retrace your steps about 0.3 mile to where the Le Mesnager Loop Trail veers right. Take this slightly longer but view-rich route back toward the start, taking advantage of two short spur trails along the way. The spurs lead to points overlooking Dunsmore Canyon and Cooks Canyon. Both afford a more distant view of the suburbs below and the rising swell of the Verdugo Mountains beyond. On the Le Mesnager Loop Trail you'll also pass the Rim of the Valley Trail, a winding footpath that crosses the stream in Cooks Canyon and ascends toward a hairpin turn on the Haines Canyon fire road above.

## trip 2 Haines Canyon

see map on p. 76

| | |
|---|---|
| **Distance** | 3.4 miles round trip, Out-and-back |
| **Hiking Time** | 2 hours (round trip) |
| **Elevation Gain/Loss** | 1100'/1100' |
| **Difficulty** | Moderate |
| **Trail Use** | Dogs allowed, good for kids |
| **Best Times** | October through June |
| **Agency** | ANF/LARD |
| **Optional Map** | USGS 7.5-min *Sunland* |
| **Notes** | Marked trails/obvious routes, moderate terrain, bushwhacking |

**DIRECTIONS** From Foothill Boulevard in Tujunga, follow Haines Canyon Avenue north for 1 mile to the end of the street. There's free parking in this residential neighborhood.

Coyotes howl, water splashes down a willow-lined creek, hummingbirds flit about in search of nectar. All of this takes place barely a mile from the grid of suburban streets on L.A.'s fringe. It's Haines Canyon we're referring to here, but it sounds a lot like dozens of other small canyon streams that give up their water to the concrete storm channels of the city below. At the mouth of almost every one yawns a debris basin, often 50 to 100 feet wide, designed to catch the slurry of silt, sand, rocks, and boulders that roar down the mountain slopes during infrequent cloudbursts.

A fire road ascends Haines Canyon and continues all the way to 5074-foot Mount Lukens. Our modest goal on this hike is merely to quickly reach a secluded middle section of Haines Canyon, removed from both the improvements of the L.A. County Flood Control District and the sight and sound of the city.

From the end of Haines Canyon Avenue, walk around the vehicle gate and bypass a typical, ugly debris basin and dam. Continue upstream on the dirt road. The sight of civilization quickly fades, except for a dozen check dams ("crib dams") down along the creek, all constructed of the same kind of precast concrete "logs." Decades of regrowth of native trees such as willows, live oaks, and sycamores have done a lot to soften their visual impact.

After 1.2 miles, the road curves abruptly right and climbs out of the canyon toward Mount Lukens. You take the old road to the left, up the main branch of the canyon. It soon becomes a trail, and then nothing but an informal, brushy path, with patches of asphalt underfoot here and there. Encroaching vegetation will slow or possibly stop you. Remnants of the old road end beneath a large live oak, 1.7 miles from the start. A seasonal stream trickles by. You can picnic at this secluded spot, or press on to explore one source of the water, a spring a couple hundred yards upstream (watch out for poison oak). Decades ago, a hiking path known as the Sister Elsie Trail climbed east from this point to join Stone Canyon Trail atop Mount Lukens. Local hikers have recently reworked this path; however, it tends to get overgrown to the point of invisibility if it is not constantly maintained.

## trip 3  La Tuna Traverse

see map on p. 76

| | |
|---|---|
| **Distance** | 9.5 miles, Loop |
| **Hiking Time** | 4½ hours |
| **Elevation Gain/Loss** | 2050'/2050' |
| **Difficulty** | Moderately strenuous |
| **Trail Use** | Dogs allowed |
| **Best Times** | October through May |
| **Agency** | SMMC |
| **Optional Map** | USGS 7.5-min *Burbank* |
| **Notes** | Marked trails/obvious routes, easy terrain |

**BASIN AND FOOTHILLS**

**DIRECTIONS** Drive to the main La Tuna Canyon Park entrance on the south side of La Tuna Canyon Road. This is 1.4 miles west of the La Tuna Canyon Road exit from Foothill Freeway, and 3.3 miles east of Sunland Boulevard in Sun Valley. Don't confuse this trailhead with a similar one, "The Grotto," which is 0.4 mile east.

The 1100-acre La Tuna Canyon Park, basically an open-space area with minimal picnic facilities, drapes over the north-facing, relatively lush slopes of the Verdugo Mountains. On this trek you'll pass through luxuriant growths of aromatic chaparral and visit a couple of surprisingly attractive oak- and sycamore-shaded mini-canyons. On clear days, the best part is the walk along the Verdugo ridgecrest. There you can "bag" 3126-foot Verdugo Peak, the tallest bump in the range.

From the trailhead follow the La Tuna Canyon Trail up along a small canyon about 100 yards to a fenced viewpoint overlooking a natural declivity, where water cascades after a good rain. From there you double back and undertake an easy switchback ascent of the canyon's east wall. Rooted to the steep slopes are a tangled assortment of mature chaparral shrubs—scrub oak, hollyleaf cherry, ceanothus, and toyon.

After about 0.6 mile the trail starts to contour across a slope immediately above La Tuna Canyon Road, and afterward drops quickly to the bottom of another small canyon, parallel to the first. (Down this canyon is the top of a 20-foot waterfall called "The Grotto.") For a while you're engulfed in a cool tunnel of overarching live oak and bay laurel limbs. Wild blackberry vines and poison oak thrive in this intimate little glen.

At 1.3 miles the narrow trail-tread joins traces of an old road that quickly gains the ridge between the two canyons and then connects with Verdugo Fire Road. A heart-pounding climb (600 vertical feet in 0.6 mile) puts you on the wide fire road. Turn left and head east toward Verdugo Peak. Much of the area ahead was scorched during a 2006 wildfire, so there's little vegetation to block views.

Next stop (worth the short side trip if the air is clear) is a 2646-foot knoll on the right, 0.6 mile from the top of the La Tuna Canyon Trail. Scramble up the fire break on the knoll's east side and enjoy what is likely the most complete view of the San Fernando Valley available from any land-based vantage point. The pseudo-aerial perspective reveals flat grids of linear streets slashed by curving freeways, huge complexes of industrial buildings that look like giant computer circuit boards, endless rows of stuccoed single-family homes half-hidden in a green haze of street trees, and spiky clusters of high rises. The valley's geographic connection to the main Los Angeles Basin is plainly revealed. In the gap where the connection is made (between the Verdugo and Santa Monica mountains), sunlight gleams on the concrete banks of the Los Angeles River flood channel.

Farther east you pass several antenna sites and skirt the Fire Warden's Grove—

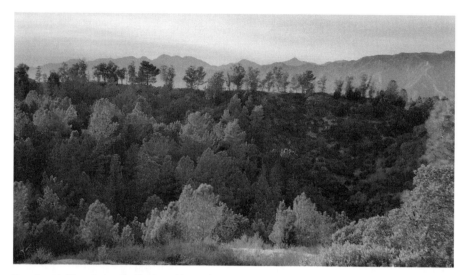

Experimental forest atop the Verdugo Mountains

scattered pine, cedar, and cypress trees planted for experimental purposes after a major fire in 1927. Clearly out of their natural element on these high and dry slopes, the trees are nonetheless a welcome addition to the scenery.

A right turn at the next fire-road junction (4.3 miles from the start) and a short climb south take you toward the high point unofficially known as Verdugo Peak. The antenna facility at the top blocks a complete 360-degree view. The San Gabriel Mountains and La Crescenta valley to the east are especially striking. On the far side of the valley, subdivisions completely cover most of the classically formed alluvial fans that spill from the foot of the San Gabriels. Debris dams at the apex of nearly every fan do their best (but sometimes fail) to catch the muddy slurry that sweeps down the canyons whenever storms unleash torrents of water on the slopes above.

After visiting the peak, backtrack to last junction, but bear right (north) on Hostetter Fire Road. Three miles of easy descent take you down to a large parking area alongside La Tuna Canyon Road. Follow the wide left (south-side) shoulder of that road to return to your car—an easy half-hour walk or a 15-minute jog.

## trip 4  Verdugo Peak Traverse

see map on p. 76

| | |
|---|---|
| **Distance** | 5.8 miles, Point-to-point |
| **Hiking Time** | 3 hours |
| **Elevation Gain/Loss** | 1500'/1750' |
| **Difficulty** | Moderately strenuous |
| **Trail Use** | Dogs allowed |
| **Best Times** | November through April |
| **Agency** | SMMC |
| **Optional Map** | USGS 7.5-min *Burbank* |
| **Notes** | Marked trails/obvious routes, moderate terrain |

**DIRECTIONS** *West End:* Drive to the trailhead at "The Grotto" on the south side of La Tuna Canyon Road. This is 1 mile west of the La Tuna Canyon Road exit from Foothill Freeway, and 3.7 miles east of Sunland Boulevard in Sun Valley. Don't confuse this trailhead with a similar one 0.4 mile west, which is the main La Tuna Canyon Park entrance. *East End:* From the south end of Pennsylvania Avenue at Honolulu Avenue, follow Whiting Woods Road west to a gate at the foot of the Whiting Woods Fire Road.

With a drop-off-and-pick-up transportation arrangement, you can enjoy a lively traverse across the north end of the Verdugo Mountains, ascending though La Tuna Canyon Park on a rough foot trail and descending toward the finish at Henderson Canyon on a wide, graded fire road. Assuming the skies are crystal clear when you go, you'll have consistently spectacular views the entire way.

From the trailhead, walk 50 yards up the deeply shaded ravine to the base of the small cliff (a waterfall in the wet season) called The Grotto. From there, find and follow the faint trail going sharply up the canyon wall to the left. This is the La Tuna Foot Trail, which quickly becomes more distinct once you get past the initial very steep stretch. The trail quickly settles into a steady and almost uninterrupted uphill

Shaggy north slopes, Verdugo Mountains

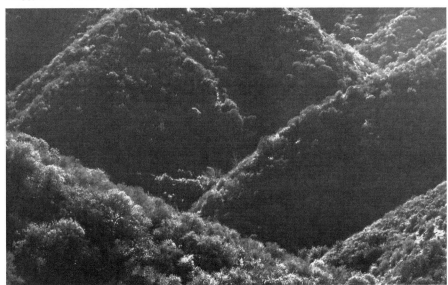

BASIN AND FOOTHILLS

grade, zigzagging when necessary to keep on or near the top of a well-defined ridge trending southeast. This hand-tooled route takes you right through mature chaparral, including manzanitas up to 15-feet tall.

After 2.0 miles and nearly 1200 feet of elevation gain, the trail arrives at a wide, graded fire road. To the left and below lies the main part of the Fire Warden's Grove, an experimental forest dating from the 1920s. You turn right, however, and climb 0.3 mile farther to the Verdugo Fire Road, where you get your first wide vistas of the vast San Fernando Valley to the west and south.

Turn left on the Verdugo Fire Road and follow it east for 1.1 miles, passing various antenna installations on the crest of the ridge, including the one on Verdugo Peak, the high point of the range. The 'dozer-scraped ridgeline, burned in 2006, doesn't look like much, but the view's the thing here—it's panoramic and stunningly spacious as seen through clear air.

Look for the Whiting Woods Fire Road intersecting at 3.4 miles into the hike. Turn left and follow its twisting course down an east-plunging ridgeline all the way into the shady depths of Henderson Canyon. The traverse ends where the fire road ends, at the western end of Whiting Woods Road, a residential street.

## trip 5  Oakmont Loop

| | |
|---|---|
| **Distance** | 2.5 miles, Loop |
| **Hiking Time** | 1½ hours |
| **Elevation Gain/Loss** | 600'/600' |
| **Difficulty** | Moderate |
| **Trail Use** | Suitable for mountain biking, dogs allowed, good for kids |
| **Best Times** | All year |
| **Agency** | SMMC |
| **Optional Map** | USGS 7.5-min *Pasadena* |
| **Notes** | Marked trails/obvious routes, easy terrain |

see map on p. 76

**DIRECTIONS** From La Crescenta Avenue, 1 mile south of Interstate 210, turn south on Oakmont View Drive. Follow this curvy residential street uphill to Oakmont View Park, where the street ends.

The pint-sized (244-acre) Verdugo Mountains Open Space Preserve covers a scruffy patch of east-facing slopes in the city of Glendale. The circular hiking/biking route described here is pieced out of fire roads and residential streets bordering the property. The route is perfect for a late afternoon outing, when you can benefit from staying in the shade, but at the same time enjoy a brightly lit valley and mountain vista to the east.

From Oakmont View Park, follow the signed Edison Road (a fire road) and climb moderately on lazy twists and turns over the chaparral-clad slopes. The view east is somewhat compromised by some high-voltage powerlines in the near distance. Still, you can look across the sloping La Crescenta valley toward the dramatically rising San Gabriel Mountains, which culminate (from this perspective) at the antenna-bewhiskered summit of Mount Lukens. The suburban landscape fills almost every reasonably flat patch of land from here to the base of the San Gabriels.

Before long, you're starting a steep descent. At 1.0 mile you reach a gorgeous oak- and sycamore-filled glade in the bottom of a ravine called Engleheard Canyon (a perfect example of how civilization and wilderness can merge at the boundary of what is known as the wildland/urban interface). Just beyond, the Edison Road ends at a narrow driveway. Follow that driveway out to the suburbs at Eilinita Avenue, take a right on Emanuel Drive, and follow Emanuel to its end, 1.7 miles into the hike, where you again pick up Edison Road (a dirt road) on the left. The remaining 0.8 mile of distance will take you some 500 feet higher to your starting point at Oakmont View Park.

## trip 6  Beaudry Loop

see map on p. 76

| | |
|---|---|
| **Distance** | 5.5 miles, Loop |
| **Hiking Time** | 3 hours |
| **Elevation Gain/Loss** | 1500'/1500' |
| **Difficulty** | Moderately strenuous |
| **Trail Use** | Suitable for mountain biking, dogs allowed |
| **Best Times** | November through May |
| **Agency** | GPR |
| **Optional Maps** | USGS 7.5-min *Pasadena, Burbank* |
| **Notes** | Marked trails/obvious routes, easy terrain |

**DIRECTIONS**  From Country Club Drive in the city of Glendale (not to be confused with Country Club Drive in Burbank), follow Beaudry Boulevard 0.4 mile west to where it ends. Park on the street.

From the south end of the Verdugos' summit ridge, your gaze takes in the San Gabriel Mountains, much of the L.A. megalopolis, and even the ocean on occasion. Do this trip late in the day if you want to enjoy both a spectacular sunset and a blaze of lights after twilight fades. At best, try this on any cloud-free, smog-free day that falls within two weeks on either side of the winter solstice (December 21). During that period, the sun sets on the flat ocean horizon behind Santa Monica Bay. At other times of year, the sun's sinking path is likely to intersect the coastal mountains. The seemingly strange fact of the sun setting over land most of the year is a consequence of the east-west orientation of California's coastline in the area "up-coast" from Los Angeles.

From the residential neighborhood at the end of Beaudry Boulevard, walk up a paved segment of fire road, bypass a vehicle gate, and continue on dirt past a debris basin to where the fire road splits (0.3 mile). Choose for your way the shadier but less viewful right branch, Beaudry North Fire Road. You'll return to this junction by way of the left branch, the Beaudry South Fire Road. About halfway up the north road you come to a trickling spring and a water tank nestled in a shady ravine, a good place for a breather.

When you reach the summit ridge (2.3 miles), turn sharply left on Verdugo Fire Road and continue climbing another 0.4 mile toward a cluster of brightly painted radio towers atop a 2656' bump—the highest point along this hike. From the towers, continue south along the ridge 0.6 mile to a road junction. The right branch descends to Sunshine Drive in Glendale; you take the left branch and return along an east ridge to the split just above the debris basin.

# trip 7  Vital Link Trail

see map on p. 76

| | |
|---|---|
| **Distance** | 3.6 miles round trip, Out-and-back |
| **Hiking Time** | 2½ hours (round trip) |
| **Elevation Gain/Loss** | 1600'/1600' |
| **Difficulty** | Moderately strenuous |
| **Trail Use** | Dogs allowed |
| **Best Times** | November through April |
| **Agency** | WCP |
| **Optional Map** | USGS 7.5-min *Burbank* |
| **Notes** | Marked trails/obvious routes, moderate terrain |

**DIRECTIONS** Exit Interstate 5 at Olive Avenue in Burbank. Follow Olive northeast 1.2 miles to Sunset Canyon Drive. Turn left, go 6 blocks northwest, then turn right on Harvard Road. Go 0.6 mile and turn right into Wildwood Canyon Park. Drive 0.3 mile to the trailhead on the left.

The nearly straight-up Vital Link Trail connects popular Wildwood Canyon Park in Verdugo foothills with the Verdugo Mountains crestline. Almost every step on the trail yields a higher vantage for the panoramic view of the plate-like San Fernando Valley floor and the pillowy Santa Monica Mountains beyond. The reverse, downhill leg of the trek is a possibly knee-banging exercise, but the view then lies directly in front of you. The entirely south-facing aspect of this hike mandates that you hike only during the coolest time of year, and preferably not in the midday sunshine.

From the trailhead 0.3 mile into Wildwood Canyon Park (actually the second of a total of four gateways to the park's trail system), head sharply up the canyon wall to the north. After a quarter mile, make a right and settle into a moderate grade that will take up along the crest of the canyon wall. Go 0.3 mile and stay left at the next trail junction. Go another 0.3 mile (not quite as far as a picnic table perched on knoll), and look for the narrow Vital Link Trail slanting left.

The real climb begins now as the trail doggedly sticks to a narrow ridge trending north and goes acutely uphill all the way to the Verdugo Fire Road on the crest of the Verdugo Mountains. Return the same way for a 3.6-mile round-trip distance.

Possible extensions include a visit to the nearby Fire Warden's Grove, a traverse west and then south into Stough Canyon, or a traverse east ending at any of several trailheads on the north or west sides of the Verdugos. The Vital Link trail truly provides a vital link for all kinds of travel possibilities.

# trip 8  West Side Loop

|  |  |
|---|---|
| **Distance** | 7.9 miles, Loop |
| **Hiking Time** | 4 hours |
| **Elevation Gain/Loss** | 2000'/2000' |
| **Difficulty** | Strenuous |
| **Trail Use** | Dogs allowed |
| **Best Times** | November through April |
| **Agency** | GPR |
| **Optional Map** | USGS 7.5-min *Burbank* |
| **Notes** | Navigation required, moderate terrain, bushwhacking |

see map on p. 76

**DIRECTIONS**  Exit Interstate 5 at Olive Avenue in Burbank. Follow Olive northeast 1.2 miles to Sunset Canyon Drive. Proceed straight across on what becomes Country Club Drive. After 0.3 mile turn right on Via Montana. Go uphill one long block to the corner of Via Montana and Camino de Villas, where you can find curbside parking.

This is one of the more adventurous trips in this book, even though when you're on it you're almost never out of sight or earshot of the suburbs below. You climb the Verdugo crest by way of an old road—abandoned and washed out in several places, but not completely ignored by hikers and even a few intrepid mountain bikers. Wear long pants, or else you'll be benignly scourged by the scratchy buckwheat and sage vegetation taking root in the road bed.

From the corner of Via Montana and Camino de Villas, head north across the street, traverse across an empty lot, and climb a bit to pick up an old dirt road bed going north. The road contours across a hillside toward some houses in the bottom of Sunset Canyon. After about 0.3 mile, turn right where another old road goes sharply up the ridge. Stay on the same for the next 1.7 miles, picking your way past bushes and occasional rock slides.

At 2.0 miles from the start you come upon a maintained dirt road, serving a water tank on the left. Keep right, and walk another 0.5 mile up to the crest of the Verdugo Mountains, where you arrive at an unmarked, four-way junction. Take the middle branch (the road on the right

quickly dead-ends), which is the wide Verdugo Fire Road. Continue another 0.3 mile to a junction with Brand Park Road, where a wooden bench on the shadeless ridgeline invites you to sit a spell (if it's not too hot) and enjoy the view.

Brand Park Road, a fairly new addition to the fire-road network, is somewhat less scenic than what you've traveled so far. Follow its turns and twists 3.3 miles south to the green lawns of Brand Park in the valley below.

In a corner of Brand Park stands Glendale's architecturally noted Brand Library, originally a Spanish-Moorish-style mansion built by early 1900s civic booster Leslie Brand. Near the library and for some distance up the canyon behind it are the remnants of the tropical gardens that once graced Brand's estate.

To complete this loop hike, walk along pleasantly shaded Mountain Street (which becomes Sunset Canyon Drive as you pass into the city of Burbank) for 1.2 miles to Tujunga Avenue. Turn right on Tujunga (which later becomes Camino de Villas) and walk 0.4 mile uphill to Villa Montana and your waiting car.

# chapter 8

# Basin and Foothills: Griffith Park

Why shouldn't one of the world's most expansive cities boast one of the world's biggest city parks? It does, in fact. Griffith Park's 4467 acres—about five times the size of New York's Central Park—rate as the nation's largest municipal park completely surrounded by urban areas.

Griffith Park is L.A.'s "park for the people," where Angelenos (and some tourists) come to spread a picnic blanket, visit the homegrown zoo or the observatory and planetarium, and explore the chaparral-covered hills and scenic vistas. Over half of the park's area consists of terrain too steep to be developed as parkland in the conventional manner, so it remains as a kind of in-city wilderness, albeit of a mostly dry and scrubby kind.

Toyon—the "holly" of Hollywood

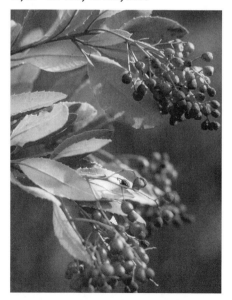

More than 50 miles of fire roads and foot trails lure those on foot and horseback; while bicyclists can explore more than 20 miles of twisting pavement, or take to the dirt wherever such use is permitted. The trails are busy on sunny weekends, yet it can be amazingly quiet here as long as you get an early start (the park's several gates swing open at 6 a.m. for access by automobile). By starting early you can also take advantage of the day's coolest temperatures and generally the cleanest air.

The sketch map of Griffith Park in this chapter, though adequate for the purposes of navigating the routes described here, omits some lesser paths and geographic details. At the ranger station and visitor center on the east side of the park, however, you can pick up a free copy of an excellent, large-scale color map/brochure showing a wealth of detail.

In the time since the first edition of this book was written, two of the park's interior paved roads—Mount Hollywood Drive and Vista del Valle Drive—have been closed to motorized traffic. This is a bit of a bother for hikers wishing to get easy access to remote parts of the park, and a blessing for bicyclists who are not allowed to ride on the park's trails but who now can enjoy biking on miles of car-free pavement.

Griffith Park occupies the eastern tip of the Santa Monica Mountains, a fact difficult to discern until you climb one of the park's high points and look west along the crest of the range. The higher and wilder parts of the Santa Monicas, west of Sepulveda Pass, are covered later in the Santa Monica Mountains section of this book.

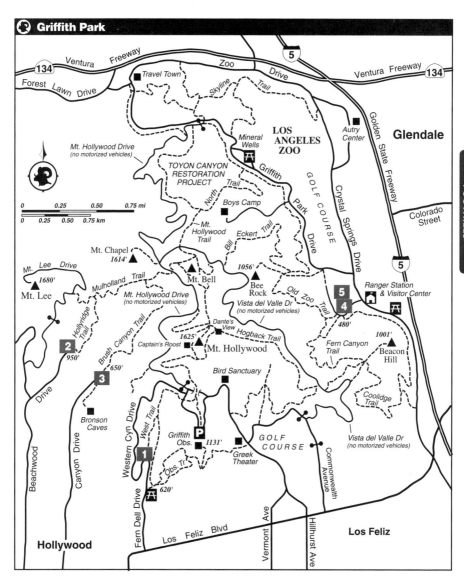

## Griffith Park

134 Ventura Freeway
Forest Lawn Drive

Travel Town
Zoo Drive
5
Ventura Freeway 134

Skyline Trail

Mineral Wells

LOS ANGELES ZOO

Autry Center

Golden State Freeway

**Glendale**

Mt. Hollywood Drive
(no motorized vehicles)

TOYON CANYON RESTORATION PROJECT

Griffith

North Trail

Boys Camp

Park Drive

G O L F   C O U R S E

Crystal Springs Drive

Colorado Street

0    0.25    0.50    0.75 mi
0    0.25   0.50   0.75 km

Mt. Hollywood Trail

Eckert Trail

Bill

5

Mt. Chapel
1614'

Mt. Lee Drive

Mt. 1680'
Mt. Lee

Mulholland Trail

Mt. Bell

1056'

Bee Rock

Ranger Station
& Visitor Center

Mt. Hollywood Drive
(no motorized vehicles)

Vista del Valle Dr
(no motorized vehicles)

Old Zoo Trail

5
4

480'

Hollyridge Trail

Brush Canyon Trail

Dante's View

Captain's Roost

1625'

Hogback Trail

Mt. Hollywood

Fern Canyon Trail

1001'
Beacon Hill

2
950'

650'

3

Bird Sanctuary

Coolidge Trail

Drive

Beachwood

Canyon Drive

Bronson Caves

Western Cyn Drive

West Trail

Griffith Obs.

P

1131'

Greek Theater

G O L F   C O U R S E

Vista del Valle Dr
(no motorized vehicles)

Commonwealth Avenue

1

Obs. Tr.

620'

Fern Dell Drive

Los Feliz Blvd

Vermont Ave

Hillhurst Ave

**Los Feliz**

**Hollywood**

## trip 1 Mount Hollywood

| | |
|---|---|
| **Distance** | 4.7 miles, Loop |
| **Hiking Time** | 2 hours |
| **Elevation Gain/Loss** | 1050'/1050' |
| **Difficulty** | Moderate |
| **Trail Use** | Dogs allowed, good for kids |
| **Best Times** | October through May |
| **Agency** | GP |
| **Optional Maps** | USGS 7.5-min *Hollywood, Burbank* |
| **Notes** | Marked trails/obvious routes, easy terrain |

see map on p. 87

**DIRECTIONS** From just east of the bend where Western Avenue becomes Los Feliz Boulevard (1 mile north of the Hollywood Freeway), go north on Fern Dell Drive into Griffith Park. Find a parking spot in the lot 0.7 mile north, or else nearby.

The bald, flattish summit of Mount Hollywood would scarcely be something to write home about except for its strategic location overlooking just about everything. Hikers approach from all directions, but the most popular starting point is the observatory parking lot. On the somewhat longer trek described here, you'll start out below the observatory so you can enjoy the exotically landscaped Fern Dell area, too. The dell features picnic tables, a year-round brook (a part of the observatory's cooling system, but appealing nonetheless), plenty of succulent plants, and shade trees.

From Fern Dell's main parking lot, walk across the lowermost horseshoe curve on Western Canyon Road and continue on the wide, dirt fire road heading uphill (north)

Griffith Observatory

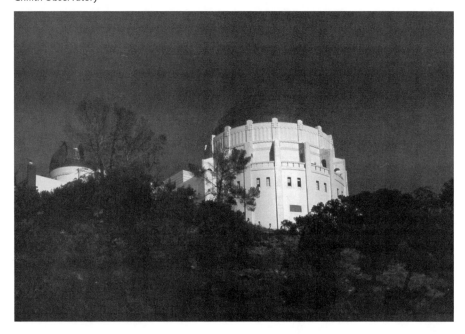

into sunny chaparral country. Dry and a bit trampled at first, the landscape improves as you climb. Along the trail are larger shrubs such as toyon, elderberry, laurel sumac, sugarbush, and ceanothus; and smaller ones such as black sage, buckwheat, and fuchsia-flowered gooseberry—all very typical of the drier, south- and west-facing slopes in the park. Here, too, are common weedy plants such as fennel, tree tobacco, and castor bean. Planted eucalyptus and pines stand high on the nearby slopes, while a handful of native live oaks tucked into the bigger creases on the sun-seared slopes draw just enough moisture from the soil to survive.

After passing under a couple of shade-giving oaks, the trail curves left and crosses the west observatory road. Soon you're on the ridgeline south of Mount Hollywood, passing high over a road tunnel. Listen for horns blaring as cars barrel through below.

A couple of long, lazy switchback legs take you to a trail junction not far below Mount Hollywood's summit. Make a sharp left, pass the shady Captain's Roost picnic area (drinking water here), and continue to a wide trail junction just north of the summit. Make a hard right there and walk over to the picnic tables on the top. Your gaze takes in (among many other things) the downtown L.A. skyline and the antenna-topped Mount Lee with its famous HOLLYWOOD sign facing south over "Tinseltown." Just beyond Mount Lee is the top of Cahuenga Peak (1820′), the highest summit in this corner of the Santa Monica Mountains.

On your return, backtrack to the wide junction and go right, circling Mount Hollywood's east side. Retrace your steps on the two switchback segments, but keep south along the ridgeline after you reach the top of the tunnel. Walk across the observatory parking lot toward the monumental, three-domed building that houses a state-of-the-art planetarium and museum (upgraded in 2002–06), a massive, antique Zeiss refractor telescope, and various solar instruments. Swing around the back side of the building to discover observation decks offering commanding views of the L.A. Basin.

For the final leg of the trip, follow the trail that descends the slope just east of the observatory. It starts from the left side of the building as you face its grand entrance. After 0.2 mile of descent, swing sharply right on the Observatory Trail. Go either way at the next junction where the trail divides into West Observatory Trail and East Observatory Trail. The two branches meet down below at Fern Dell. After winding past golden-blossomed silk oak trees, you arrive at Fern Dell's bubbling brook. Your starting point is just up the road to the right.

## trip 2 Mount Lee

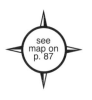

see map on p. 87

| | |
|---|---|
| **Distance** | 3.0 miles round trip, out-and-back |
| **Hiking Time** | 1½ hours (round trip) |
| **Elevation Gain/Loss** | 750'/750' |
| **Difficulty** | Moderate |
| **Trail Use** | Suitable for mountain biking, dogs allowed, good for kids |
| **Best Times** | All year |
| **Agency** | GP |
| **Optional Map** | USGS 7.5-min *Burbank* |
| **Notes** | Marked trails/obvious routes, easy terrain |

**DIRECTIONS** From Franklin Avenue, just east of the Hollywood (101) Freeway, turn north on Beachwood Drive. Follow Beachwood all the way to its north end deep in the Hollywood Hills. Park (if you can find space there) in the dirt lot just shy of the Sunset Ranch Stables. There's more space for parking a quarter mile below, along Beachwood Drive or along residential streets parallel to it.

At 1680 feet above sea level, the summit of Mount Lee perches high above the Los Angeles Basin on the western edge of Griffith Park. In addition to hosting the iconic HOLLYWOOD sign, the summit area offers one of the most stupendous views of the Southland's real estate—carpets of houses, shopping centers, industrial buildings, and office towers that roll out miles and miles toward distant snow-flecked peaks and the blue Pacific Ocean.

From the dirt lot, climb briefly south of the Hollyridge Trail to a hillside vantage point where you can gaze south over the Hollywood Hills and the L.A. Basin to the Palos Verdes Peninsula, Long Beach, and (when clear enough) Santa Catalina Island. From there, swing left and continue uphill (north) on the Hollyridge Trail. Horses and riders from the nearby stables are sometimes in view ahead; behind you is an ever-widening view of the L.A. Basin. Eventually,

Hollywood Reservoir vista from Mount Lee

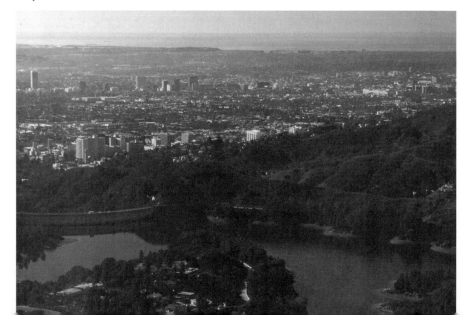

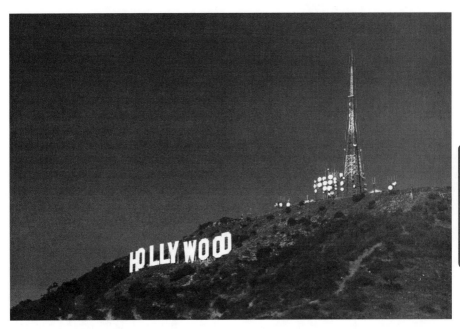

Mount Lee and the iconic HOLLYWOOD sign

the tops of L.A. downtown office towers come into view.

At about 0.5 mile you reach a junction. Go left on Mulholland Trail, and follow its curvy course west until you reach the paved (but closed to motorized traffic) service road called Mount Lee Drive. Follow that road uphill to a crest where a full, 180-degree sweep of the San Fernando Valley comes into view. Keep climbing, and don't give up until you reach the summit.

A formidable fence divides the topmost part of Mount Lee from the sheer slope below, which precariously supports the spindly-looking whitewashed letters of the famous sign. Climb a rocky peaklet at the end of the service road (just shy of a fenced antenna installation) to get a nearly 360-degree view of the landscape. Serene Lake Hollywood lies right below, and far beyond it the ocean is sometimes visible. From December through about March you'll probably notice a prominent mantle of snow on a rounded peak far to the east. That's Mount San Antonio, or Old Baldy, 10,064 feet above sea level—the highest point in Los Angeles County.

# trip 3 Mulholland Ridge

| | |
|---|---|
| **Distance** | 3.6 miles round trip, Out-and-back |
| **Hiking Time** | 2 hours (round trip) |
| **Elevation Gain/Loss** | 1000'/1000' |
| **Difficulty** | Moderate |
| **Trail Use** | Dogs allowed |
| **Best Times** | All year |
| **Agency** | GP |
| **Optional Map** | USGS 7.5-min *Burbank* |
| **Notes** | Marked trails/obvious routes, easy terrain |

see
map on
p. 87

**DIRECTIONS**  From Franklin Avenue, a half mile east of the Hollywood (101) Freeway, turn north on Canyon Drive. Follow Canyon Drive all the way to its far end. There's room for parking in a small lot here or back a little way alongside Canyon Drive itself.

If the scenic highway following the crest of the Santa Monica Mountains (Mulholland Drive/Highway) were ever extended eastward, it would probably snake along the sharply defined ridge between Mount Lee and Mount Chapel. But for now, and probably forever, the phenomenal views both north and south from this ridge remain the privilege of self-propelled travelers only.

From the end of Canyon Drive, proceed on foot past a gate and up the dirt-road extension of Canyon Drive, which climbs steadily up the east slope of a ravine known as Brush Canyon. After 1.1 miles (and 600 feet of elevation gain) you come to an intersection of a fire road known as the Mulholland Trail (Mulholland Highway on some older maps). Turn right, and continue climbing a little until you reach the paved, but closed-to-auto-traffic Mount Hollywood Drive. Make a sharp left there, walk on pavement for another 0.2 mile, and then cut left on the wide path going up along the southeast slope of Mount Chapel. The path leads to a water tank just north of the peak itself, and you can improvise a route to the 1614-foot summit itself.

On Mount Chapel you almost feel like you're flying as you gaze a thousand feet down on the Hollywood foothills to the south and the tidy green spaces of Forest Lawn Memorial Park to the north. When you're satisfied with the complete view, return to Mount Hollywood Drive and head back the same way you came.

**trip 4**  # Beacon Hill

| | |
|---|---|
| **Distance** | 2.5 miles round trip, Out-and-back |
| **Hiking Time** | 1½ hours (round trip) |
| **Elevation Gain/Loss** | 550'/550' |
| **Difficulty** | Moderate |
| **Trail Use** | Dogs allowed, good for kids |
| **Best Times** | All year |
| **Agency** | GP |
| **Optional Map** | USGS 7.5-min *Burbank* |
| **Notes** | Marked trails/obvious routes, easy terrain |

see
map on
p. 87

**DIRECTIONS** Exit Interstate 5 at Los Feliz Boulevard. Go west a short distance and then turn right (north) on Crystal Springs Drive. After 1.3 miles (next to the visitor center/ranger station) turn left on Griffith Park Drive. Go 0.2 mile to the large parking lot on the right, near the merry-go-round.

**BASIN AND FOOTHILLS**

Sharply terminated by the Los Angeles River flood channel and Interstate 5, Beacon Hill stands as the last eastward gasp of a 50-mile-long mountain range—the Santa Monicas. Back in the early 20th Century it served a utilitarian purpose as the site of an illuminated beacon for Grand Central Airport in Glendale. Today it presides over flatlands overrun by industrial buildings. Commercial air operations have long since shifted to LAX and four other big airports around the L.A. Basin. On this looping trip up to Beacon Hill's summit, you'll have a unique view of Glendale's industrial tracts, its medium-rise downtown skyline, and the looming Verdugo Mountains beyond.

From the merry-go-round parking lot, head southwest across Griffith Park Drive, and find and follow the Fern Canyon Trail. Ascend moderately up along a ravine called Fern Canyon, whose vegetation (including ferns) is recovering from a 2007 wildfire that burned 800 acres. Prior to the fire this area featured the park's densest growths of vegetation: native chaparral, oaks, toyons, and various non-native trees. It remains to be seen how much of this will thrive in the future.

After 1.0 mile of gentle ascent, you'll come to a five-way intersection of trails. Turn left on the Upper Beacon Trail, which follows a slightly rounded ridgeline for a quarter mile and takes you to Beacon Hill's 1001-foot summit. The summit dome is fairly clear of vegetation due to the fire, but likely it will fill in with tall laurel sumac shrubs eventually. Descend a little to the east for an unobstructed view of Glendale.

When it's time to go, return the same way you came.

## trip 5  East Side Loop

| | |
|---|---|
| **Distance** | 5.9 miles, Loop |
| **Hiking Time** | 3½ hours |
| **Elevation Gain/Loss** | 1350'/1350' |
| **Difficulty** | Moderately strenuous |
| **Trail Use** | Dogs allowed |
| **Best Times** | October through June |
| **Agency** | GP |
| **Optional Maps** | USGS 7.5-min *Hollywood, Burbank* |
| **Notes** | Marked trails/obvious routes, easy terrain |

see map on p. 87

**DIRECTIONS** Exit Interstate 5 at Los Feliz Boulevard. Go west a short distance and then turn right (north) on Crystal Springs Drive. After 1.3 miles (next to the visitor center/ranger station) turn left on Griffith Park Drive. Go 0.2 mile to the large parking lot on the right, near the merry-go-round.

Botanically and geologically, this is perhaps Griffith Park's most interesting hike. It's no slouch when it comes to good views either. The route tops out on the very crest of the park at Mount Hollywood.

The large 2007 Griffith Park wildfire burned large sections of the park's east side, destroying certain specimens of live oak, pine, eucalyptus, and California walnut trees. In these burned areas you are likely to see the recovery of chaparral vegetation first. This includes both blue and white varieties of blooming ceanothus, and four relatives in the family of sumacs that frequent the Southern California chaparral—laurel sumac, lemonade berry, sugarbush, and poison oak.

From the merry-go-round parking lot, cross Griffith Park Drive and start heading southwest up Fern Canyon Trail. Just 0.1 mile ahead turn right on Old Zoo Trail. In the next 0.7 mile you pass the site of the old L.A. Zoo, and a side trail leading left (west) toward Bee Rock, an impressive outcrop of cavernous sandstone poking out of the ridge above. Bee Rock is a good example of the types of marine sedimentary rock that are widely exposed throughout the middle and eastern Santa Monica Mountains. Up around Mount Hollywood, the bedrock consists of volcanic rocks more characteristic of the west end of the Santa Monicas.

Just past the Bee Rock trail, turn sharply left on the Bill Eckert Trail (aka East Trail). You zigzag around a chaparral-covered ridge overlooking the Griffith Park Boy's Camp and arrive, after 1.2 miles, at Vista del Valle Drive. Swing right, walk about 0.1 mile down the pavement, then veer left on the wide trail that ascends sharply up the slope to the south. Turn sharply left at the next junction and continue south along the ridge between Mount Bell and Mount Hollywood.

From the wide intersection just below Mount Hollywood's summit, you will eventually go east along the sunny ridgeline. But first pay a visit to the summit itself, and later cool off and refill your water bottle at the irrigated spot east of the summit known as Dante's View. Eucalyptus trees and succulent plants frame a view to the south at this little hideaway.

The view-rich but sometimes steep trail along the ridgeline to the east, Hogback Trail (aka East Ridge Trail), meanders down to meet Vista del Valle Drive. Cross the pavement there, walk down along the shoulder for about 100 feet, and pick up the trail going left past a water tank and down into the upper reaches of Fern Canyon. When you reach the five-way junction near Beacon Hill, make a hard left and descend Fern Canyon Trail to your starting point below.

# chapter 9

# Basin and Foothills: Hollywood Hills

The scraggly ridges and precipitous canyons separating San Fernando Valley from Hollywood and Beverly Hills harbor more than just a tangled net of serpentine streets and the homes of the rich and famous. Here and there a few pockets of open space remain where one can roam over sage-scented trails and partake, however briefly, of some of the perks—like great vistas on a clear day—afforded to Hollywood's most privileged residents.

The patchwork of parks and open spaces covered here are included within the sinuous boundaries of the Santa Monica Mountains National Recreation Area, a mosaic of federal, state, and local parkland, and private lands stretching from Cahuenga Pass above Hollywood to Point Mugu in Ventura County. The remainder of the national recreation lands will be treated separately in the Santa Monica Mountains section of this book. Here on the east end of the Santa Monicas, even diminutive parcels of land mean a lot for an area whose last unprotected ridges and canyons have for decades been cut and filled in by massive development.

Literally minutes away from L.A.'s most congested districts, the hikes described below offer remarkable opportunities to escape noise, traffic, and low-lying smog.

Lupines in springtime, Hollywood Hills

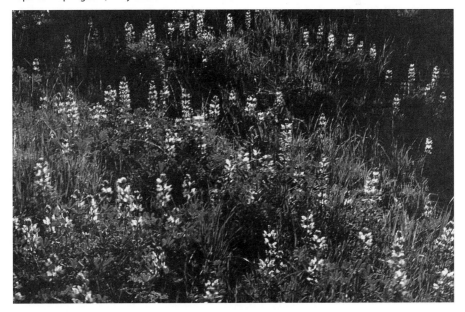

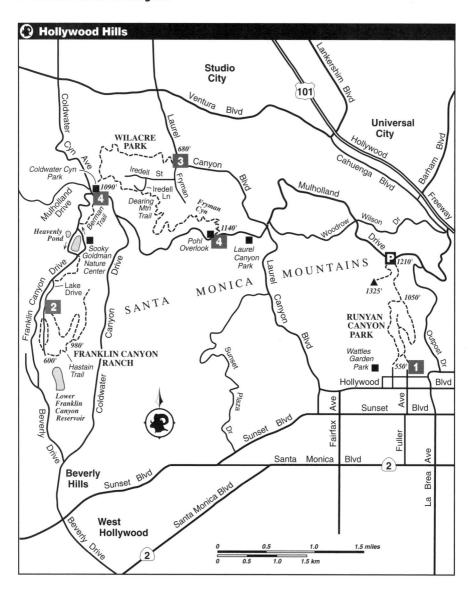

Hollywood Hills

## `trip 1` **Runyan Canyon**

|  |  |
|---|---|
| **Distance** | 2.0 miles, Loop |
| **Hiking Time** | 1 hour |
| **Elevation Gain/Loss** | 500'/500' |
| **Difficulty** | Moderate |
| **Trail Use** | Dogs allowed, good for kids |
| **Best Times** | All year |
| **Agency** | LACRPD |
| **Optional Map** | USGS 7.5-min *Hollywood* |
| **Notes** | Marked trails/obvious routes, easy terrain |

see map on p. 96

**DIRECTIONS** From Hollywood Boulevard, 2 miles west of the 101 Freeway, turn north on Fuller Avenue. Go 0.3 mile to the north end of Fuller, where you will find the Pines entrance to Runyan Canyon Park.

Runyan Canyon Park, a narrow strip of open space rising into the hills just a couple of miles from the heart of Hollywood, counts among its former residents the actors John McCormick and Errol Flynn. The now-quiet canyon site was long threatened by proposals to transform it into either a massive resort or a luxury housing development. In 1984, the property was purchased as parkland by the City of Los Angeles. Its popularity has grown among those seeking a little peace from the pressure-cooker pace of life in the metropolis below. The park is extremely popular for dog-walking.

In the 1930s, McCormick built a mansion here and began to landscape the area around it. Despite the later razing of the mansion and the effects of fire, flood, and general neglect, plenty of palms, pines, eucalyptus, and other exotic vegetation still grow on the site. Native chaparral vegetation thrives as well—dry and unappealing during summer's drought, but verdant and aromatic in the springtime.

From the Pines Trailhead at the north end of Fuller Avenue, start by following, on the left, an old asphalt road up along Runyan Canyon's west slope. Eventually you circle to the right and reach the east ridge near the head of the canyon. There you meet a north-south trail, the left branch leading toward Mulholland Drive, and the right going south along the east ridge. Make a right, and pass over a viewpoint called Cloud's Rest, where the view of the L.A. Basin is spectacular and panoramic. Continue descending about 300 feet of elevation to a second, lower viewpoint called Inspiration Point and the sketchy ruins of a "pool house" designed by Frank Lloyd Wright. Continue your descent all the way back to the Pines Trailhead.

You can also enter Runyan Canyon Park by way of its uppermost end. On Mulholland Drive, you'll find a small dirt parking area 1.6 miles west of Highway 101 at Cahuenga Pass. From there, you can descend toward the Cloud's Rest viewpoint, or else take a short spur trail to the west that leads to the park's 1325-foot high point atop a small summit.

## trip 2 Franklin Canyon

| | |
|---|---|
| **Distance** | 1.8 miles, Loop |
| **Hiking Time** | 1 hour |
| **Elevation Gain/Loss** | 400'/400' |
| **Difficulty** | Easy |
| **Trail Use** | Dogs allowed, good for kids |
| **Best Times** | All year |
| **Agency** | NPS |
| **Optional Map** | USGS 7.5-min *Beverly Hills* |
| **Notes** | Marked trails/obvious routes, easy terrain |

see map on p. 96

**DIRECTIONS** From Sunset Boulevard and Beverly Drive in Beverly Hills, go north on Beverly Drive. After 0.7 mile, be careful to fork left on the lesser-traveled north end of Beverly Drive at the intersection where the main road (Coldwater Canyon Drive) goes straight. After another 0.8 mile, bear right on narrow Franklin Canyon Drive. Go 1.2 miles farther along the canyonside to Lake Drive. Turn right and backtrack 0.3 mile south to a small parking area. The Hastain Trail begins there, on the left. (You can also reach Lake Drive and the Hastain Trail by driving south from Mulholland Drive on Franklin Canyon Drive.)

The Franklin Canyon Ranch park site, a part of the Santa Monica Mountains National Recreation Area, belongs to a complex of open-space units straddling the Santa Monica Mountains crest. The other units include Upper Franklin Canyon Reservoir, Coldwater Canyon Park, Wilacre Park, and the Fryman Canyon Natural Area. The Franklin Ranch itself was owned by the family of pioneering Angeleno Edward Doheny, who discovered oil in Los Angeles in 1892. The 400-acre ranch property was acquired as parkland in 1981.

From the parking area, walk the twisting Hastain Trail (a fire road) 0.9 mile along chaparral-covered slopes to a hairpin turn (980 feet elevation) with a panoramic view of the city. Looking over green-mantled Beverly Hills estates and the office towers and condominiums of the Wilshire corridor, you can sometimes see a blue horizon beyond.

Amphitheater at Franklin Canyon Ranch

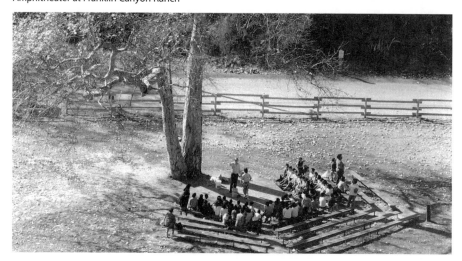

From the hairpin turn, the fire road continues climbing toward Coldwater Canyon Drive. You veer right on the narrow switchback trail descending to the green lawn and Doheny ranch house below. Somehow the old Doheny spread has managed to retain its rustic, rural charm.

From the ranch house you can walk back to your car on either of two trails that parallel Lake Drive. The trail on the right passes under a shady canopy of live oak, while the trail on the left meanders among scattered oaks and sycamores down along Franklin Canyon's usually dry stream bed.

For additional hiking in the area, try following the Berman Trail, which leads 1 mile north to Mulholland Drive. You can also walk or drive around placid Upper Franklin Canyon Reservoir, visit a tiny duck pond adjoining it on the west dubbed "Heavenly Pond," and/or check out the exhibits at the nearby Sooky Goldman Nature Center.

## trip 3  Wilacre & Coldwater Loop

see
map on
p. 96

| | |
|---|---|
| **Distance** | 2.7 miles, Loop |
| **Hiking Time** | 1½ hours |
| **Elevation Gain/Loss** | 500'/500' |
| **Difficulty** | Moderate |
| **Trail Use** | Dogs allowed, good for kids |
| **Best Times** | All year |
| **Agency** | SMMC |
| **Optional Map** | USGS 7.5-min *Van Nuys* |
| **Notes** | Marked trails/obvious routes, easy terrain |

**DIRECTIONS** Exit Highway 101 at Laurel Canyon Boulevard in Studio City. Drive south 1.4 miles to where Fryman Road diverges to the right. Go right and park in the small lot on the right (west) side of Fryman Road.

A 129-acre island of open space in the midst of Studio City's more lavish residential areas, Wilacre Park (the former estate of silent movie star Will Acres) offers a wide-ranging view of San Fernando Valley and a peaceful, quiet atmosphere. This loop route goes up through Wilacre Park and visits Coldwater Canyon Park, which is the headquarters of TreePeople, a grassroots organization that is spearheading efforts to plant millions of trees in the urban Los Angeles area.

From the trailhead parking lot, walk west up the gated Dearing Mountain Trail (aka Betty B. Dearing Trail), named in honor of the late advocate of Santa Monica Mountains trails. At first, you are on a curving, hardtopped driveway flanked by pine and cypress trees. After passing the slab foundation of Acres' old house, the road turns to dirt. You ascend, more easily now, along north-facing slopes dotted with live oak and native walnut trees. After a while you turn south, descend slightly, and arrive at a wide junction (1.4 miles) on the edge of Coldwater Canyon Park. Take the Magic Forest Trail on the right, or use some steps a little way to the left to reach the old fire station above that serves as headquarters for TreePeople. Pick up a brochure at the parking lot and make your own self-guided tour of TreePeople's exhibits and nursery.

Return to the wide junction and continue east (downhill) on the Dearing Mountain Trail. After 0.5 mile you hit pavement at Iredell Lane, a cozy, residential cul-de-sac. The last 0.6 mile is along lightly traveled streets—down Iredell Lane to Iredell Street, down Iredell Street to Fryman Road, and down Fryman Road to the starting point.

# trip 4  Coldwater to Fryman Canyon

see map on p. 96

|  |  |
|---|---|
| **Distance** | 2.5 miles, Point-to-point |
| **Hiking Time** | 1½ hours |
| **Elevation Gain/Loss** | 500'/450' |
| **Difficulty** | Moderate |
| **Trail Use** | Dogs allowed |
| **Best Times** | All year |
| **Agency** | SMMC |
| **Optional Maps** | USGS 7.5-min *Van Nuys, Beverly Hills* |
| **Notes** | Marked trails/obvious routes, easy terrain |

**DIRECTIONS** *West End:* Start the hike at Coldwater Canyon Park, located at the intersection of Coldwater Canyon Avenue and Mulholland Drive. *East End:* Finish the hike at the Nancy Hoover Pohl Overlook (formerly known as the Fryman Canyon Overlook) on Mulholland Drive 0.8 mile west of Laurel Canyon Boulevard.

The Dearing Mountain Trail commemorates Betty B. Dearing (1917–77), a conservationist who foresaw a trail stretching from Los Angeles along the mountain crests to the sea. Today's nearly completed Backbone Trail through the Santa Monica Mountains is the realization of her dream.

The Dearing Mountain Trail, which is not a part of the Backbone Trail or even near it, runs roughly parallel to the motorist's equivalent of the Backbone Trail—Mulholland Drive. Mulholland Drive, and Mulholland Highway to the west, stretches 50 miles through the Santa Monica Mountains National Recreation Area.

Do this as a car-shuttle trip by leaving cars at both Coldwater Canyon Park (parking 9 a.m. to dusk) and Pohl Overlook; or leave one car and go out and back on the same route for a rugged 5 miles of ups and downs. Another alternative would be to make a loop by walking or jogging over or back along Mulholland Drive—a good option if you can do the road-walking part very early on a Sunday morning to avoid traffic.

Pay careful attention to the following directions. In places this poorly marked trail is like a rabbit run through the brush, with plenty of intersecting roads and false paths to lead you astray.

From the east side of the TreePeople complex in Coldwater Canyon Park, descend a stone staircase and hook up with the dirt road—Dearing Mountain Trail—below. Go downhill 0.5 mile to where you meet Iredell Lane. Walk 100 yards down the sidewalk there and then veer off on the fire road that slants up to the right. After only 0.1 mile, turn left and follow a foot trail. You soon bend right and begin climbing straight up a slope over wooden water bars. The trail levels along a brushy slope and soon intersects a disused dirt road bed overlooked by some towering, opulent residences. Turn left on the road bed, curve past a private, fenced exercise yard and descend into the eucalyptus-shaded upper reaches of Fryman Canyon. This shady little ravine is a part of the small Fryman Canyon Natural Area between Mulholland Drive and the edge of the residential area below. Part of the year a tiny stream enhances this cool and appealing spot.

After curving sharply left to cross the ravine, you ascend gradually on an old road bed another 0.3 mile, then take the steep foot trail (Dearing Mountain Trail) going up the slope to the right. This meanders generally eastward, staying about 150–200 feet of elevation below Mulholland Drive. Near the end you settle into switchbacks leading up to a fire road just east of the Nancy Hoover Pohl Overlook.

# chapter 10

# Basin and Foothills: Puente Hills

The rambling Puente Hills, overlooking the San Gabriel Valley to the north and Orange County to the south, interrupt what would otherwise be a continuous spread of flat, nondescript suburbs. Rising no higher than 1500 feet in elevation, they host a collection of hillside homes; the sprawling, mostly undeveloped Rose Hills Memorial Park; the huge Puente Hills Landfill; and several large open-space areas for habitat preservation and public recreation. L.A. County's Skyline equestrian trail skips over the west end of the Puente Hills from one rounded summit to the next, joining a number of spur trails that connect to suburbs below.

Whenever the L.A. Basin is swept clear of smog and moisture by offshore winds, the upper elevations of the Puente Hills offer truly mind-blowing views of almost everything from the mountains to the sea. Don't miss the spectacular sunrises over the San Bernardino and San Jacinto mountains, and sunsets over the Pacific Ocean.

Sycamores, Sycamore Canyon, Puente Hills

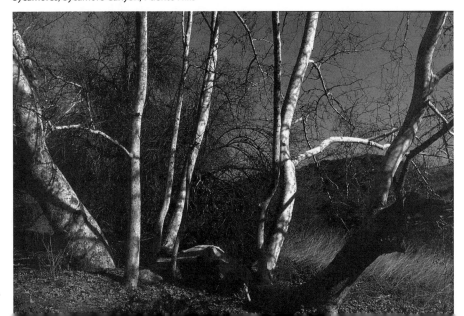

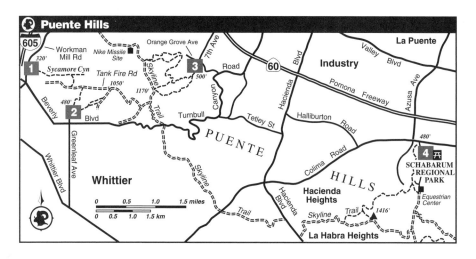

Early-morning sun rays over the Puente Hills

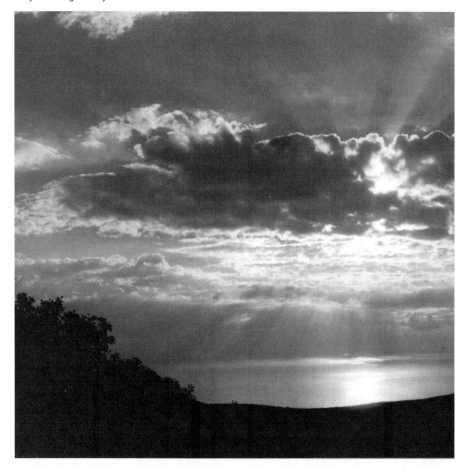

see map on p. 102

# trip 1 Sycamore Canyon

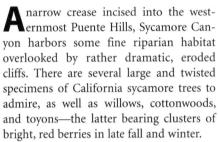

| | |
|---|---|
| **Distance** | 2.0 miles, Out-and-back |
| **Hiking Time** | 1 hour (round trip) |
| **Elevation Gain/Loss** | 200'/200' |
| **Difficulty** | Easy |
| **Trail Use** | Good for kids |
| **Best Times** | All year |
| **Agency** | PHPA |
| **Optional Map** | USGS 7.5-min *El Monte* |
| **Notes** | Marked trails/obvious routes, easy terrain |

**DIRECTIONS** Exit Interstate 605 at Beverly Boulevard in Whittier. Go east on Beverly for 0.6 mile and turn left (north) on Workman Mill Road. Go 0.4 mile north to the entrance to Sycamore Canyon on the right. There is no parking lot, but you can park alongside the curb.

**BASIN AND FOOTHILLS**

A narrow crease incised into the westernmost Puente Hills, Sycamore Canyon harbors some fine riparian habitat overlooked by rather dramatic, eroded cliffs. There are several large and twisted specimens of California sycamore trees to admire, as well as willows, cottonwoods, and toyons—the latter bearing clusters of bright, red berries in late fall and winter.

From the curbside trailhead, bypass the vehicle gate and proceed up the narrow trail, following signs. You pass a groaning oil well and bend left to join a wider path, which is an old roadbed that currently functions as the Sycamore Canyon Trail. Note the contrast between the sheer and barren south-facing canyon wall on the left, which bears the full force of sunlight, and the more gently sloping, north-facing, grassy slopes on the right.

After 1.0 mile of travel, the main trail turns sharply right and wastes no time in ascending those grassy slopes. Straight ahead (east) lies a sketchy trail that continues up Sycamore Canyon toward a tributary ravine called Dark Canyon. This juncture is a good place to turn around and return if your hike is going to be a casual one. If you decide to hike farther into Sycamore Canyon, then watch out for poison oak.

Sycamore Canyon

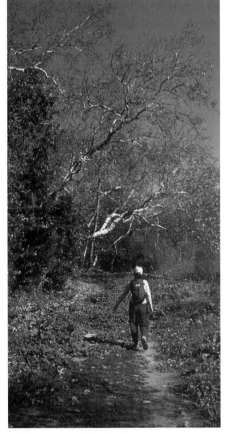

## trip 2  Hellman Wilderness Park

see map on p. 102

| | |
|---|---|
| **Distance** | 1.8 miles, Loop |
| **Hiking Time** | 1 hour |
| **Elevation Gain/Loss** | 500'/500' |
| **Difficulty** | Moderate |
| **Trail Use** | Dogs allowed, good for kids |
| **Best Times** | All year |
| **Agency** | PHPA |
| **Optional Map** | USGS 7.5-min *Whittier* |
| **Notes** | Marked trails/obvious routes, easy terrain |

**DIRECTIONS** Exit Interstate 605 at Beverly Boulevard in Whittier. Go east on Beverly for 2 miles and turn left (north) on Greenleaf Avenue. Go 0.2 mile north to the Hellman Wilderness Park Trailhead on the right.

Hellman Wilderness Park is a patch of open space perched on steep hillsides overlooking the city of Whittier. Whenever crystal-clear skies prevail, a vast sweep of L.A Basin landscape stretching from skyscrapers of downtown L.A. to Palos Verdes comes into vivid view, along with nearly all of Orange County. At times a distinct Pacific Ocean horizon can be seen, interrupted by the rambling profile of Santa Catalina Island.

It doesn't take much of a lengthy hike to achieve such vistas, but the route is so steep in places it has been nicknamed "cardiac hill." From the Hellman Wilderness Park Trailhead on Greenleaf Avenue, start up the fire road going straight up the ridge to the east. Ignore lesser paths that diverge right. After 0.4 mile the trail dips slightly and you are faced with two alternatives: a more gradual ascent on a curvy trail to the left, or a continuing steep climb along the spine of the ridge. Pick the left fork (you will return on the steep path to the right) and thread alongside slopes overlooking a yawning chasm to the north.

At 1.0 mile, you reach a wide fire road. To the left (north) is the ridge-running Tank Fire Road, and plenty of other possible routes to hike all over the Puente Hills if you have the time and inclination. Our briefer, looping route, though, goes sharply right. After a short stint on the wide fire road, veer right and go uphill briefly on the path that follows the spine of the ridge. Pass over the ridge crest and continue steeply downhill all the way to the trailhead.

# trip 3  West Skyline Loop

see map on p. 102

|  |  |
|---|---|
| **Distance** | 4.3 miles, Loop |
| **Hiking Time** | 2½ hours |
| **Elevation Gain/Loss** | 1100'/1100' |
| **Difficulty** | Moderate |
| **Trail Use** | Suitable for mountain biking, dogs allowed |
| **Best Times** | October through May |
| **Agency** | PHPA |
| **Optional Maps** | USGS 7.5-min *Baldwin Park, El Monte* |
| **Notes** | Marked trails/obvious routes, easy terrain |

**DIRECTIONS** Exit the Pomona Freeway at 7th Avenue near the city of Industry. Drive 0.7 mile south to the intersection of Orange Grove Avenue. Park anywhere in the surrounding neighborhood.

On this looping hike, you'll explore hardy little pockets of oak woodland, and also get a close look at the marine sedimentary bedrock of the Puente Hills, which dates back 15–30 million years. Mostly this consists of silty, layered deposits, but you'll also find some conglomerate rock in the ravines. Some newer alternate trails have recently been added to the trail network in this area; however, our route described here stays on the older trails that are open to both hiking and mountain biking.

This is an especially fun trip to take on an evening lit by the full moon. You'll make your way along spooky ravines where moonbeams filter through the twisted oaks and glance off the cobbled rock formations.

From the informational kiosk at the intersection of 7th Avenue and Orange Grove Avenue, start hiking south on the unpaved roadway—a would-be extension of 7th Avenue. The trail ahead used to be named 7th Avenue Trail, but it is now called the Ahwingna Trail.

After 0.3 mile you veer right up an asphalt strip that leads to an abandoned hillside reservoir. From there, you ascend on switchbacks going up the ridge. At 0.8 mile you reach a small flat with a hitching post. Keep going straight up the ridge

(you'll later return to this spot by way of the Native Oak Trail coming up from the right). At 1.3 miles you arrive at the Skyline Trail, which at this point follows the wide Puente Hills crest. The trail traces, more or less, the route of the Juan Bautista de Anza expedition of 1775–76.

Turn right and follow the Skyline Trail's right-of-way, fenced on both sides, roughly paralleling some high-voltage powerlines. Long views (clear air allowing) west toward downtown L.A.'s Oz-like skyline and the blue Pacific atone for the rather harsh and barren-looking foreground.

At 1.8 miles, turn right on the Native Oak Trail. It goes briefly up a little hill and then steadily down along oak-dotted slopes overlooking a deep ravine. After several switchbacks you arrive at the mouth of that ravine (2.7 miles) and traverse to the right around a hillside just above the edge of a subdivision. The trail steers you into another shade-dappled ravine, similar to the first. You ascend moderately along the bottom, veer left (south) up a tributary, and climb switchbacks to the hitching post on the ridge above (3.5 miles). From there retrace your earlier steps past the hillside reservoir to your starting point at 7th Avenue.

# trip 4  Schabarum Trail

see map on p. 102

| | |
|---|---|
| **Distance** | 5.2 miles, Loop |
| **Hiking Time** | 2½ hours |
| **Elevation Gain/Loss** | 900'/900' |
| **Difficulty** | Moderate |
| **Trail Use** | Dogs allowed |
| **Best Times** | October through May |
| **Agency** | LADPR |
| **Optional Map** | USGS 7.5-min *La Habra* |
| **Notes** | Marked trails/obvious routes, easy terrain |

**DIRECTIONS** Exit the Pomona Freeway at Azusa Avenue in the city of Industry. Drive 0.4 mile south to Colima Road, and turn left (east). Just ahead, turn right into Schabarum Regional Park.

Schabarum Regional Park features a green-grass strip extending nearly a mile into the Puente Hills, and lots of steep, brushy hillsides affording some great panoramas of the San Gabriel Valley and the San Gabriel Mountains. You'll share these views with hawks and ravens who ride the hillside thermals.

After parking in any of the park's spacious lots (open during daylight hours), start your hike on the signed Schabarum Trail. It starts near the park entrance and twists and turns along dry, prickly-pear-covered slopes west of the park's long strip of green turf. At 0.8 mile from the park

Old Baldy from the Schabarum Trail

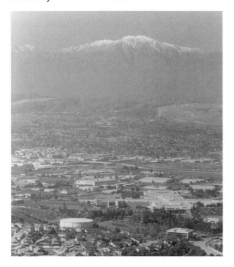

entrance you come to a split; the left branch goes over to an equestrian ring at the south end of the turf strip, while the right branch, your route, takes you up through dense chaparral toward the Puente Hills crest. The panorama below includes nearby subdivisions in Hacienda Heights, the linear city of Industry (which, it is manifestly clear, specializes in industry), and assorted other suburban sprawl stretching to the foot of the San Gabriel Mountains. The winter-white-capped summit of Mount San Antonio (Old Baldy) floats serenely above it all.

As you approach the ridgeline, you contour below an antenna-topped, 1416-foot peak. A shortcut to the ridge-running Skyline Trail is possible up and around this.

After 2.5 miles from the park entrance, bear left as you approach a water tower and antenna site served by a paved service road coming up from below. Follow the dirt road going east, which is the Skyline Trail. You climb some more, passing the 1416-foot peak, and then descend. To the south you look over the wooded community of La Habra Heights, and across the coastal plains of Orange County.

After winding down a steep hillside, you reach a north-south dirt road in a saddle (3.8 miles). Go left and continue 0.7 mile down a draw to the equestrian ring. From there you can follow an asphalt walkway down the middle of the turf area to reach the park entrance.

# chapter 11

# Basin and Foothills: San Gabriel Valley

The million-plus residents of the greater San Gabriel Valley area are fortunate to have easy access to dozens of higher-country trails in the San Gabriel Mountains. This chapter, however, focuses on seven worthy hikes on the rim of the valley itself—five right along the base of the San Gabriel Mountains, and two in the San Jose Hills not far from Cal Poly Pomona. Four more low-land hikes, in the Puente Hills, are described in the previous chapter. All 11 of these hikes make fine winter and spring additions to your repertoire of favorite hiking spots—especially if you're a local resident.

Trail to Vista Point, Claremont Hills Wilderness Park

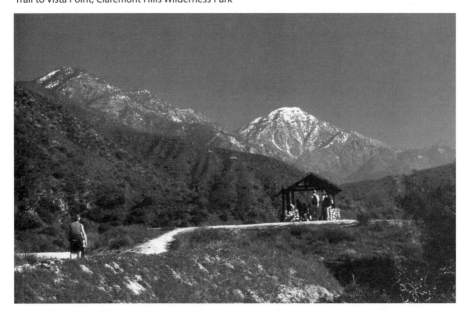

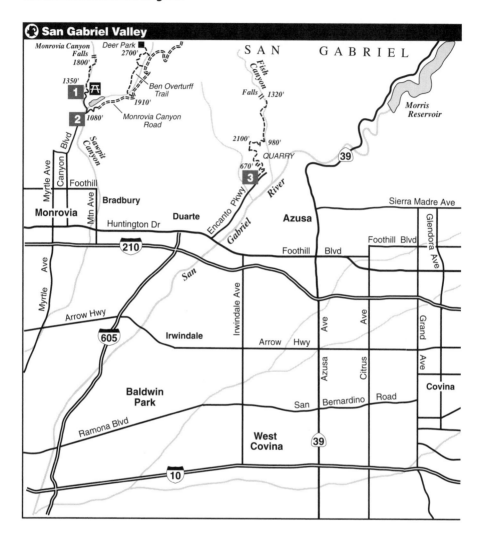

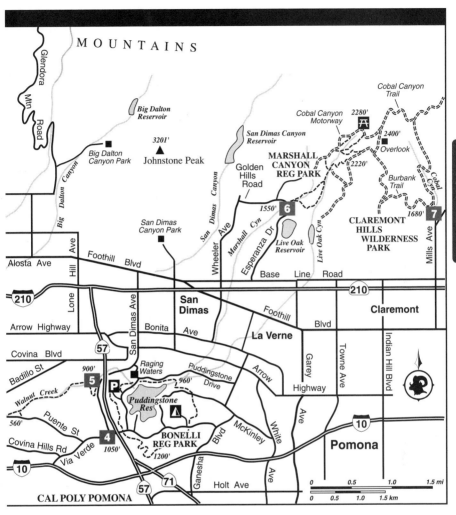

## trip 1 Monrovia Canyon Falls

see map on p. 108

|   |   |
|---|---|
| **Distance** | 1.6 miles round trip, Out-and-back |
| **Hiking Time** | 1 hour (round trip) |
| **Elevation Gain/Loss** | 500'/500' |
| **Difficulty** | Easy |
| **Trail Use** | Dogs allowed, good for kids |
| **Best Times** | All year |
| **Agency** | MCP |
| **Optional Map** | USGS 7.5-min *Azusa* |
| **Notes** | Marked trails/obvious routes, easy terrain |

**DIRECTIONS** Exit Interstate 210 at Myrtle Avenue in Monrovia, and drive north for 1.9 miles to where Myrtle Avenue ends at Scenic Drive. Turn right and follow Scenic Drive on a meandering eastward course for three blocks, then keep straight as Canyon Boulevard joins from the right. Proceed uphill on Canyon Boulevard, which crookedly ascends alongside the Sawpit Canyon wash to the park entrance. After paying a small fee, drive an additional 0.5 mile to the nature center parking lot. (*Note:* The park is closed on Tuesdays.)

Tucked away obscurely in two shady canyons behind the foothill community of Monrovia is one of the most beautiful parks in the Los Angeles area: Monrovia Canyon Park. Adding spice to the rich profusion of the riparian vegetation in these canyons is 40-foot-high Monrovia Canyon Falls, which runs with frothy exuberance for weeks or months after the rainy season ends.

From the nature center, start walking up Monrovia Canyon to the north on a trail that mostly sticks close to the canyon's sparkling stream. Sometimes the trail gets narrow, eroded, and slippery enough to cause some difficulty with footing—a cautionary note for those with small kids. Alder, oak, and bay trees cluster in the canyon bottom so densely that hardly any sunlight is admitted, even at midday. After 0.8 mile the sound of splashing water heralds your arrival at the falls, where the stream either leaps or dribbles down two distinct declivities on a water-worn cliff face.

The trail ends there; so your return will be a retracing of your steps.

Monrovia Canyon Falls

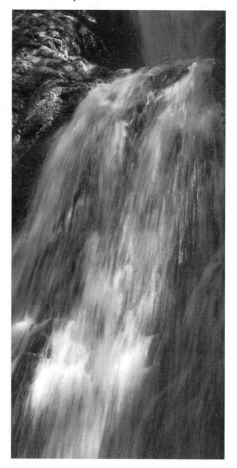

`trip 2` # Ben Overturff Trail

| | |
|---|---|
| **Distance** | 7.1 miles, Loop |
| **Hiking Time** | 4 hours |
| **Elevation Gain/Loss** | 2000′/2000′ |
| **Difficulty** | Moderately strenuous |
| **Trail Use** | Dogs allowed |
| **Best Times** | October through May |
| **Agency** | MCP |
| **Optional Map** | USGS 7.5-min *Azusa* |
| **Notes** | Marked trails/obvious routes, easy terrain |

see map on p. 108

**DIRECTIONS** Exit Interstate 210 at Myrtle Avenue in Monrovia, and drive north for 1.9 miles to where Myrtle Avenue ends at Scenic Drive. Turn right and follow Scenic Drive on a meandering eastward course for three blocks, then keep straight as Canyon Boulevard joins from the right. Proceed uphill on Canyon Boulevard, which crookedly ascends alongside the Sawpit Canyon wash to the park entrance. After paying a small fee, park near the entrance. (***Note:*** The entire park is closed on Tuesdays, and the Overturff Trail specifically is closed on Wednesdays.)

**BASIN AND FOOTHILLS**

The more lengthy trek in Monrovia Canyon Park takes you up the Sawpit Canyon drainage to Deer Park, the site of a tourist lodge popular during the early 20th Century. There you'll see the remains of a stone lodge built by Monrovia building contractor Ben Overturff in 1911. Torrential rainfall in 1938 wiped out large sections of Overturff's access trail to the lodge, and by 1948 the lodge and the trail were

Large Whipple Yucca in bloom, Sawpit Canyon

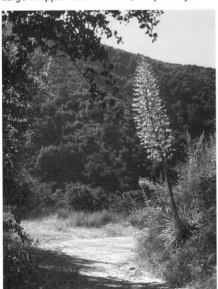

effectively abandoned. Not until the 1990s would the access trail again come into use; by this time the entire area had become a Monrovia city park.

For variety, it's best to follow what remains of the old Overturff Trail to the lodge and return by way of a newer fire road. About 200 yards uphill from the park entrance, the gated Monrovia Canyon fire road goes right. Walk uphill on this road (paved initially), climbing on zigzags to a point overlooking the small Sawpit dam and reservoir. Pavement ends and you continue climbing, more moderately now, past a turnoff for a Boy Scout reservation (1.3 miles) to a very sharp hairpin turn to the left (1.7 miles), where a sign announces OVERTURFF JUNCTION.

At the junction, start descending into the ravine on the left using the narrow Ben Overturff Trail. You now experience a terrific 2-mile stretch of narrow footpath densely shaded by live oaks and mature chaparral so thick that it frequently forms a canopy overhead. About halfway through the stretch, the trail delicately threads a narrow ridge known as "Razorback." Three-fourths of the way through you traverse a soggy, oak-shaded draw known as Twin Springs Canyon, passing a spur trail on the right leading over to the nearby fire road. Up and over the next

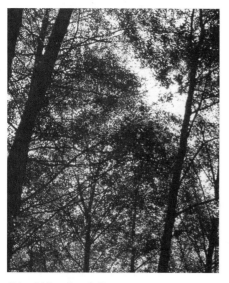

Alder thicket, Sawpit Canyon

ridge, you come to a second trail junction. Go left and hike the final 0.1 mile to the stone cabin ruins. So serene are the surroundings that it's hard to believe the site was once teeming with tourists.

When it's time to go, retrace your steps 0.1 mile—but turn left to get access to the nearby fire road, where a restroom has been thoughtfully placed. Follow the fire road all the way back (3.2 miles of easy walking), passing a Monrovia Police shooting range and later the aforementioned Overturff Junction. Target practice occurs at the shooting range on Tuesdays and Wednesdays, which is why the route is unavailable to the public on those days.

## trip 3  Fish Canyon Falls

see map on p. 108

| | |
|---|---|
| **Distance** | 8.8 miles round trip, Out-and-back |
| **Hiking Time** | 6 hours (round trip) |
| **Elevation Gain/Loss** | 3000'/3000' |
| **Difficulty** | Strenuous |
| **Trail Use** | Dogs allowed |
| **Best Times** | November through May |
| **Agency** | ANF/SGRD |
| **Optional Map** | USGS 7.5-min *Azusa* |
| **Notes** | Navigation required, difficult terrain |

**DIRECTIONS** From the northernmost end of Interstate 605 in Duarte, turn east on Huntington Drive. Proceed 0.6 mile east to Encanto Parkway. Turn left and follow Encanto Parkway (and its extension, Fish Canyon Road) northeast for 1.4 miles. Turn left into the dirt parking lot, which is just short of the Vulcan Materials rock quarry entrance.

Time-traveling visitors from nearly a century ago would have a hard time recognizing Fish Canyon today. Long gone are the dozens of vacation cabins lining the canyon and the dance hall at the canyon's mouth. For the past quarter-century, the lower canyon has been chewed apart on an astounding scale by rock quarrying operations. These operations, however, extend only as far into the canyon as the Angeles National Forest boundary. Beyond lies the perennially green

Fish Canyon, its sparkling stream, and its magnificent, multi-tiered waterfall.

During the 1980s and most of the '90s, public access to the canyon was made difficult or impossible by operations at the quarry. The access issue was finally resolved in 1998, when the city of Duarte opened a new trail bypassing the quarry on the canyon's steep, west wall. Unfortunately, the devilish climb and descent on this trail—which must be accomplished twice during the round trip to and from the falls—occupies almost three-fourths of the time and energy expended on the entire hike. To make matters worse, this quarry bypass trail hasn't been properly maintained in recent years. Be aware of the uncertain state of trail maintenance if you intend to try to follow it.

The alternative to following the bypass trail is to join one of the periodic "Family Wilderness Day" events sponsored by the City of Duarte Parks and Recreation Department (626-357-7931). These events feature a shuttle-bus ride through the quarry, and let you avoid completely the brutally steep and rough bypass route.

Here's a description of the route to the falls using the bypass trail: Start hiking north from the parking area, and start climbing in earnest on the primitive, switchbacking trail that at times barely gains purchase on the soft dirt of the 40-degree slopes. Relief from the heart-pounding effort comes at a flat spot on the ridge above (1.3 miles) where you may catch one last panoramic glance behind you of nearly the entire San Gabriel Valley. There's a patch of tall chaparral just ahead where you may take a breather in the shade.

Next, the trail follows a watershed divide, staying just outside the quarry fenceline for a while. Then it veers left (west) to follow an old firebreak for 0.2 mile. Next comes a sharp right turn (north) up Van Tassel Ridge. Further climbing takes you to a point on the ridge (elevation 2100 feet, 1.9 miles from the start), just inside the Angeles National Forest boundary.

Thereafter, you descend a series of knee-banging switchback segments, nearly as steep as those you climbed, down along an east-facing slope liberally sprinkled with poison oak. At 3.0 miles you reach bottom, and the trail turns abruptly left (north), following the west wall of Fish Canyon. The uppermost end of the quarry lies a short distance to the right.

Now comes the payoff. The remainder of the trail is delightful with its gentle ascent, superb scenery, and historical reminders. Notice the old cabin foundations, rock and mortar walls, and rusty household equipment. Check out the botanical evidence: nonnative ivy, vinca, trees-of-heaven, agaves, and ornamental yuccas. Plenty of native vegetation thrives here, too. Live oaks, big-leaf maples, and bay laurels cling tenaciously to the canyon's precipitous walls, helping to hold together the structurally precarious miscellany of smashed-up granitic and metamorphic rock.

Fish Canyon Falls

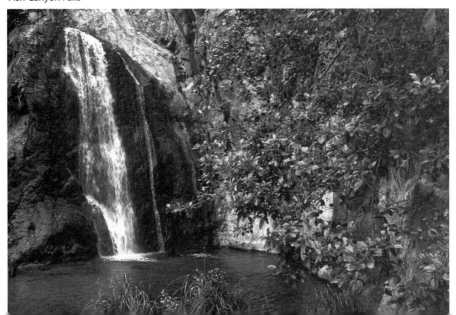

After 1.1 miles in the canyon, the trail crosses over the creek to the east bank—a foot- and leg-wetting exercise when the water's running high. A final 0.3-mile stretch leads to a point on the canyon wall offering a fine but not intimately close view of Fish Canyon Falls. The water tumbles nearly 100 feet down a cliff with four separate tiers, slides through riparian vegetation a short way, and makes a final, small leap into a crystalline pool just below the trail.

On the return, you must retrace your steps exactly and refrain from taking a short cut through the quarry—unless, of course, you are on an officially sanctioned tour.

## trip 4  Bonelli Regional Park

see map on p. 108

| | |
|---|---|
| **Distance** | 7.0 miles, Loop |
| **Hiking Time** | 3½ hours |
| **Elevation Gain/Loss** | 1050'/1050' |
| **Difficulty** | Moderately strenuous |
| **Trail Use** | Suitable for mountain biking, dogs allowed |
| **Best Times** | November through May |
| **Agency** | LADPR |
| **Optional Map** | USGS 7.5-min *San Dimas* |
| **Notes** | Marked trails/obvious routes, easy terrain |

**DIRECTIONS** Exit the 57 freeway at Via Verde in San Dimas, just north of Interstate 10. Immediately west of the freeway is a Park & Ride lot, which on weekends has plenty of space (and no fee to pay).

Girded by freeways and busy streets, the trails around Puddingstone Reservoir in Bonelli Regional Park are hardly the place to get away from it all—unless, perhaps, you arrive early on a Saturday or Sunday morning. During those quiet times you can get a sense of how peaceful a spot this was before World War II. In those distant days, the reservoir nestled among serene hills overlooking a patchwork quilt of citrus groves.

Today, the reservoir and the surrounding Los Angeles County-operated regional park are quite popular, with attractions such as the Raging Waters aquatic amusement park, a golf course, acres of RV camping and picnic grounds, horse stables, hot tubs, and even motorboat drag races on occasion. For hikers, what remains of the dry, grassy hills above the reservoir can be very attractive in March and April, especially if California poppies brighten the velvety green slopes.

Although many of the trails at Bonelli Park were designed to serve equestrians, they are popular with hikers, mountain bikers, and leashed dogs, too. About 14 miles of dirt roads and bridle trails lace the outer perimeter of the park, not even including some pedestrian and bike paths that follow parts of the reservoir's shoreline.

This 7-mile "grand tour" of the park circles Puddingstone Reservoir in a roundabout but scenic way. From the Park & Ride lot, walk east on Via Verde over the freeway toward Bonelli Park's west entrance booth and nearby administration center, where you can obtain a trail map. Just after crossing the overpass you'll see a trail, passing through a tunnel under Via Verde, going southeast up onto a grassy hillside dotted with planted pines. Take it, and let the EQUESTRIAN TRAIL signs be your guide for the next couple of miles. The trail dips momentarily, almost touching Via Verde, and then swings right and later left as it climbs to the top of the ridge. Keep climbing and ignore

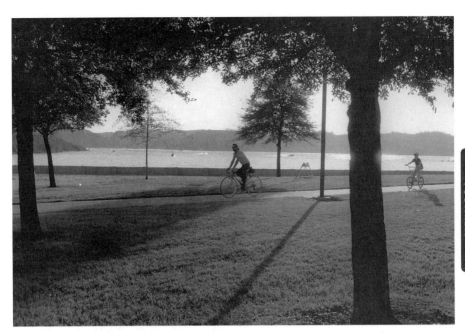

North shore, Puddingstone Reservoir

side trails to the left. Topping out at about 1200 feet elevation (1.4 miles from where you parked), there's a fine view over the Puente Hills to the south and across the flat lands stretching interminably east toward San Bernardino and Riverside.

Continue following the ridge, generally east, for the next mile. You'll arrive at a road intersection close to the park's east entrance booth. Cross the pavement and climb north and east around some horse stables to a gap in the ridge to the north (restrooms here). Continue north down a draw, and bear left to join McKinley Avenue (3.5 miles), which is gated to the left. Near the gate pick up a signed bridle trail that briefly follows a shoreline access road. The trail soon swings north, follows a fence delimiting Brackett Field (a small airport), and then crosses a muddy creek (Live Oak Wash) to join a paved walkway through grassy picnic and play areas along the reservoir's north shore.

Continue west on the walkway—or across the lawns—to the boat-launching area. Just beyond that, climb up over the spillway, cross a paved road, and descend sharply into a shady ravine (Walnut Creek) below the spillway's snout. Like Sisyphus you immediately start a steep, zigzagging ascent back up the far wall—but at least that passage takes you through an enchanting little grove of live oaks.

After topping out, follow a paved road west to a large parking lot (equestrian staging area) below. From there, head generally south (parallel to the 57 Freeway), up and over an oak and walnut-dotted ridge, and down to the tunnel beneath Via Verde at Bonelli Park's west entrance.

# trip 5  Walnut Creek

see map on p. 108

| | |
|---|---|
| **Distance** | 5.0 miles, Out-and-back |
| **Hiking Time** | 2½ hours |
| **Elevation Gain/Loss** | 350'/350' |
| **Difficulty** | Moderate |
| **Trail Use** | Suitable for mountain biking, dogs allowed, good for kids |
| **Best Times** | All year |
| **Agency** | LADPR |
| **Optional Map** | USGS 7.5-min *San Dimas* |
| **Notes** | Marked trails/obvious routes, easy terrain |

**DIRECTIONS**  Exit the 57 Freeway at Via Verde in San Dimas. Go a short distance west to San Dimas Avenue, and turn right. Continue 1.0 mile north to a roadside parking area on the left (west) side of San Dimas Avenue.

Walnut Creek County Park is a secluded ribbon of open space stretching through the cities of San Dimas and Covina. A wide and well-traveled bridle trail goes the length of the park, crossing the Walnut Creek stream several times (you'll get your feet wet in winter and spring). Plenty of oaks, sycamores, willows, and assorted non-native ornamental trees—but relatively few walnut trees—line the banks.

Steep south walls along most of this stretch of Walnut Creek make it a cool haven on all but the hottest days. Often on winter mornings the canyon bottom is a frosty wonderland, since it acts as a sink for cold, dense night air slinking down along the slopes of the nearby San Gabriel Mountains.

From the parking lot, the Walnut Creek Trail zigzags west down the road embankment and arrives at the shady canyon floor. You then go down alongside the creek, where there are several splits in the trail. The first three are merely alternate routes that go along the opposite bank or up onto the steep south slope before returning to the main trail. The fourth splitting trail to the left connects with Puente Street.

Beyond Puente Street there's not much of a trail at all, though the strip of county park land continues about a mile farther to Covina Hills Road. Therefore, Puente Street is a good place to turn around and return the way you came.

Walnut Creek Trail

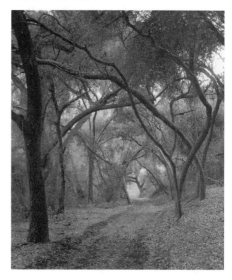

# trip 6  Marshall Canyon Trail

see map on p. 108

| | |
|---|---|
| **Distance** | 5.0 miles, Loop |
| **Hiking Time** | 2½ hours |
| **Elevation Gain/Loss** | 1100'/1100' |
| **Difficulty** | Moderately strenuous |
| **Trail Use** | Suitable for mountain biking, dogs allowed |
| **Best Times** | October through June |
| **Agency** | LADPR |
| **Optional Map** | USGS 7.5-min *Mt. Baldy* |
| **Notes** | Marked trails/obvious routes, easy terrain |

**DIRECTIONS** From Baseline Road in La Verne, drive north on Esperanza Drive 1.7 miles to the Marshall Canyon Regional Park staging area on the right.

**BASIN AND FOOTHILLS**

The multi-use trails of Marshall Canyon Regional Park (for hikers, mountain bikers, and equestrians) thread through Marshall and Live Oak canyons in the foothills of the San Gabriel Mountains. The inner recesses of both canyons are smothered by a leafy canopy of live oak, sycamore and alder trees. In some areas luminescent curtains of poison oak and wild grape cling to the trees, while carpets of blackberry vines and vinca (an ornamental groundcover gone wild) coat the stream banks. Steep, chaparral-covered slopes, dotted here and there with planted pines and eucalyptus, round out the scene.

On the intricate figure-eight route described here you'll explore parts of both canyons and pay a visit to a shady picnic spot. Many shorter routes are possible, as well as a longer extension, which could take you farther east into the recently opened, adjoining Claremont Hills Regional Park.

As you start off from the staging area, after only a few steps you're enveloped in a shade-dappled milieu—Marshall Canyon. Bear left at the first split at 0.1 mile. You'll return to this point later on the fork to the right.

In a little while, you leave Marshall Canyon's shady creek bed and climb to the perimeter of a fenced nursery (0.7 mile), atop the low ridge that divides Marshall and Live Oak canyons. You contour into the latter, where you hook up with a trail coming up along its bottom. Continue upstream to another trail junction (1.2 miles). Stay right and go another 0.1 mile to yet another junction. Take the equestrian trail on the left, ignoring the dirt road that curves right up the hillside. After gaining a sweaty 400 vertical feet on switchbacks, you reach a dirt road atop a ridge-running fire break (1.7 miles, 2220 feet elevation) offering rare, clear-day vistas extending all the way to downtown L.A.'s skyscrapers.

Turn left, continue on the fire break 0.2 mile, and then veer sharply left on a trail that takes you back down into the shady depths of Live Oak Canyon (2.2 miles). Swing right at the bottom (remaining on the trail) and continue uphill 0.4 mile to a dirt road. Turn left and follow the road 200 yards down to the picnic area (2.8 miles), which sits in a shady draw at the head of Live Oak Canyon.

From the picnic area, keep descending along the dirt road, which at this point follows Live Oak Canyon's mostly sun-exposed northside slope. About 0.3 mile farther, don't miss the pleasant trail that conveniently shortcuts a couple of curves in the road. On the road again you pass above the point where you turned uphill a mile earlier. Farther ahead, at 3.7 miles, you

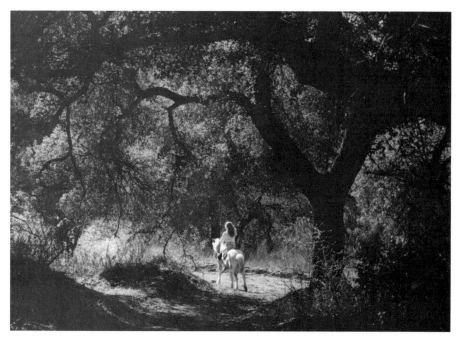

Live Oak Canyon

leave the road and veer left on a path going down a shallow draw. This soon hooks up with the trail through Live Oak Canyon. Retrace your earlier steps for 0.2 mile, then fork left, remaining in Live Oak Canyon. A murmuring stream swishes through here most of the year. At 4.5 miles, the trail abruptly switches back and climbs to an open flat with two large water tanks. Pass to the left of the first, to the right of the second, and pick up the path that descends into Marshall Canyon. You arrive back at the first split you encountered, and just beyond, your starting point.

## trip 7 Cobal Canyon Loop

| | |
|---|---|
| **Distance** | 5.0 miles, Loop |
| **Hiking Time** | 2½ hours |
| **Elevation Gain/Loss** | 900'/900' |
| **Difficulty** | Moderate |
| **Trail Use** | Suitable for mountain biking, dogs allowed, good for kids |
| **Best Times** | November through April |
| **Agency** | CHWP |
| **Optional Map** | USGS 7.5-min *Mt. Baldy* |
| **Notes** | Marked trails/obvious routes, easy terrain |

see map on p. 108

**DIRECTIONS** Exit the 210 Freeway at Baseline Road on the border between the cities of Claremont and Upland. Go west on Baseline for 0.7 mile, then turn right (north) on Mills Avenue. After 1.1 mile the main road (signed Mount Baldy Road) veers sharply right, while the dead-end Mills Avenue continues straight. Follow Mills Avenue to its end, which is where you find the trailhead for Claremont Hills Wilderness Park.

Adjoining the vast spaces of Angeles National Forest, Claremont Hills Wilderness Park spreads over foothills spilling down toward the college town of Claremont. The Cobal Canyon Loop, the one significant hike and popular in the park, is particularly rewarding during the cool-air/cleaner-air months of late fall and winter. That's when the views over the San Gabriel Valley assume cinemascopic proportions. The route is entirely on wide fire roads, so there's plenty of room for leashed dogs and mountain bikes, as well as walkers and runners.

From the trailhead parking area, proceed up the bottom of Cobal Canyon on the Cobal Canyon Trail (aka Cobal Canyon Motorway). You quickly plunge into the deep shade of coast live oaks, the hearty survivors of repeated wildfires, including the 2003 Grand Prix Fire. Large brown mileage signs tick off the half-miles along the route, but they count backward from 5.0 on the counterclockwise loop you are following. This direction is preferred, since you get to go uphill and slower on the more scenic Cobal Canyon piece of the loop.

By 1.0 mile you're rounding a horseshoe curve and climbing out of Cobal Canyon. Looking back you can see a handful of bigcone Douglas-firs clinging to the north-facing slope. They are about as low (1800 feet in elevation) as these evergreen trees can grow in their native habitat.

Continue a steady climb on sunny slopes to an unmarked fire road on the right (1.8 miles), which connects with fire roads in Angeles National Forest. Stay left. After another half mile of climbing you reach a crest; right afterward there's another fire road (the continuation of Cobal Canyon Motorway) branching right (2.5 miles). This leads to the fire roads and trails of Marshall Canyon Regional Park. Stay left again.

Just ahead, off to the left side, is an elaborate shade ramada perched atop a knoll for maximum panoramic impact. The view from there stretches from the relatively nearby summit of Mount San Antonio to distant features such as San Jacinto Peak, the Santa Ana Mountains, and Santa Catalina Island.

The remainder of the loop hike is somewhat anticlimactic. Continue south along the fire road, ignoring yet another wide fire road on the right that leads toward Marshall Canyon Regional Park. Stay with the main, undulating ridge on the wide, south-going fire road called Burbank Trail (aka Burbank Motorway), and stick with that route as it curls down dry, brushy slopes overlooking Burbank Canyon. At 5.0 miles you arrive back in Cobal Canyon very close to the trailhead parking lot.

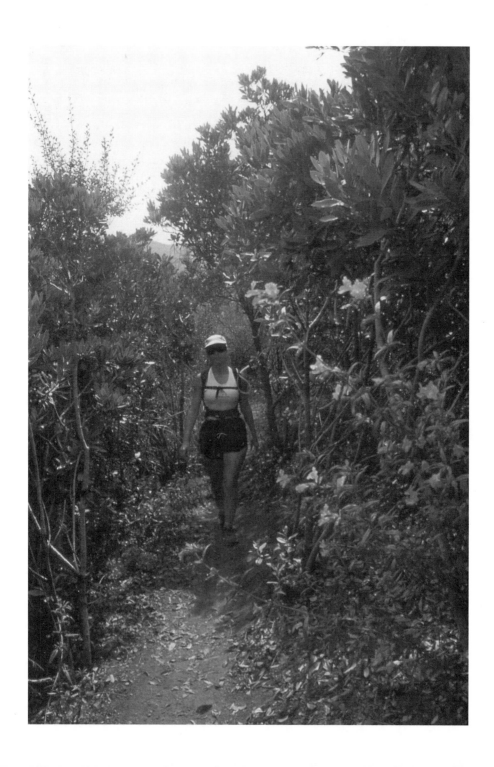

# chapter 12

# Santa Monica Mountains: Pacific Palisades & Topanga

*opanga*—"The place where the mountains meet the sea." That simple and descriptive Gabrielino Indian name aptly applies to the famous canyon and community, and to the big state park sprawling along the canyon's east rim. The ocean is your almost perpetual companion here, if not in sight, at least in the feel of the cool marine air flowing up along the sunny slopes and through the dark, wooded canyons.

Assembled from purchases of public and private lands in the late 1960s and early '70s, Topanga State Park's 9000 acres (which are almost entirely within the Los Angeles city limits) rate as one of the world's largest wildlands adjacent to an urban area. The park also serves as a key anchor in the patchwork quilt of public and private lands known as the Santa Monica Mountains National Recreational Area. (The next four chapters in this book cover the somewhat more remote middle and western sections of the SMMNRA.)

Perhaps nowhere else in Southern California is the attack on the integrity of large open spaces so graphically illustrated as right here. The park's ragged boundary necessarily excluded lands earmarked for development in two of the coastal canyons—Santa Ynez and Pulga. Over the past two or three decades, massive grading and construction

in and along the walls of these canyons marred the otherwise open vistas. (On the flip side, of course, you need only look east to the Hollywood Hills to imagine how these mountains would probably look decades hence if they lacked any protection at all.)

Topanga State Park's only area developed specifically for drive-in visitors centers around the Trippet Ranch, off Topanga Canyon Boulevard on Entrada Road. The ranch (open during daylight hours) was originally one of the many second-home and resort properties developed in the Topanga Canyon area early in the century. There you'll find a tiny administrative office, a pond, oak-shaded picnic tables, a 1-mile self-guiding nature trail, and trailheads for several of the wide-ranging routes described in this chapter. The trail system is also accessible from several other points on or near the periphery of the park.

A number of additional hikes outside the state park itself are included here. This chapter's sketch map includes fire roads and established trails, but does not show dozens of miles of firebreaks and informal paths threading some of the canyons and going up or along most of the ridges. Some of these seldom-trod pathways have become overgrown; others pass through private lands for which there is no public access.

Hiking through chaparral, Rivas Canyon

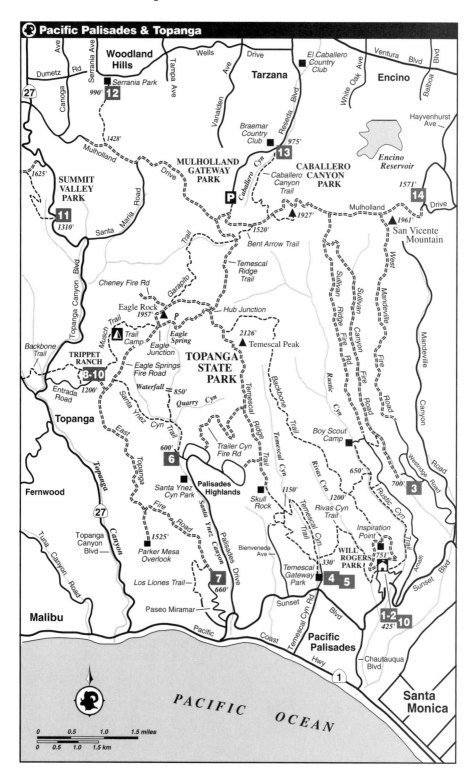

## Pacific Palisades & Topanga

## trip 1 Will Rogers Park

| | |
|---|---|
| **Distance** | 2.0 miles, Loop |
| **Hiking Time** | 1 hour |
| **Elevation Gain/Loss** | 350'/350' |
| **Difficulty** | Easy |
| **Trail Use** | Suitable for mountain biking, dogs allowed, good for kids |
| **Best Times** | All year |
| **Agency** | WRSHP |
| **Optional Map** | USGS 7.5-min *Topanga* |
| **Notes** | Marked trails/obvious routes, easy terrain |

see map on p. 122

**DIRECTIONS** The entrance to Will Rogers State Historic Park is located on the north side of Sunset Boulevard about 4 miles west of Interstate 405 and midway between Chautauqua Boulevard and Amalfi Drive in Pacific Palisades. The entrance road curls up a hillside to the park itself, which features abundant parking space (fee charged). The park is open daily, except certain holidays, from 8 a.m. to 5 p.m.

Drive up a short mile from the speedway known as Sunset Boulevard toward Will Rogers State Historic Park, and you'll instantly leave the rat race behind. Especially on weekdays or early on weekend mornings, this quiet spot is perfect for getting some exercise and taking advantage of multimillion-dollar views of Santa Monica, West L.A., and downtown.

Newspaperman, radio commentator, movie star and pop-philosopher Will Rogers purchased this 182-acre property in 1922 and lived with his family here from 1928 until his death in 1935. Historic only by Southern California standards, his 31-room mansion is nevertheless interesting to tour.

Our main goal, however, is to reach Inspiration Point, a flat-topped bump on a ridge overlooking the entire spread. Follow the main, wide, riding and hiking trail that makes a 2-mile loop, starting at the north end of the big lawn adjoining the Rogers home. Or use any of several shorter, more direct paths. You may want to obtain a copy of the detailed hikers' map, available at the gift shop in a wing of the home. Printed on the map is one of Will's memorable aphorisms, ". . . if your time is worth anything, travel by air. If not, you might just as well walk."

Relaxing on the benches at the top on a clear day, you can admire true-as-advertised, inspiring vistas stretching east to the front range of the San Gabriel Mountains and southeast to the Santa Ana Mountains. South past the swelling Palos Verdes peninsula you can sometimes spot Santa Catalina Island, rising in ethereal majesty from the shining surface of the sea.

**SANTA MONICA MOUNTAINS**

L.A.'s amazing skyline seen from Inspiration Point

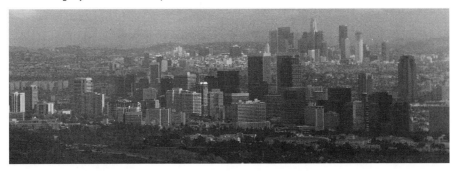

# trip 2 Rustic Canyon

see map on p. 122

|  |  |
|---|---|
| **Distance** | 4.6 miles, Loop |
| **Hiking Time** | 3 hours |
| **Elevation Gain/Loss** | 900'/900' |
| **Difficulty** | Moderately strenuous |
| **Best Times** | October through June |
| **Agency** | TSP |
| **Optional Map** | USGS 7.5-min *Topanga* |
| **Notes** | Marked trails/obvious routes, moderate terrain |

**DIRECTIONS** Drive to the entrance to Will Rogers State Historic Park, which is located on the north side of Sunset Boulevard, about 4 miles west of Interstate 405 and midway between Chautauqua Boulevard and Amalfi Drive in Pacific Palisades. Continue uphill on the entrance road, which leads to the park itself. A fee is charged for parking.

Rustic Canyon, now almost fully reverted to wilderness condition after Nature's one-two punches of fire and flood, was quite lively in the past. Pop-philosopher Will Rogers and his associates used it as a retreat back in the 1930s, and it even held the makings of a hideout for Nazi sympathizers later in the 20th Century.

Your exploration by foot in Rustic Canyon begins and ends at the historic Will Rogers country home. Take the eucalyptus-lined east branch of the Inspiration Point loop trail 0.8 mile to a signed junction with the Backbone Trail (aka Rogers Trail), just north of Inspiration Point.

As soon as you start climbing the well-defined ridge, you'll realize how appropriate the name "Backbone" is. The trail skips up, over, or around cobbled sandstone "vertebrae" along a stretch known variously as Chicken Ridge and Gobbler's Knob. It is also the easternmost small piece of the nearly completed Backbone Trail that will soon stretch the length of the Santa Monica Mountains.

At 1.5 miles you cross a bridge overlooking a knife-edge saddle between Rivas Canyon on the west and Rustic Canyon on the east. Just ahead at another saddle (1.8 miles) you turn right on a trail that wastes no time descending into Rustic Canyon.

On the descent you make your way through a mini-forest of chaparral, including green-bark ceanothus, mountain mahogany, chamise, manzanita, toyon, sumac, and buckwheat. After another 0.7 mile you reach a secluded glade in the bottom of Rustic Canyon, where you might spook a deer if no one else is around to have done it already.

Upstream, to the left, lies the Boy Scouts' Camp Josepho, named after Will Rogers' friend Anatol Josepho, inventor of the pay telephone. Our route turns south (down-canyon) past the site of one of Rogers' cabins and an assortment of other structures, burned or abandoned. Plenty of ornamental trees and shrubs mix with the native live oak and sycamores along the trickling stream.

On the left a way down stands the concrete shell of a power-generator building. This, along with a diesel-fuel bunker and sheet-metal buildings, was part of the pre-World-II "Murphy Ranch," which was protected by a high fence and patrolled by armed guards. Short-wave broadcasts beamed to Germany from the site finally convinced authorities of its true nature and led to the arrest of a German spy. The spy, it seems, had duped a wealthy couple and convinced them to finance construction of this stronghold, which was to serve as a haven for true believers in the Third Reich. After the war, this section of the canyon became an artists' colony, until ravaged by fire and flood. Today it is owned by the City of Los Angeles.

Past an old flood-control dam (3.6 miles) the canyon narrows and the trail becomes merely a muddy track through a tight constriction in the canyon. Walls of conglomerate rock soar eerily on both sides. Watch out for poison oak and slippery rocks. At 4.1 miles, the canyon abruptly widens. On the right a wide trail curves uphill toward the polo field across from the Will Rogers home, your starting point.

Lower Rustic Canyon

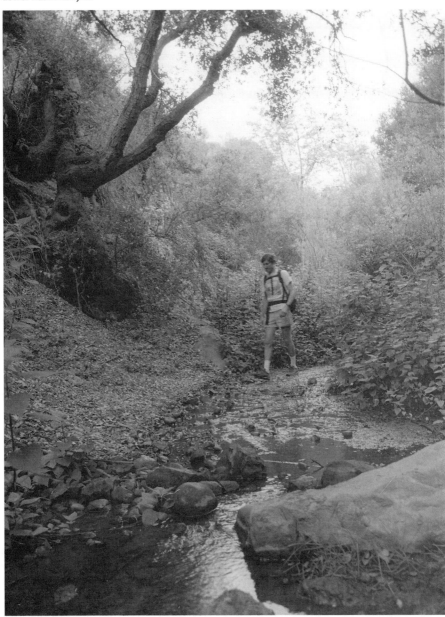

# trip 3  Sullivan Canyon

| | |
|---|---|
| **Distance** | 10.0 miles, Loop |
| **Hiking Time** | 4½ hours |
| **Elevation Gain/Loss** | 1600'/1600' |
| **Difficulty** | Moderately strenuous |
| **Trail Use** | Suitable for mountain biking, dogs allowed |
| **Best Times** | October through May |
| **Agency** | SMMC |
| **Optional Maps** | USGS 7.5-min *Topanga, Canoga Park* |
| **Notes** | Marked trails/obvious routes, easy terrain |

see
map on
p. 122

**DIRECTIONS** Drive 2.3 miles west on Sunset Boulevard from Interstate 405, and turn right (north) onto Mandeville Canyon Road in Brentwood. Make a left on the first intersecting street, Westridge Road, and go 1.2 miles to Bayliss Road. Turn left on Bayliss and continue 0.3 mile to Queensferry Road, a dead-end street on the left. Find any convenient parking space on Bayliss or Queensferry.

In serene Sullivan Canyon you can hike for at least an hour without catching sight of any manmade improvements, save for a gravelly service road and some markers indicating a buried pipeline. For a long time it appeared as though Sullivan and neighboring upper Rustic Canyon would become a huge dump site for solid waste. But that threat seems to have passed now, and much of the land here may eventually come into state ownership.

This comprehensive tour goes up along Sullivan Canyon's sycamore-lined bottom and touches upon Mulholland Drive, where on clear days a hiker can view the ocean and the San Fernando Valley from a single stance. It concludes with an easy descent on the long, sinuous ridge just east of the canyon. The route, and variations of it, is ideally suited for long-distance runners, mountain bikers, and horse riders, as well as walkers.

The route lies almost entirely on a geologic formation called Santa Monica Slate, a gray, bluish-gray or black rock. These 150 million-year-old rocks of marine origin, the oldest found in the Santa Monica Mountains, are exposed in a broad area stretching almost continuously from Coldwater Canyon and Franklin Canyon behind Beverly Hills into the east half of Topanga State Park.

Since the road in Sullivan Canyon is at best only semi-shaded, you may want to choose a time that takes advantage of early-morning or late-afternoon shadows. You could, for example, walk up the canyon late in the day, catch the setting sun from Mulholland, and watch the city lights twinkle on as you walk down the east ridge.

Start off by stepping around a gate at the end of Queensferry Road and walk down to the service road going up along the bottom of Sullivan Canyon. Oaks, willows, and sycamores cluster along the usually dry creek bed. At 0.7 mile a narrow path comes down from the left, giving access to Sullivan Canyon's west-ridge fire road, an alternate route used by some people.

The almost imperceptible climb on the canyon-bottom road takes you past thinning sycamores to a fork in the canyon (3.4 miles), where the main canyon branch heads northeast. You follow the road up a smaller, steeper ravine going northwest. Climbing in earnest, you swing around some sharp turns and then hook up with the west-ridge fire road (4.3 miles). Continue north to unpaved Mulholland Drive, then follow Mulholland east along the Santa Monica Mountains divide toward San Vicente Mountain (5.5 miles). When you reach that high point, you'll discover the interpretive site known as San Vicente Mountain Park, which centers on a Cold-War-era Nike missile base. The view from here, when not compromised by smog or haze, is undeniably spectacular. Look north to glimpse the Tehachapi Mountains, 70 miles distant, through the gap between the Santa Susana and San Gabriel mountains.

From San Vicente Mountain Park, head south along the West Mandeville Fire Road. It curves around several rounded bumps on the ridge between Mandeville and Sullivan canyons, climbing on occasion, but mostly descending. You'll have outstanding views of the L.A. Basin to the east and south, marred only by some foreground powerlines.

At 9.0 miles you hook up with Westridge Road in a suburban housing development. Walk 0.5 mile down Westridge, turn right on Bayliss, and continue another 0.5 mile down to Queensferry.

## trip 4 Temescal Canyon

see map on p. 122

|  |  |
|---|---|
| **Distance** | 2.8 miles |
| **Hiking Time** | 1½ hours |
| **Elevation Gain/Loss** | 850'/850' |
| **Difficulty** | Moderate |
| **Trail Use** | Good for kids |
| **Best Times** | All year |
| **Agency** | TSP |
| **Optional Map** | USGS 7.5-min *Topanga* |
| **Notes** | Marked trails/obvious routes, easy terrain |

**DIRECTIONS** The trail begins at Temescal Gateway Park, just north of the intersection of Sunset Boulevard and Temescal Canyon Road in Pacific Palisades. Park for a fee inside the park, sunrise to sunset, or find a curbside space in the commercial district of Pacific Palisades across Sunset Boulevard.

A favorite of west-side L.A. hikers, this short loop includes both wonderful views from high places and a shady passage through riparian and oak woodland.

Using directional signs on the Temescal Gateway Park property, head north toward several buildings that comprise the former Presbyterian conference grounds. On the left side find and follow the Temescal Ridge Trail, which vigorously ascends the scrubby canyon wall to the west. After several twists and turns, the trail gains a moderately ascending crest and sticks to it. Pause often so you can turn around and look at the ever-widening view of the coastline curving from Santa Monica Bay to Malibu. Ahead, two short trails (the Leacock and Bienveneda trails) strike off to the left toward a trailhead at the end of Bienveneda Avenue. Ignore those paths and continue a junction (1.3 miles from the start) with the old Temescal Fire Road—signed TEMESCAL RIDGE

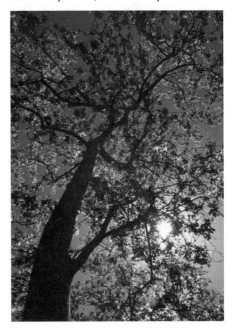
California sycamore, Temescal Canyon

SANTA MONICA MOUNTAINS

TRAIL to the north and TEMESCAL CANYON TRAIL to the south. (At this point you have the option of making a side trip north 0.5 mile to a wind-carved, sandstone outcrop known as Skull Rock.)

Staying on the loop route, turn right and head downhill on the Temescal Canyon Trail. When you hit the shady canyon bottom (1.7 miles), you'll cross over Temescal Canyon's creek and pick up a smoother section of the old fire road on the far side. Above and below this crossing are small, trickling waterfalls and shallow, limpid pools. Poke around the creek a bit for a look at its typical denizens—water striders and newts.

The final stretch follows the canyon bottom, then contours along a slope to the right of the conference buildings. Lots of live oak, sycamore, willow, and bay trees—their woodsy scents commingling on the ocean breeze—highlight your return.

## trip 5  Rivas Canyon

| | |
|---|---|
| **Distance** | 2.0 miles, Point-to-point |
| **Hiking Time** | 1½ hours |
| **Elevation Gain/Loss** | 600'/600' |
| **Difficulty** | Moderate |
| **Best Times** | October through June |
| **Agency** | SMMC |
| **Optional Map** | USGS 7.5-min *Topanga* |
| **Notes** | Navigation required, moderate terrain |

see map on p. 122

**DIRECTIONS** *West End:* The trail begins at Temescal Gateway Park, just north of the intersection of Sunset Boulevard and Temescal Canyon Road in Pacific Palisades. Park for a fee inside the park, sunrise to sunset, or find a curbside space in the commercial district of Pacific Palisades across Sunset Boulevard. *East End:* Drive to the entrance to Will Rogers State Historic Park, which is located on the north side of Sunset Boulevard, midway between Chautauqua Boulevard and Amalfi Drive in Pacific Palisades. Continue uphill on the entrance road, which leads to the park itself. A fee is charged for parking.

Temescal Canyon and Will Rogers State Historic Park in Pacific Palisades are just two of the many units of parkland and open space that make up the sprawling Santa Monica Mountains National Recreation Area. The Rivas Canyon Trail, of relatively recent origin, now connects these two park units. This hand-tooled route at times resembles a rabbit run in the brush, so you can be assured of close encounters with the native vegetation. This is exciting and feels like adventurous hiking, but be aware that the encounters may involve poison oak. Be certain you can identify the plant and avoid any physical contact with it.

From any parking lot in Temescal Gateway Park, head north on pavement toward some institutional buildings that make

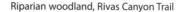
Riparian woodland, Rivas Canyon Trail

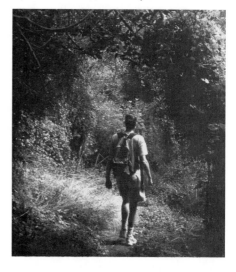

up the former Presbyterian conference grounds. On the right, look for a small sign indicating the Rivas Canyon Trail, and start following the obscure path indicated.

You make your way circuitously up the east wall of Temescal Canyon, gaining a ridgeline after about 0.5 mile. You then go up along the ridgeline itself, pass over a crest, and descend sharply and crookedly to the shady bottom of Rivas Canyon. A delightfully gradual downhill promenade ensues, taking you through riparian and oak woodland vegetation. Several private residences lie within the canyon; take care to stay in the canyon bottom and not take a wrong turn into anyone's back yard.

By about 1.8 mile into the hike, you're approaching the dead end of a residential street. Once you hit pavement, find and follow the path to the left that enters the grounds of Will Rogers State Historic Park. Proceed east into the main park area, which includes parking spaces, a polo field, and the historic ranch home of famed radio personality and pop-philosopher Will Rogers.

If you have arranged for someone to fetch you there, your hike is over. Otherwise, you have two options. You can return the way you came, or you can follow busy Sunset Boulevard back to Temescal Gateway Park—a possibly faster but not inspiring walk.

## trip 6  Santa Ynez Waterfall

see map on p. 122

| | |
|---|---|
| **Distance** | 2.4 miles round trip, Out-and-back |
| **Hiking Time** | 1½ hours (round trip) |
| **Elevation Gain/Loss** | 250'/250' |
| **Difficulty** | Moderate |
| **Trail Use** | Good for kids |
| **Best Times** | All year |
| **Agency** | TSP |
| **Optional Map** | USGS 7.5-min *Topanga* |
| **Notes** | Marked trails/obvious routes, moderate terrain |

**DIRECTIONS** From Pacific Coast Highway in Pacific Palisades, take Sunset Boulevard north 0.5 mile to Palisades Drive. Follow Palisades north for 2.4 miles into the Palisades Highlands housing development and to the street called Vereda de la Montura. Turn left and within a long block find the Santa Ynez Canyon Trailhead on the right—a narrow gate unlocked during daylight hours. There's abundant free curbside parking in the surrounding neighborhood.

Twisted live oaks, sycamores, and pungent bay laurel trees highlight the brief trek up the L.A. coast's most easily accessible waterfall-bearing canyon. The goal is an 18-foot cascade tucked into an upper branch of Santa Ynez Canyon. The flow of water in these falls is usually significant from winter through early summer. Both the trail and the falls, however, may be rendered inaccessible if too much rain arrives at one time.

After a short descent from the trailhead on Vereda de la Montura, follow the trail going up along Santa Ynez Canyon. Before long, you're dodging stray branches of willow and bay trees, stepping across the soggy creek, and forgetting about the civilized world behind you. The California bay (bay laurel) trees here are commonly found in shady, moist canyons throughout coastal California. Crush one of the dark, elongated leaves and sniff it to get a whiff of the minty/pungent scent.

After 0.5 mile, the wide mouth of Quarry Canyon, site of an old limestone quarry, opens to the right. Stay left and go another 100 yards to a second canyon on the right.

The main trail going straight leads to the Trippet Ranch headquarters of Topanga State Park. Take the lesser-traveled trail right (north) up the second canyon, which is actually the major fork of Santa Ynez Canyon.

After some foot-wetting creek crossings and a slippery scramble over some conglomerate boulders, you arrive at a grotto below the falls. With their orientation subject to deep shadow, the falls are difficult to photograph properly—unless the day is cloudy-bright, in which case the lighting is fine. The cool, damp air here is always refreshing, whether or not the falls are whispering or hissing loudly.

On your return, utilizing the same way back, near the two canyon mouths mentioned earlier, look for the stone chimney of a burnt-out cabin and a sandstone boulder pocked by Indian *morteros* (mortar holes used centuries ago for the grinding of acorns and other foodstuffs).

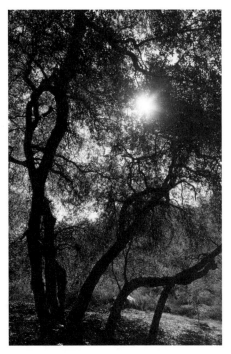

Live oaks, Santa Ynez Canyon

## trip 7  Topanga Overlook

see map on p. 122

| | |
|---|---|
| **Distance** | 5.0 miles round trip, Out-and-back |
| **Hiking Time** | 2½ hours (round trip) |
| **Elevation Gain/Loss** | 1200'/1200' |
| **Difficulty** | Moderate |
| **Trail Use** | Suitable for mountain biking |
| **Best Times** | All year |
| **Agency** | TSP |
| **Optional Map** | USGS 7.5-min *Topanga* |
| **Notes** | Marked trails/obvious routes, easy terrain |

**DIRECTIONS** From Pacific Coast Highway in Pacific Palisades, take Sunset Boulevard north 0.3 mile to the street called Paseo Miramar, on the left. Drive up narrow Paseo Miramar to its end, where limited parking is available just short of a vehicle gate.

From the perch known as Topanga Overlook, Parker Mesa Overlook, or simply the "Overlook," you get a bird's-eye view of surfers off Topanga Beach, the crescent shoreline of Santa Monica Bay, L.A.'s westside cityscape—and much, much more if the air is really transparent. You can reach the overlook by walking south along Topanga Canyon's east ridge from Trippet Ranch, but we'll describe a shorter and more interesting route from a street called Paseo Miramar, west of Pacific Palisades.

This trip is especially rewarding when done early on certain fall or winter mornings, when tendrils of fog fill the canyons, leaving the mountains to rise above a cottony sea. It's also excellent as a sunset or night hike. For a special treat, do it on any clear, full-moon evening between May and August. In the fading twilight you'll watch the moon's pumpkin-like disk silently materialize in the east or southeast, hovering over a million glittering lights.

From the end of Paseo Miramar, walk along the dirt fire road that continues up along a ridge, passing after 0.2 mile a foot trail coming up from Los Liones Drive.

Farther ahead you briefly traverse a cool, north-facing slope overlooking Santa Ynez Canyon and neighboring ridges. You arrive at a road junction (2.0 miles) overlooking Topanga Canyon to the west. Turn south and walk out along the bald ridge to Topanga Overlook. Down below are Parker and Castellammare mesas, parts of a striking marine-terrace structure that continues east into Pacific Palisades. When it's time to go back, return the way you came.

## trip 8  Eagle Rock Loop

see map on p. 122

|  |  |
|---|---|
| **Distance** | 6.7 miles |
| **Hiking Time** | 3½ hours |
| **Elevation Gain/Loss** | 1200'/1200' |
| **Difficulty** | Moderately strenuous |
| **Trail Use** | Suitable for backpacking, good for kids |
| **Best Times** | October through June |
| **Agency** | TSP |
| **Optional Map** | USGS 7.5-min *Topanga* |
| **Notes** | Marked trails/obvious routes, easy terrain |

**SANTA MONICA MOUNTAINS**

**DIRECTIONS** Take Topanga Canyon Boulevard (Highway 27) south from the San Fernando Valley, or north from Pacific Coast Highway. About midway along the highway's twisty 12-mile course from valley to sea, turn east on Entrada Road (signs for Topanga State Park on the highway alert you to this turnoff). Follow winding Entrada Road, carefully observing directional signs for the park, for 1 mile to Trippet Ranch, which is the headquarters for Topanga State Park. Pay the day-use fee at the entrance station (open 8 a.m.), and park in the large lot beyond.

Eagle Rock, the most impressive landmark in all of Topanga State Park, affords hikers an airy perch overlooking the upper watershed of Santa Ynez Canyon and the ocean beyond. Make it your destination for lunch during a lazy day's hike, but do it on a cooler day—there's little shade on the route. This is a figure-eight route, so if you have smaller kids along, you can cut the distance to about 4 miles by avoiding the far loop.

From the large parking lot at Trippet Ranch, walk north on a paved drive about 100 yards to where the signed Musch Trail slants to the right across a grassy hillside. You soon plunge into the shade of oak

and bay trees. Enjoy the shade—there's not much more ahead. After contouring around a couple of north-flowing ravines, the trail rises to meet a trail campground at the former Musch Ranch (1.0 mile). This camp, and others along the Backbone Trail, serves equestrians and through-hikers. With an advance reservation, you could use it as part of this hike.

Beyond the campground, the trail soon starts climbing through sun-blasted chaparral. After a crooked ascent you reach a ridgetop fire road at Eagle Junction (2.5 miles), from which Eagle Rock can be seen looming over the headwaters of Santa Ynez Canyon. This layered sandstone outcrop, pitted with small caves, is an outstanding example of the 15-million-year-old Topanga Canyon Formation. Turn left and follow the fire road up to the gentler north side of Eagle Rock. Walk to the top for the best view.

Back on the fire road, continue east up along a ridgeline and then down to a four-way junction of fire roads at 3.9 miles, called "Hub Junction" because of its central location in the park. On a side trip south from here you could visit Cathedral Rock and Temescal Peak, but our way goes sharply right on the Backbone Trail (a fire road) leading west under Eagle Rock and back to Eagle Junction. Before you reach the junction, there's a side path on the right to Eagle Spring, where water trickles out of the sandstone bedrock beneath oaks and sycamores.

When you reach Eagle Junction again (5.3 miles), turn left and return to Trippet Ranch the fast and direct way: Go 1.2 miles down the Eagle Springs Fire Road to the south, and then 0.2 mile northwest on the wide trail leading down to the picnic area and parking lot at Trippet Ranch.

## trip 9  Garapito Loop

see map on p. 122

| | |
|---|---|
| **Distance** | 9.6 miles, Loop |
| **Hiking Time** | 5 hours |
| **Elevation Gain/Loss** | 1600'/1600' |
| **Difficulty** | Moderately strenuous |
| **Best Times** | November through May |
| **Agency** | TSP |
| **Optional Map** | USGS 7.5-min *Topanga* |
| **Notes** | Marked trails/obvious routes, easy terrain |

**DIRECTIONS** Take Topanga Canyon Boulevard (Highway 27) south from the San Fernando Valley, or north from Pacific Coast Highway. About midway along the highway's twisty 12-mile course from valley to sea, turn east on Entrada Road (signs for Topanga State Park on the highway alert you to this turnoff). Follow winding Entrada Road, carefully observing directional signs for the park, for 1 mile to Trippet Ranch, which is the headquarters for Topanga State Park. Pay the day-use fee at the entrance station (open 8 a.m.), and park in the large lot beyond.

In springtime, the "elfin forest" of chaparral in the Santa Monica Mountains takes on dozen shades of green and bursts forth with nectar-bearing blossoms that are often more attractive to the sense of smell than to the sense of sight. The loop described here, which includes the chaparral-draped upper reaches of Garapito Creek (a tributary of Topanga Canyon) will expose you to plenty of these heavenly scents.

From the large parking lot at Trippet Ranch, walk north on a paved drive about 100 yards to where the signed Musch Trail slants to the right across a grassy hillside.

You soon plunge into the shade of oak and bay trees. Enjoy the shade—there's not much more ahead. After contouring around a couple of north-flowing ravines, the trail rises to meet a trail campground at the former Musch Ranch (1.0 mile). This camp, along with others along the Backbone Trail, serves equestrians and through-hikers.

Beyond the campground, the trail soon starts climbing through sunny chaparral. After a crooked ascent you reach a ridgetop fire road at Eagle Junction (2.5 miles), from which Eagle Rock can be seen looming over the headwaters of Santa Ynez Canyon. This layered sandstone outcrop, pitted with small caves, is an outstanding example of the 15-million-year-old Topanga Canyon Formation. Turn left and follow the fire road up to the gentler north side of Eagle Rock. If you want to make a side trip for the view from the top, go ahead and do so.

Back on the fire road, you quickly pass the dead-end Cheney Fire Road on the left. Just beyond, on the left again, find and follow the narrow Garapito Trail as it darts through a continuous carpet of chaparral—mostly mountain mahogany and ceanothus. The blossoms of the ceanothus exude a wild-honey scent in spring, attractive to bees as well as humans. You contour along a west-facing slope, then descend along a sharply falling ridgeline, crisscrossing on many tight switchbacks. At the bottom, the trail swings around to cross a south fork of

Garapito Creek, and then contours a short distance over to an east fork. A steady climb up along this east fork takes you to a wide dirt road, the Temescal Ridge Trail (5.5 miles into the hike).

Make a right turn on the Temescal Ridge Trail and commence a crooked, gradually rising, viewful traverse on top of or somewhat below the Temescal ridgeline itself. At 6.9 miles, you reach the four-way "hub junction" of fire roads, where the view opens broadly toward the ocean.

Choose the middle road at Hub Junction—the route to Eagle Spring—which is a segment of the Backbone Trail. You pass under Eagle Rock and arrive back at Eagle Junction (8.2 miles). Turn left there and return to Trippet Ranch by way of 1.2 miles of downhill hiking on Eagle Springs Fire Road, and another 0.2 mile on the wide trail leading down to the picnic area and parking lot at Trippet Ranch.

Eagle Rock, landmark of Topanga State Park

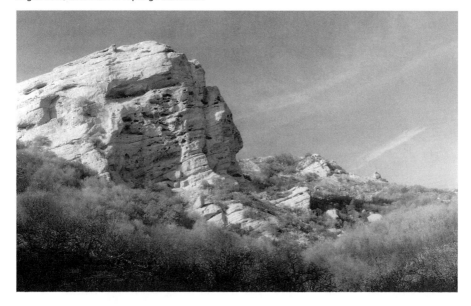

# trip 10 East Backbone Trail

see
map on
p. 122

| | |
|---|---|
| **Distance** | 9.2 miles, Point-to-point |
| **Hiking Time** | 4½ hours |
| **Elevation Gain/Loss** | 1700'/2500' |
| **Difficulty** | Moderately strenuous |
| **Best Times** | October through May |
| **Agency** | TSP |
| **Optional Map** | USGS 7.5-min *Topanga* |
| **Notes** | Marked trails/obvious routes, easy terrain |

**DIRECTIONS** *North End:* Take Topanga Canyon Boulevard (Highway 27) south from the San Fernando Valley, or north from Pacific Coast Highway. About midway along the highway's twisty 12-mile course from valley to sea, turn east on Entrada Road (signs for Topanga State Park on the highway alert you to this turnoff). Follow winding Entrada Road, carefully observing directional signs for the park, for 1 mile to Trippet Ranch, which is the headquarters for Topanga State Park. Pay the day-use fee at the entrance station (open 8 a.m.), and park in the large lot beyond. *South End:* Drive to the entrance to Will Rogers State Historic Park, which is located on the north side of Sunset Boulevard, midway between Chautauqua Boulevard and Amalfi Drive in Pacific Palisades. Continue uphill on the entrance road, which leads to the park itself. A fee is charged for parking.

On a cool, clear day, the easternmost section of the Backbone Trail—Trippet Ranch to Will Rogers State Historic Park—yields dazzling and ever-changing perspectives of the meeting of mountains and sea. A lesser benefit of this one-way trip is that you get to walk downhill most of the time. Arrange a car shuttle, or better yet, have someone drop you off at Trippet Ranch (opens at 8 a.m.) and later pick you up in front of the Rogers home or at some other agreed-upon spot in Will Rogers Park (closes at 5 p.m.).

From the picnic area at Trippet Ranch, head southeast on the fire road going up the hill to the Santa Ynez Fire Road. Turn

Polo Grounds at Will Rogers State Historic Park

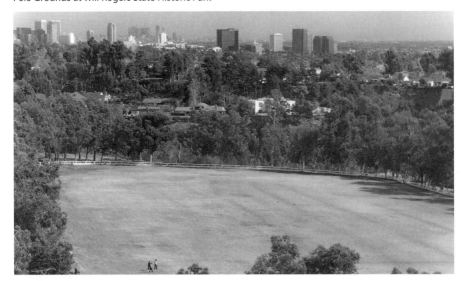

left at the top and climb to Eagle Junction (1.4 miles). Go right there, pass under Eagle Rock, climb some more, and arrive at Hub Junction (2.7 miles). Turn right on the Temescal Ridge Trail and walk 0.5 mile south, passing a cavernous sandstone outcrop on the left called Cathedral Rock, to another junction. The Backbone Trail goes left here on an old fire road. Nearby Temescal Peak, whose summit can be reached by way of a short, steep fire break on its west side, is worth climbing if the visibility is good. This somewhat undistinguished looking bump on the Temescal Ridge holds the distinction of being the highest peak in the Santa Monicas east of Topanga Canyon.

The Backbone Trail (originally the Rogers Trail from here on down to Will Rogers Park) goes east for about 1 mile, then veers south to loosely follow an undulating ridgeline that always lies west and well above Rustic Canyon and its tributaries. For a couple of miles the upper reaches of Temescal Canyon lie to the west, but then you bear left (southeast) to join the ridge between Rivas and Rustic canyons. On a flat overlooking the head of Rivas Canyon at 6.5 miles, there's a live oak tree that provides welcome shade.

Past the oak, 2 more miles of foot trail lead down to a junction just above Inspiration Point in Will Rogers Park. Turn right on the wide trail. After about 0.3 mile, make a left on the shortcut path signed BACKBONE TRAIL. That will take you straight down to the big lawn above Will Rogers' home.

**trip 11  Summit Valley**

| | |
|---|---|
| **Distance** | 2.2 miles round trip, Out-and-back |
| **Hiking Time** | 1 hour (round trip) |
| **Elevation Gain/Loss** | 500'/500' |
| **Difficulty** | Moderate |
| **Trail Use** | Dogs allowed, good for kids |
| **Best Times** | November through June |
| **Agency** | SMMC |
| **Optional Map** | USGS 7.5-min *Canoga Park* |
| **Notes** | Marked trails/obvious routes, easy terrain |

see map on p. 122

**DIRECTIONS** From Topanga Canyon Boulevard's intersection with Mulholland Drive, drive south 2.6 miles to a sweeping, 180-degree curve. On the inside of this curve (west side of Topanga Canyon Boulevard) is a dirt parking area for Summit Valley.

**S**ummit Valley, aka Edmund D. Edelman Park (named in honor of a county supervisor) spreads across both sides of Topanga Canyon Boulevard south of Woodland Hills, and features one easily accessible trail on the west side. Come and see Summit Valley at its best when it's spring green and burgeoning with wildflowers—most likely in April.

From the parking area, head west down a ravine for 0.2 mile to a south-flowing drainage (an upper tributary of Topanga Canyon) adorned with a number of giant coast live oaks and many stream-hugging willows. Eucalyptus and California walnut trees dot the slopes higher up in this bowl-like valley.

You cross a little stream at the bottom, turn north, and climb around a couple of switchbacks so as to gain the top of a linear ridge. Following this ridge nearly a half mile farther takes you to the boundary of the Summit Valley property at the edge of a wide fire road known as the Summit Motorway. Enjoy the commanding view from this spot, then return the way you came.

SANTA MONICA MOUNTAINS

# trip 12 Woodland Ridge

see map on p. 122

| | |
|---|---|
| **Distance** | 2.2 miles round trip, Out-and-back |
| **Hiking Time** | 1 hour (round trip) |
| **Elevation Gain/Loss** | 500'/500' |
| **Difficulty** | Moderate |
| **Trail Use** | Dogs allowed |
| **Best Times** | All year |
| **Agency** | SMMC |
| **Optional Map** | USGS 7.5-min *Canoga Park* |
| **Notes** | Marked trails/obvious routes, easy terrain |

**DIRECTIONS** Turn south at the De Soto Avenue exit from the Ventura Freeway (U.S. 101) in Woodland Hills, and continue 1 mile south on Serrania Avenue to where Serrania Avenue becomes Wells Drive. There you'll find Serrania Park and the trailhead.

**A**t sunset the weird chorus of sharp-pitched shrieks and howls started up, with echoes that reverberated off the walls of the houses below. The coyotes were defiantly laying claim (so it seemed when I was there) to one of the dwindling number of open spaces remaining on San Fernando Valley's south rim.

That little patch of public land, known variously as Woodland Ridge and Serrania Ridge, features a ridge-running trail connecting Serrania Park with Mulholland Highway.

The trail climbs along the park's east boundary, tops a couple of rises offering nice views across the valley, and finally arrives at Mulholland Drive a little below the Santa Monica Mountains crest. To the right as you climb are views of the Woodland Hills Country Club golf course and hillside housing developments characteristic of the 1950s and '60s. On the left is a more recent version of suburbia—a small canyon jam-packed with hulking pseudo-mansions, ridiculously out of proportion to the postage-stamp-sized lots on which they sit. Behind that development, the clay hills have been elaborately graded and stabilized to protect against mudslides. The contrast between the older and the newer illustrates how valuable even marginally buildable land has become in this well-to-do corner of the valley.

## trip 13  Caballero Canyon

| | |
|---|---|
| **Distance** | 4.2 miles round trip, Out-and-back |
| **Hiking Time** | 2 hours (round trip) |
| **Elevation Gain/Loss** | 1000'/1000' |
| **Difficulty** | Moderate |
| **Trail Use** | Suitable for mountain biking |
| **Best Times** | October through June |
| **Agency** | TSP |
| **Optional Map** | USGS 7.5-min *Canoga Park* |
| **Notes** | Marked trails/obvious routes, easy terrain |

see map on p. 122

**DIRECTIONS**  Exit the Ventura Freeway (U.S. 101) at Reseda Boulevard in Tarzana, and drive south on Reseda to the trailhead on the left, opposite the Braemar Country Club clubhouse.

Caballero Canyon's convenient trailhead allows San Fernando Valley hikers to gain easy access to the trails of Topanga State Park without having to drive either the curvy Topanga Canyon Boulevard or the notoriously rutty dirt section of Mulholland Drive. Mountain bikers may travel the Caballero Canyon route as well, but they are not allowed on the Bent Arrow Trail at the top.

From the trailhead, walk up sycamore-dotted Caballero Canyon on an old fire road. After 1.5 miles and about 600 feet of elevation gain, you arrive at a saddle traversed by unpaved Mulholland Drive. The view is good there—but it's much better if you climb a little farther. To the east you'll notice a very steep fire break going up a ridge. Go up this a short distance, then contour to the right to pick up a segment of the Bent Arrow Trail. This narrow path takes you on a winding route up a south-facing slope, crosses a wide fire break, and finally tops out on a rounded, nearly flat ridge. There's a 1927-foot knoll immediately to the east, and a slightly higher point overlooking Mulholland Drive 0.4 mile east. Late in the day you can watch evening shadows elongate across the San Fernando Valley, and clouds form along the coast as the chill of evening descends upon the land.

SANTA MONICA MOUNTAINS

Caballero Canyon at twilight

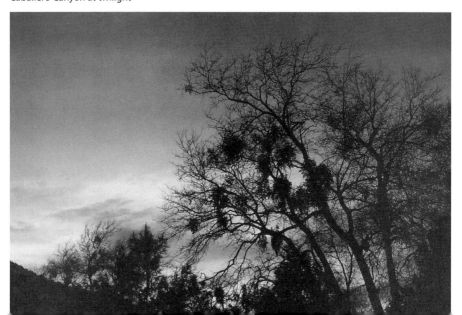

## trip 14  San Vicente Mountain

see map on p. 122

|  |  |
|---|---|
| **Distance** | 2.0 miles round trip, Out-and-back |
| **Hiking Time** | 1 hour (round trip) |
| **Elevation Gain/Loss** | 400'/400' |
| **Difficulty** | Easy |
| **Trail Use** | Suitable for mountain biking, dogs allowed, good for kids |
| **Best Times** | October through June |
| **Agency** | SMMC |
| **Optional Map** | USGS 7.5-min *Canoga Park* |
| **Notes** | Marked trails/obvious routes, easy terrain |

**DIRECTIONS** Drive west from Interstate 405 near Encino on a paved section of Mulholland Drive. The blacktop ends after 2.1 miles at an intersection where Encino Hills Drive descends north toward the San Fernando Valley. Park along the roadside here.

Perched above the San Fernando Valley on one of the more prominent bumps of the Santa Monica Mountains, the Cold-War-era Nike missile site at San Vicente Mountain has become a destination for hikers, mountain bikers, and passing drivers maneuvering over the unpaved section of famed Mulholland Drive. On occasions when "dirt Mulholland" closes to motor vehicles (likely during the wet season), it can still be used by hikers willing to hoof it a mile or so. You shake off most of the crowds and enjoy an extraordinary view from the mountain itself.

Walk or bike past the sturdy gate (open or closed) on dirt Mulholland, heading steeply up the wide, rutted dirt roadway. The steady ascent takes you to the old Nike missile installation, which is now a popular interpretive site within the Santa Mon-

ica Mountains National Recreation Area. Between 1956 and 1968 soldiers from the LA96C battalion manned the site, which was part of a continental system of defensive missile-launch sites.

At best, the view from San Vicente Mountain Park includes the Tehachapi Mountains to the north, a distant Pacific Ocean horizon to the southwest, and the urban sprawl of the Los Angeles Basin and San Fernando Valley lapping at the Santa Monica Mountain foothills. The park also serves as a primary trailhead into spacious parcels of undeveloped land to the south: the Mulholland Gateway Park, and a spread of canyons and ridges becoming known as the "Big Wild"—20,000 acres of wilderness and wildlife habitat practically on the edge of the West L.A. metropolis.

# chapter 13

# Santa Monica Mountains: Malibu Creek

Nosing its way around an obstacle course of upraised and tilted sandstone, conglomerate and volcanic rock formations, Malibu Creek clearly has been successful in adapting to the tectonic creaks and groans of Mother Earth. It's the only stream that has managed to cut entirely through the Santa Monica Mountains. Its tentacle-like tributaries reach far west and north, draining parts of the north edge of the Santa Monicas, as well as about one-third of the Simi Hills. Lower Malibu Creek has cut an impressively deep gorge, followed most of the way by the fast, two-lane highway called Malibu Canyon Road.

Hikers and other self-propelled travelers can enjoy 6000-acre Malibu Creek State Park, which features a quiet stretch of Malibu Creek and picturesque outcrops of sandstone and volcanic rock. Several newer parcels of park and open-space land lie adjacent to the state park, and these are included as well in the 20 trips that belong to this chapter.

In contrast to the area covered in last chapter (Topanga), full-blown urbanization is not as much of a factor here. Still, urban-style housing developments have crept into the mountain valleys along Las Virgenes Road and along Mulholland Highway near San Fernando Valley. Timely efforts by park advocates in the 1960s and '70s resulted in the present substantial inventory of park and open-space areas, and these efforts continue today. A quick historical review will be helpful in understanding the area's value as parkland and open space:

Bedrock mortars (grinding holes) and other archaeological evidence indicate thousands of years of prehistoric use of the Malibu Creek area, most recently by the coast-dwelling Chumash. These Indians maintained a presence here up to at least the mid-1800s. Some say that Chumash descendants cast the adobe bricks for construction of the Sepulveda Adobe (still standing near Mulholland Highway and Las Virgenes Road) in 1863.

At the turn of the century, a group of wealthy individuals bought property along Malibu Creek and formed the exclusive Crag's Country Club. A clubhouse and several private homes were built, but a more lasting effort involved the erection of a dam across a rocky defile on Malibu Creek. The 7-acre lake created by the dam was later named Century Lake by the succeeding owner of the property, Twentieth Century Fox.

By the mid-1900s, much of Malibu Creek country was a kind of annex for Hollywood studios, with sets strategically placed to take advantage of a great variety of exotic backdrops. A vestige of this activity continues today, though most of the sets in Malibu Creek State Park and elsewhere have been removed.

The land owned by Twentieth Century Fox was purchased by the state in 1974, and adjoining parcels acquired soon after. In 1976 Malibu Creek State Park was opened to the public. Then, in 1978, Congress established the Santa Monica Mountains National Recreation Area to "preserve and enhance its scenic, natural, and historical setting and its public health value as an airshed for the Southern California metropolitan area

*continued on page 142*

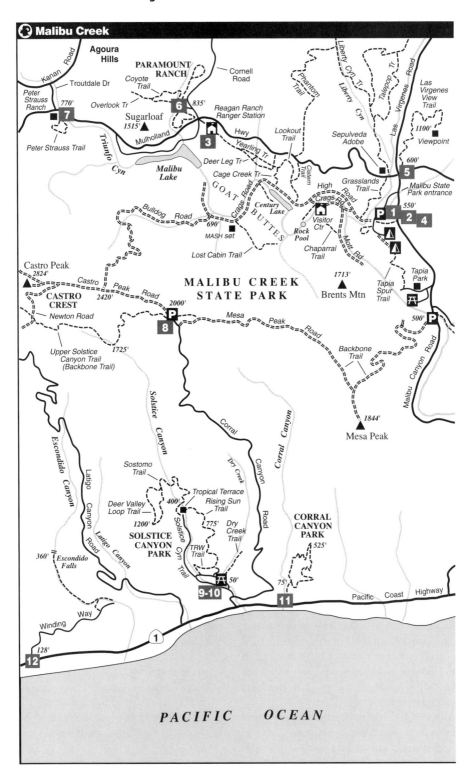

**Malibu Creek**

Agoura
Hills

PARAMOUNT
RANCH

Cornell
Road

Coyote
Trail

Kanan
Road

Troutdale Dr

Peter
Strauss
Ranch        770'

7

Overlook Tr        835'        6

Sugarloaf
1515'

Reagan Ranch
Ranger Station

Mulholland        Hwy

3

Peter Strauss Trail

Triunfo Cyn

Malibu
Lake

Yearling Tr

Deer Leg Tr

Cage Creek Tr

Lookout
Trail

Phantom Trail

Liberty Cyn Tr

Liberty Cyn

Talepop Tr

Las Virgenes Road

Las
Virgenes
View
Trail

Sepulveda
Adobe

1100'

Viewpoint

600'

5

Malibu State
Park entrance

GOAT BUTTES

Bulldog        Road

690'

MASH set

Lost Cabin Trail

Century
Lake

Cistern Trail

High
Crags

Rock
Pool

Visitor
Ctr

Grasslands
Trail

Crags Rd

Chaparral
Trail

Mott Rd

550'

1        P

2        4

Castro Peak
2824'

CASTRO
CREST

Newton Road

Castro        Peak        Road
2420'

2000'

P

8

MALIBU CREEK
STATE PARK

1713'

Brents Mtn

Tapia
Spur
Trail

Tapia
Park

500'        P

Mesa        Peak        Road

Backbone
Trail

Malibu Canyon Road

1725'

Upper Solstice
Canyon Trail
(Backbone Trail)

Solstice Canyon

Corral

Corral        Canyon

Canyon

1844'

Mesa Peak

Escondido Canyon

Latigo Canyon

Sostomo
Trail

Deer Valley
Loop Trail

400'

1200'

SOLSTICE
CANYON
PARK

Tropical Terrace
Rising Sun
Trail

775'

Dry
Creek
Trail

Dry Creek

Corral        Canyon        Road

CORRAL
CANYON
PARK

525'

Latigo        Canyon        Road

360'        Escondido
Falls

TRW
Trail

Solstice Cyn Trail

50'

9-10

75'

11

Pacific        Coast        Highway

Winding        Way

1

128'

12

PACIFIC        OCEAN

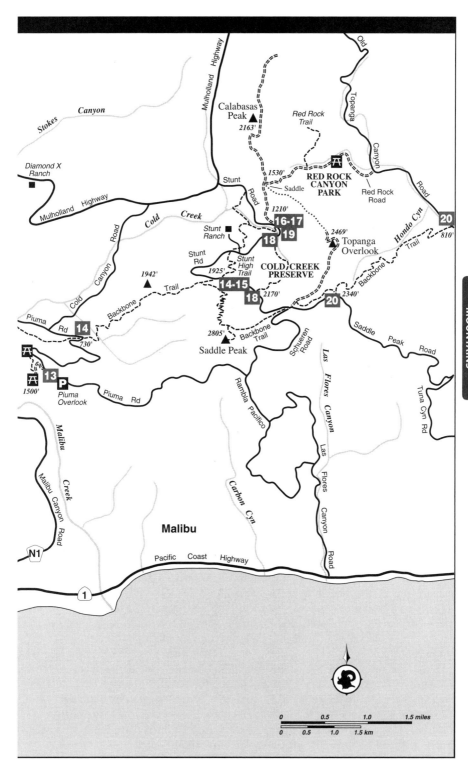

while providing for the recreational and educational needs of the visiting public." To date these goals have been partially realized through the cooperation of several government agencies as well as private landowners. Malibu Creek State Park grew to encompass more than 7000 acres. All the while, the state-funded Santa Monica Mountains Conservancy, the National Park Service, and private organizations have been busily buying key parcels of land in the Malibu Creek area and beyond for use as open space and parkland. About half of the land shown on our map of the Malibu Creek area is in public ownership so far.

The state park (and nearby Paramount Ranch) harbors some of the southernmost valley-oak habitat in California. You can see beautiful specimens of this sprawling, deciduous tree in Liberty Canyon north of Mulholland Highway, and along the Nature Trail, located near the state park's main entrance off Las Virgenes Road.

Malibu Creek State Park also features a large, tidy campground with cold showers, quiet in the off-season but often full on spring and summer weekends. Even if you live rather close by in the L.A. area, you can stay overnight here and use the campground as a base for early morning or evening hikes. The park's hours for day users are 8 a.m. until dusk.

## trip 1  Century Lake

|  |  |
|---|---|
| **Distance** | 3.0 miles round trip, Out-and-back |
| **Hiking Time** | 1½ hours (round trip) |
| **Elevation Gain/Loss** | 250′/250′ |
| **Difficulty** | Easy |
| **Trail Use** | Suitable for mountain biking, good for kids |
| **Best Times** | All year |
| **Agency** | MCSP |
| **Optional Map** | USGS 7.5-min *Malibu Beach* |
| **Notes** | Marked trails/obvious routes, easy terrain |

see map on p. 140

**DIRECTIONS** From Highway 101 take Las Virgenes Road 3 miles south to Mulholland Highway (traffic light here). Continue on Las Virgenes 0.2 mile farther to the Malibu Creek State Park entrance on the right. Pay the state park day-use fee, and drive to the main parking lot, open 8 a.m. until dusk.

If you only have time for a single hike at Malibu Creek State Park, this is the one to take. In 3 miles of easy walking you can explore the park's main attractions, and also drop by the visitor center (open on the weekends), which is not accessible by car. Picnic tables and water are available along the route.

From the main parking lot, walk west on unpaved Crags Road. After 0.5 mile you come to a concrete-ford crossing of Malibu Creek. Youngsters come here to toss in a line for bass, bluegill, and catfish. A right at the fork in the road just beyond leads you most directly to the visitor center. (A more interesting, roundabout and arduous alternative is to turn south at the fork, make a left at Mott Road, and then follow Chaparral Trail up and over a saddle to reach the visitor center. At that saddle you're rewarded with a great view of the Goat Buttes.)

The visitor center is housed in a grand old home once occupied by a member of the Crag's Country Club, and later by the groundskeeper for Twentieth Century Fox. Even if the center isn't open, you can peruse the interpretive panels set up outside beneath the oaks.

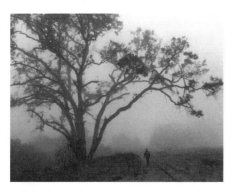

Valley oak on a foggy morning, Malibu Creek State Park

From the visitor center, cross over Malibu Creek on a sturdy bridge and continue up the hill on Crags Road, gaining about 200 feet in elevation. When you reach the crest, look for the Forest Trail descending left. In a minute or two, you'll reach the shady east shoreline of Century Lake, created in 1901 by damming Malibu Creek with a tall concrete structure. Subsequent silting-in has allowed a freshwater marsh to overtake much of what was previously open water. Ducks, coots and herons frequent the lake, their squallings and callings reverberating off the weathered, honeycombed volcanic cliffs rising from the reservoir's far shore. Redwing blackbirds flit among the cattails and rushes.

When you've had your fill of these engaging sights and sounds, backtrack to the bridge over Malibu Creek. Just before you reach it, though, turn south onto a footpath signed GORGE TRAIL. In a few minutes you'll come upon the Rock Pool, a placid stretch of water framed by volcanic cliffs. This generically wild-looking site has served as a backdrop for outdoor sequences filmed for *South Pacific, Tarzan, Swiss Family Robinson*, and many other productions.

To return to the starting point, simply backtrack to Crags Road, and walk east on it for a scant mile until you reach the main parking lot.

Rock Pool on Malibu Creek

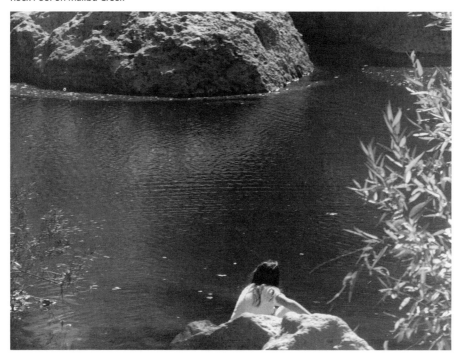

# trip 2  Lost Cabin Trail

see map on p. 140

|  |  |
|---|---|
| **Distance** | 6.2 miles round trip, Out-and-back |
| **Hiking Time** | 3 hours (round trip) |
| **Elevation Gain/Loss** | 700'/700' |
| **Difficulty** | Moderate |
| **Best Times** | October through June |
| **Agency** | MCSP |
| **Optional Map** | USGS 7.5-min *Malibu Beach* |
| **Notes** | Marked trails/obvious routes, easy terrain |

**DIRECTIONS** From Highway 101 take Las Virgenes Road 3 miles south to Mulholland Highway (traffic light here). Continue on Las Virgenes 0.2 mile farther to the Malibu Creek State Park entrance on the right. Pay the state park day-use fee, and drive to the main parking lot, open 8 a.m. until dusk.

It's been said that the number of people on a wilderness trail diminishes in proportion to the square of the distance and the cube of the elevation gain from the nearest road. Perhaps that explains why only about one in every hundred visitors to Malibu Creek State Park bothers to check out the dead-end Lost Cabin Trail.

In truth, when you reach the end, there's no "there" there—just a trickling brook, a line of willows and oaks, lots of fragrant chaparral on the hillsides, plus the overarching dome of the blue sky. (The cabin, if there ever was one, seems to be truly lost.) This placid scene, however, lies in the heart of the 1900-acre Kaslow Natural

Goat Buttes from the Chaparral Trail

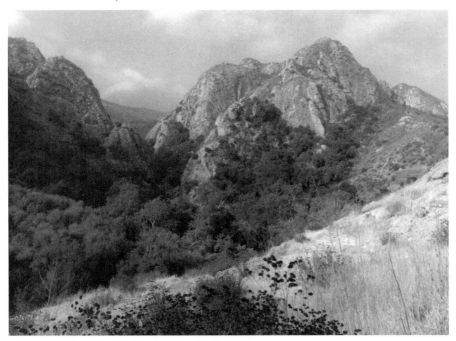

Preserve, the largest of three areas in the park managed for research and low-level public use. The Kaslow (meaning golden eagle in the language used by the Chumash Indians) Preserve harbors mountain lions, golden eagles, and a rare native plant—the Santa Susana tarweed. (The other natural preserves, incidentally, cover the valley oak habitat in Liberty Canyon, and a small amount of oak-and-chaparral country along Udell Creek, north of Crags Road and south of the Reagan Ranch.)

From the main parking lot, walk west on unpaved Crags Road. After 0.5 mile you come to a concrete-ford crossing of Malibu Creek. On the far side, stay right to remain on Crags Road, which takes you straight to the visitor center (open weekends).

From the visitor center itself, cross over Malibu Creek on a sturdy bridge and continue up the hill on Crags Road, gaining about 200 feet in elevation. When you start descending note, on the right, the marine sedimentary Calabasas Formation, consisting of light-colored, easily eroded rocks roughly 15 million years old. On the left are the dramatically sheer Goat Buttes, which consist of the erosion-resistant Conejo Volcanics, also about 15 million years old. Ahead on the Lost Cabin Trail you'll get a look at the south side of those buttes, which features a weird assortment of pock-marked outcrops and boulders.

At 1.7 miles you come to a bridge over Malibu Creek. There's a water fountain on the near side—the last water available until you return to this point on your way back. (Just ahead, the Forest Trail goes left, providing access to Century Lake's south shore.)

From the Forest Trail intersection, follow Crags Road another 0.6 mile, to where an old bulldozed road goes left up along a

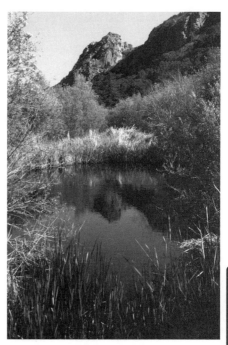

Malibu Creek at Malibu Creek State Park

draw. This is the Lost Cabin Trail, formerly an access road for sites used in the filming of the *M\*A\*S\*H* television series. The main *M\*A\*S\*H* site, dismantled upon the conclusion of filming in 1982, is marked by a sign along Crags Road. Little remains of the site of the fictional 4077th tent hospital other than an old burned-out jeep amid the encroaching brush.

Follow the Lost Cabin Trail up to a divide and then down to the bank of Lost Cabin Creek, a small tributary of Malibu Creek. At the trail's end a sign advises you to go no farther. Downstream, the trickling creek tumbles over a precipice to join Malibu Creek in the gorge between Century Lake and the Rock Pool.

SANTA MONICA
MOUNTAINS

# trip 3  Lookout Loop

see map on p. 140

| | |
|---|---|
| **Distance** | 3.8 miles, Loop |
| **Hiking Time** | 2 hours |
| **Elevation Gain/Loss** | 500'/500' |
| **Difficulty** | Moderate |
| **Trail Use** | Good for kids |
| **Best Times** | November through June |
| **Agency** | MCSP |
| **Optional Map** | USGS 7.5-min *Malibu Beach* |
| **Notes** | Marked trails/obvious routes, easy terrain |

**DIRECTIONS** From Highway 101 take Las Virgenes Road 3 miles south to Mulholland Highway (traffic light here). Turn right on Mulholland and proceed another 3 miles to the intersection of Cornell Road, where on the left you will find the entrance to the Reagan Ranch Ranger Station, which serves as state park headquarters. Limited roadside parking is available there, and there's virtually unlimited parking space at Paramount Ranch, just 0.3 mile north.

If it's springtime, you'll want to have your camera, plus macro lens or close-up attachment, with you on this hike. After a wet winter, these gentle meadows and oak-dotted hillsides can muster quite a showing of wildflowers from March into May or June. Keep an eye out for lupine, larkspur, California poppy, wild pansy, Chinese houses, goldfields, creamcups, wallflower, wild rose, and the ever-present, but weedy mustard. You're seldom out of sight or sound of nearby Mulholland Highway, but there's plenty of botanical variety to make the trip an enjoyable one.

From the intersection of Mulholland Highway and Cornell Road, walk southeast on the eucalyptus-lined, unpaved driveway to the park headquarters buildings, which are on the site of the ranch owned by former president Ronald Reagan prior to his election as California governor in 1966. Bypassing the ranch buildings, pick up the signed Yearling Trail, which runs for more than a half mile through a grassy meadow. After a short distance, bear right on the Deer Leg Trail (later you'll return to this intersection on the Yearling Trail, the path to the left). The Deer Leg Trail rambles through a strip of oak woodland and then descends to cross tiny Udell Creek.

A side path slants left to reconnect with the Yearling Trail, but you stay right on the narrow path that climbs up a brushy slope. In a few minutes, you arrive on top of a ridge overlooking Century Lake and Malibu Creek. In the background, the Goat Buttes soar into a milky blue sky. Strong backlight during most of the day makes this a difficult landscape to capture photographically. Late afternoon side-light, however, does justice to the majesty of the scene.

From the ridgetop, the trail veers north to join the Yearling Trail in the meadow below. Turn right at the bottom, go 0.1 mile east, and go right again on the Cage Creek Trail. After an abrupt 250-foot loss of elevation, you arrive at Crags Road. Turn left, and continue 0.3 mile east past Century Lake to the Lookout Trail, on the left. The Lookout Trail swings up a dry ridge to the north, offering more views of the lake and the buttes to the south. You pass the Cistern Trail on the right, which goes to a turnout along Mulholland Highway (an alternate starting point for this hike), and then contour through patches of cool oak woodland and toasty chaparral. Leaving the chaparral, you traverse a grassy saddle and rejoin the Yearling Trail. Follow it back toward the Reagan Ranch and your starting point.

# trip 4  Bulldog & Backbone Loop

| | |
|---|---|
| **Distance** | 13.7 miles, Loop |
| **Hiking Time** | 7 hours |
| **Elevation Gain/Loss** | 2700'/2700' |
| **Difficulty** | Strenuous |
| **Trail Use** | Suitable for mountain biking |
| **Best Times** | November through May |
| **Agency** | MCSP |
| **Optional Maps** | USGS 7.5-min *Malibu Beach, Point Dume* |
| **Notes** | Marked trails/obvious routes, easy terrain |

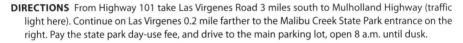

see map on p. 140

**DIRECTIONS**  From Highway 101 take Las Virgenes Road 3 miles south to Mulholland Highway (traffic light here). Continue on Las Virgenes 0.2 mile farther to the Malibu Creek State Park entrance on the right. Pay the state park day-use fee, and drive to the main parking lot, open 8 a.m. until dusk.

This is the classic grand tour of Malibu Creek State Park's rugged backcountry. Along the way you'll tramp along the crestline of the Santa Monicas, circling high above the park's most conspicuous landmarks. Mountain bikers, who use a slight variation of the route, typically make this a 3- or 4-hour task, but you'd better allow about double that amount of time on foot. There's little shade, so be prepared with plenty of water (a half gallon or more on a warm day) and sun protection.

From the main parking lot, head west on unpaved Crags Road. After 0.4 mile you come to a concrete-ford crossing of Malibu Creek. A right at the fork in the road just beyond leads you most directly to the park's visitor center, open on weekends.

From the visitor center, cross over Malibu Creek on a sturdy bridge and continue

SANTA MONICA MOUNTAINS

Sandstone cave above Corral Canyon Road

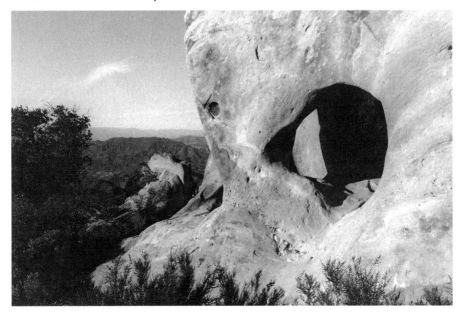

up the hill on Crags Road, gaining about 200 feet in elevation. Press on past silted-in Century Lake on the left; the Goat Buttes, also on the left; and through the M*A*S*H site, where outdoor scenes for the *M*A*S*H* television series were shot. Bird life is abundant along this stretch, where the trail parallels Malibu Creek.

After a total of 2.7 miles, bear left on Bulldog Road (Bulldog Motorway), a fire road that also serves as a powerline access road. The road ascends along a small, oak-shaded creek, then rises crookedly along slopes thickly clothed in chaparral. As you climb, you'll pass side roads leading to electrical transmission towers. The physical effort of negotiating the last, steep, uphill mile on Bulldog Road is rewarded by ever-expanding views over and beyond the now-shrunken-looking Goat Buttes. You'll also pass close to some interesting outcrops of sandstone, looking much like gigantic incisor teeth. Turn left when you reach Castro Peak Road (Castro Motorway) at 5.8 miles, and start a descent east. The Malibu shoreline soon comes into view, with a clear-air vista that includes several of the Channel Islands, Palos Verdes, and the west and south parts of the L.A. Basin.

As you approach the Corral Canyon Road Trailhead parking lot (6.6 miles), stay left on the footpath that goes up a hogback ridge bristling with sandstone pinnacles. (Bikers should stay on the roadways instead of taking the footpath.) Going east along this ridge for 0.5 mile, passing an old homesite and several gargantuan sandstone outcrops—worth climbing if you want to take the time. On the east end of the ridge, you drop down to the Mesa Peak Fire Road, which doubles as a segment of the Backbone Trail.

At 9.4 miles there's a junction. The road to Mesa Peak goes right; you bear left, staying on the Mesa Peak Fire Road. You now begin a steady descent along the precipitous west wall of Malibu Canyon. Malibu Creek and the curving highway through it come into view occasionally, seemingly straight down. At 11.2 miles, the fire road abruptly ends at a locked gate just above a water-treatment plant. You sidestep this closure by going right (east) on a more primitive road, again a part of the Backbone Trail. After contouring a while, the trail descends very sharply to the Backbone Trailhead parking area along Malibu Canyon Road (11.8 miles). This is a potentially knee-banging drop for runners, and a tricky descent for mountain bikes.

Follow Malibu Canyon Road north, over Malibu Creek, and enter Tapia Park on the left, picking up the single-track Tapia Spur Trail (closed to bikers; they must use Malibu Canyon Road and Las Virgenes Road). The Tapia Spur Trail skirts some picnic sites, passes the entrance to a private Salvation Army camp, and continues up and over a scruffy ridge to Malibu Creek State Park's group campground. From there, simply walk out the access road and over to your car in the valley ahead.

# trip 5 Upper Las Virgenes View Trail

see map on p. 140

| | |
|---|---|
| **Distance** | 4.0 miles round trip, Out-and-back |
| **Hiking Time** | 2 hours (round trip) |
| **Elevation Gain/Loss** | 650'/650' |
| **Difficulty** | Moderate |
| **Trail Use** | Suitable for mountain biking, dogs allowed |
| **Best Times** | October through June |
| **Agency** | SMMC |
| **Optional Map** | USGS 7.5-min *Malibu Beach* |
| **Notes** | Marked trails/obvious routes, easy terrain |

**DIRECTIONS** From Highway 101 take Las Virgenes Road 3 miles south to Mulholland Highway (traffic light here). The small trailhead parking area is on the left, at the northeast corner of the intersection.

The view alluded to in this trail's name is the upper drainage of Las Virgenes Creek, a tributary of Malibu Creek whose tentacles reach north into the Simi Hills west of the San Fernando Valley. The trail climbs through a varied landscapes consisting of grassland, chaparral, oak woodland, and a touch of riparian woodland. The overlook at the end of the trail is a worthwhile destination, especially when the air is clean and dry enough to afford distant vistas. Although the trail is open to mountain bikers (and equestrians as well), there are a couple of sections cut sharply into a sheer hillside that may prove hazardous to anyone in the saddle.

From the Las Virgenes Road/Mulholland Highway junction, the trail starts by heading crookedly north through weedy grasses, more or less parallel to Las Virgenes Road. After a not-very-promising half mile, the scenery improves greatly as the trail cuts east across a lushly vegetated, north facing slope, gains elevation, and pulls away from the somewhat noisy sounds of traffic. Before long, you're curling uphill on an oak-dotted ridge and enjoying ever-widening views. At the top of that ridge, the trail turns south and meanders over to an 1100-foot knoll that serves as an informal viewpoint. There, you can look out over the Las Virgenes Creek floodplain, flanked by sensuously rolling hills, and spot various high points in the Santa Monica Mountains: Saddle Peak, Goat Buttes, Castro Crest, and San Vicente Mountain (with its signature abandoned Nike missile base).

SANTA MONICA MOUNTAINS

## trip 6  Paramount Ranch

| | |
|---|---|
| **Distance** | 1 to 3 miles, various routes |
| **Hiking Time** | ½ to 1½ hours |
| **Elevation Gain/Loss** | Up to 300′/300′ |
| **Difficulty** | Easy |
| **Trail Use** | Dogs allowed, good for kids |
| **Best Times** | All year |
| **Agency** | NPS |
| **Optional Map** | USGS 7.5-min *Point Dume* |
| **Notes** | Marked trails/obvious routes, easy terrain |

see map on p. 140

**DIRECTIONS** Exit the 101 Freeway at Kanan Road in Agoura Hills. Drive south for 0.5 mile, and turn left on Cornell Way. Immediately ahead, stay right and continue on Cornell Road. Proceed 2.4 miles south to Paramount Ranch on the right.

For most of the 20th Century, Paramount Ranch served the needs of an entertainment industry always hungry for rustic outdoor scenery. Since 1980, however, the core of this property has been in the hands of the National Park Service. The park service set about restoring Western Town, a set where exteriors for hundreds of TV western episodes were shot in the 1950s and '60s. Today the false fronts and dusty streets serve both as an interpretive facility and sometimes as a working set for television productions.

Owl's clover

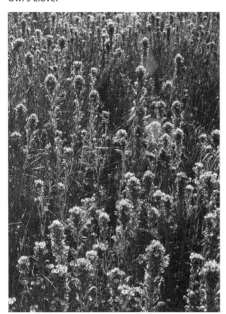

Paramount Ranch is a popular spot for guided walks, but you can explore on your own just as easily. About 4 miles of trails lace the 326-acre property. A nice route to follow during the springtime is the combination of the Coyote and Overlook trails. You start behind Western Town, go up a ravine, and circle back along a chaparral-dotted slope. Wildflowers abound in a good year—woolly blue curls, owl's clover, verbena, mallow, and more. About halfway along the trail, there's a short spur leading up to a single picnic table perched on a spot with a commanding view of Western Town, the brooding Goat Buttes, and the dark summit ridge of the Santa Monica Mountains.

Several shorter trails, plus portions of a former auto racetrack, have been linked together in the 5-km Run Trail, identified in several places by logo-like markers. From a scenic standpoint, the southern part of the Run Trail is more worthwhile. There's a passage along the bank of Medea Creek, and an easy climb of a hillock near the intersection of Cornell Road and Mulholland Highway. At the top of that hillock you can look upon the soaring profile of Sugarloaf Peak, which is made of the same stuff as the Goat Buttes—Conejo Volcanics. Hearsay has it that Sugarloaf Peak was the inspiration for the familiar mountain in the Paramount Pictures logo.

**trip 7**  **Peter Strauss Trail**

| | |
|---|---|
| **Distance** | 1.0 mile, Loop |
| **Hiking Time** | ½ hour |
| **Elevation Gain/Loss** | 200'/200' |
| **Difficulty** | Easy |
| **Trail Use** | Dogs allowed, good for kids |
| **Best Times** | All year |
| **Agency** | NPS |
| **Optional Map** | USGS 7.5-min *Point Dume* |
| **Notes** | Marked trails/obvious routes, easy terrain |

see map on p. 140

**DIRECTIONS**  Exit the 101 Freeway at Kanan Road in Agoura Hills. Drive 2.8 miles south and turn left on Troutdale Drive. Proceed 0.4 mile south to Mulholland Highway and turn left. Just ahead, on the right, is the parking lot for Peter Strauss Ranch, open 8 a.m. to sunset.

The 65-acre Peter Strauss Ranch (owned by actor-producer Peter Strauss prior to its purchase for inclusion in the national recreation area in 1983) has an interesting past. In the 1930s and '40s this was Lake Enchanto, a popular resort and amusement park, boasting the largest swimming pool west of the Rockies, a terrazzo dance floor, and amusement rides. The upper reaches of Malibu Creek (known here as Triunfo Can-

Along the Peter Strauss Trail

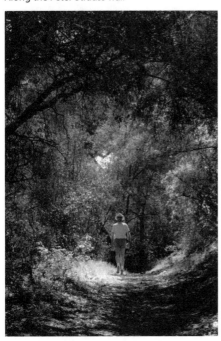

yon) were dammed to create the lake itself, a popular draw for boaters and fishermen. During the 1960s—long after Lake Enchanto's commercial demise—plans were afoot to develop the property as an elaborate Disneyland-style park, but they were never realized.

Today's Lake Enchanto bears scant resemblance to the resort it used to be. The dam washed out in 1960 and has not been rebuilt. The great swimming pool lies unfilled. A picturesque stone-and-wood bath house remains. Other than guided walks, and occasional special events such as dances, plays, art shows, and musical performances held on the grounds, this quiet refuge caters to a relatively small number of hikers, picnickers, and curious folk.

Kids will find plenty to keep them busy here. From spring into early summer the shallow, sluggish stream is alive with thousands of tadpoles. Careful investigation may reveal crayfish, newts, and pond turtles. Just south of the ranch house, there's a playground in a eucalyptus grove overlooking the remains of Lake Enchanto's dam. The Peter Strauss Trail, probably the most attractive short trail in the Santa Monica Mountains, begins here. Shaded by live oaks and flanked by a ground-hugging carpet of ferns and poison oak, the easy-to-follow path zigzags up a hillside and loops back toward the ranch house.

**SANTA MONICA MOUNTAINS**

# trip 8  Upper Solstice Canyon

see map on p. 140

| | |
|---|---|
| **Distance** | 5.0 miles, Loop |
| **Hiking Time** | 2½ hours |
| **Elevation Gain/Loss** | 1000'/1000' |
| **Difficulty** | Moderately strenuous |
| **Trail Use** | Dogs allowed |
| **Best Times** | October through June |
| **Agency** | NPS |
| **Optional Map** | USGS 7.5-min *Point Dume* |
| **Notes** | Marked trails/obvious routes, easy terrain |

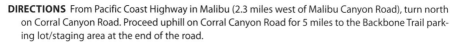

**DIRECTIONS** From Pacific Coast Highway in Malibu (2.3 miles west of Malibu Canyon Road), turn north on Corral Canyon Road. Proceed uphill on Corral Canyon Road for 5 miles to the Backbone Trail parking lot/staging area at the end of the road.

A splendid sense of isolation pervades the upper reaches of Solstice Canyon—thanks to the purchase of lands along the Castro Peak crest years ago by the National Park Service. This brushy and dry country may look a bit unfriendly under harsh midday sunshine, but it's really quite intriguing when soft morning or evening shadows drape the hillsides and hollows.

Ideally you would start this loop hike in the late afternoon, and go clockwise to take advantage of evening shadows while climbing through the canyon below. If you can leave about 2 hours before sunset, you'll hit the Castro crest by sundown. The distant lights of L.A. will be in view by the time you arrive back at your car.

From the west edge of the parking lot, follow on foot the Backbone Trail, which switchbacks downward along the rim of a bowl drained by several upper tributaries of Solstice Canyon. Mostly the trail makes use of old roads, but some of it is newer trail tread. After about a mile of indecisive descent, you join a ravine bottom and then descend decisively to the main tributary of Solstice Canyon (1.3 miles). Turn sharply right and walk up-canyon 200 yards to a small meadow. Ahead, you're going to face a gain of about 900 feet of elevation, so take a generous pull or two from your water bottle.

Onward from the meadow, the trail passes under the fire-scarred limbs of live oaks. Then, as the oaks thin, you start climbing out of the canyon bottom. After rounding some switchbacks you come up to Newton Road (2.8 miles), a dirt road crossing a saddle south of, and well below, Castro Peak. The Backbone Trail contours west toward Latigo Canyon Road at this point, but you go uphill on Newton Road, traversing Castro Peak's south slope.

When you reach the top of the grade (atop Castro Peak's east ridge) walk east about 50 yards on a side path to the top of a barren knoll. On clear days, the view encompasses almost the entire coastline from Ventura County to Palos Verdes. At least four of the Channel Islands can be seen poking out of the sea offshore. Near the winter solstice, the sun sinks to an ocean horizon as seen from here. Because the California coastline trends east-west in this area, the sun sets over land during most of the year.

Just past the knoll you'll hook up with Castro Peak Road (3.6 miles). Turn right and let gravity repay you for your previous efforts. Within a half hour your car in the parking lot should be in view.

## trip 9  Lower Solstice Canyon

see map on p. 140

|  |  |
|---|---|
| **Distance** | 2.4 miles round trip, Out-and-back |
| **Hiking Time** | 1½ hours (round trip) |
| **Elevation Gain/Loss** | 350'/350' |
| **Difficulty** | Easy |
| **Trail Use** | Dogs allowed, good for kids |
| **Best Times** | All year |
| **Agency** | NPS |
| **Optional Maps** | USGS 7.5-min *Malibu Beach, Point Dume* |
| **Notes** | Marked trails/obvious routes, easy terrain |

**DIRECTIONS** Solstice Canyon Park's gateway is located on Corral Canyon Road, 0.2 mile north of Pacific Coast Highway in Malibu. There's overflow parking space for several cars right at the entrance, and a more spacious lot 0.3 mile farther inside at the main trailhead. Park hours are 8 a.m. to sunset.

The easy-going but superbly scenic Solstice Canyon Trail takes you through the grounds of the former Robert's Ranch—now Solstice Canyon Park, a site administered by the National Park Service. The canyon once hosted a private zoo where giraffes, camels, deer, and exotic birds roamed. At trail's end you come to Tropical Terrace, the site of an architecturally noted grand home that burned in a 1982 wildfire.

Since the Solstice Canyon Trail is paved, it accommodates road bikes as well as mountain bikes and all travel by foot. Starting at the main trailhead, pass through a gate and continue upstream alongside the canyon's melodious creek. You travel through a fantastic woodland of alder, sycamore, bay, and live oak—the latter with trunks up to 18 feet in circumference. After 15 minutes or so, you pass an 1865 stone cottage on the right—thought to be the oldest existing stone building in Malibu.

At 1.2 miles, you arrive at Tropical Terrace, 90 percent burned in the 1982 fire. In a setting of palms and giant bird-of-paradise, curved flagstone steps sweep toward the roofless remains of what was for 26 years one of Malibu's grand homes. Beyond the house, crumbling stone steps and pathways lead to what used to be elaborately decorated rock grottoes, and a waterfall on Solstice Canyon's creek. Large chunks of sandstone have cleaved from the canyon walls, adding to the rubble. For all its perfectly natural setting, Tropical Terrace's destiny was that of a temporary paradise, defenseless against both fire and flood.

When it's time to return, simply go back the way you came. And if you have a little energy to spare back at the start, take a mile-long (round trip) side hike up the Dry Creek Trail. An outrageously cantilevered "Darth Vader" house overlooks the Dry Creek ravine, as well as a 150-foot-high precipice that on rare occasions becomes a spectacular waterfall.

SANTA MONICA MOUNTAINS

## trip 10  Rising Sun & Sostomo Loop

see map on p. 140

|  |  |
|---|---|
| **Distance** | 7.1 miles, Loop |
| **Hiking Time** | 4 hours |
| **Elevation Gain/Loss** | 2000'/2000' |
| **Difficulty** | Moderately strenuous |
| **Trail Use** | Dogs allowed |
| **Best Times** | October through May |
| **Agency** | NPS |
| **Optional Maps** | USGS 7.5-min *Malibu Beach, Point Dume* |
| **Notes** | Marked trails/obvious routes, easy terrain |

**DIRECTIONS** Solstice Canyon Park's gateway is located on Corral Canyon Road, 0.2 mile north of Pacific Coast Highway in Malibu. There's overflow parking space for several cars right at the entrance, and a more spacious lot 0.3 mile farther inside at the main trailhead. Park hours are 8 a.m. to sunset.

This rollercoaster-like ramble over the hillsides overlooking lower Solstice Canyon is a nearly complete tour of the entire Solstice Canyon Park. It's a sweaty affair if the day is sunny and warm. However, with an early-enough start, you can finish in time for lunch under the oaks in the cool, shady canyon bottom.

From the main trailhead, start off on the paved Solstice Canyon Trail. After 0.3 mile, veer right on the TRW Trail, which passes by some former TRW (defense contractor) research buildings. Continue climbing on an old fire road curving up the hillside—the Rising Sun Trail. With every step, a

wider slice of the ocean comes into view. After 400 feet of ascent, the signed Rising Sun Trail (a footpath) veers left, while the old road continues about 200 yards to a chain gate—private property beyond. There's a fine view of the coastline up near the gate; if you're there by 8:30 a.m. on or near winter solstice, the risen sun should be gleaming above the Palos Verdes peninsula, its light scattering into a thousand watery pinpoints on the ocean's surface below.

Resuming your travel on the Rising Sun Trail, you contour above a snaggle-toothed outcrop called Lisa's Rock, and then descend sharply to the Tropical Terrace site (2.1

The remains of Tropical Terrace

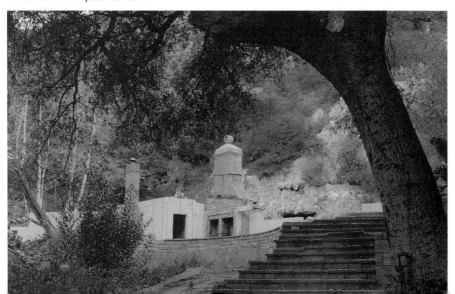

miles). Cross Solstice Canyon's creek, walk down past the ruins of the house, and pick up the Sostomo Trail on the right.

On the Sostomo Trail, which is an old road to start with, you ascend the west wall of Solstice Canyon, cross the creek (2.4 miles), and then start up the east wall. About 0.1 mile beyond the creek crossing, take the side trail to the left. This little shortcut across a bend in the road visits a tiny, burnt-out cabin, its forlorn brick chimney bravely poking above the encroaching chaparral. Starting at 2.8 miles, you drop down and cross the creek again. Going up the west bank you pass another cabin fatality—a roofless stone-and-mortar shell. Looming over the canyon ahead is a spectacular outcrop of sedimentary rock, but our trail route circles south away from it and climbs to a trail junction (3.2 miles). Ahead lies the Deer Valley Loop Trail; go either way around the loop, covering a distance of 1.3 miles. About midway along

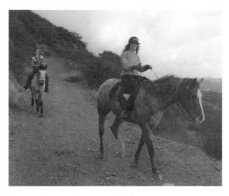
Equestrians on Sostomo Trail

the loop you reach the shoulder of a ridge at 1200 feet elevation where you can look down on Point Dume and the coastline. That view is made less dramatic by some high-voltage powerlines in the foreground.

To return to the starting point, descend Sostomo Trail back to Tropical Terrace and then take the easiest way back—downhill on the paved Solstice Canyon Trail.

**SANTA MONICA MOUNTAINS**

## trip 11 Corral Canyon

| | |
|---|---|
| **Distance** | 2.2 miles, Loop |
| **Hiking Time** | 1½ hours |
| **Elevation Gain/Loss** | 500'/500' |
| **Difficulty** | Moderate |
| **Trail Use** | Dogs allowed, good for kids |
| **Best Times** | All year |
| **Agency** | SMMC |
| **Optional Map** | USGS 7.5-min *Malibu Beach* |
| **Notes** | Marked trails/obvious routes, easy terrain |

see map on p. 140

**DIRECTIONS** To get to the trailhead, you'll need to be going westbound through Malibu on Pacific Coast Highway (there is no eastbound access to the trailhead). At a point 0.6 mile west of Puerco Canyon Road, there's a parking lot on the right for the Malibu Seafood and Deli restaurant, 25623 Pacific Coast Highway, which doubles as the Corral Canyon Trailhead. If you reach Corral Canyon Road, you have gone 0.3 mile too far.

**D**iminutive Corral Canyon Park is one of the newer parcels of open space to be added to the archipelago of public lands known as the Santa Monica Mountains National Recreation Area. A lazily looping hiking trail traverses the park's grass- and chaparral-covered slopes, inviting your exploration on foot.

Check out the interpretive plaques at the trailhead and then take off on the trail, which begins by crossing a small area of willow scrub in the often-marshy bottom of Corral Canyon. On the far side, swing left. After 0.1 mile choose the trail on the right which will take you immediately uphill and counterclockwise on a 2-mile loop. The beautifully graded pathway curls up a grassy hillside swept by fresh Pacific breezes. Hang-gliding humans on parasailing craft can often be seen drifting lazily to and fro along the shoreline, utilizing those same sea breezes.

At 0.8 mile, you reach a narrow ridge. A false trail goes right up along the top of that ridge, but you stay left, following a more gently graded trail that continues gaining elevation, going north, parallel to the canyon bottom below. By about 1.1 miles, at an elevation of 550 feet above sea level, there's a sharp switchback. You swing left and initiate a zigzagging descent down into the canyon and then alongside the canyon bottom. Keep an eye on the sky for ravens, hawks, or vultures swooping, soaring and gliding.

Nearing the end of the hike you pass a homesite—a cabin burned like so many others in this wildfire-prone region—with its forlorn chimney still standing. Shortly ahead, you come to the aforementioned split in the trail, a short distance shy of the trailhead.

Corral Canyon ocean vista

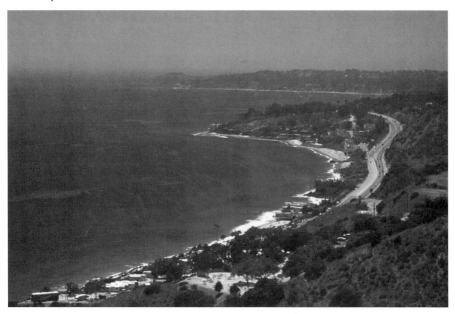

# trip 12  Escondido Canyon

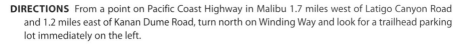

see map on p. 140

| | |
|---|---|
| **Distance** | 3.4 miles round trip, Out-and-back |
| **Hiking Time** | 2 hours (round trip) |
| **Elevation Gain/Loss** | 500'/500' |
| **Difficulty** | Moderate |
| **Trail Use** | Dogs allowed |
| **Best Times** | December through July |
| **Agency** | SMMC |
| **Optional Map** | USGS 7.5-min *Point Dume* |
| **Notes** | Marked trails/obvious routes, easy terrain |

**DIRECTIONS** From a point on Pacific Coast Highway in Malibu 1.7 miles west of Latigo Canyon Road and 1.2 miles east of Kanan Dume Road, turn north on Winding Way and look for a trailhead parking lot immediately on the left.

Escondido ("hidden" in Spanish) Canyon conceals one of the natural treasures of the Santa Monica Mountains: a shimmering waterfall leaping more than 200 feet over a broken cliff. Only during times of rare flood do the falls resemble anything thunderous, but even during an average rainy season the intricate dribblings of water are an inspiration.

On foot, follow the shoulder of Winding Way (a private road signed as a public access trail) for 0.8 mile to a summit, passing palatial newer houses perched on rounded hilltops and ocean-facing slopes. Continue 0.1 mile past the summit, then follow a narrow trail descending to the left. After another 0.1 mile you cross Escondido Canyon's stream amid oaks, sycamores, and willows. Turn left when you reach the trail on the far side, heading upstream. Fine displays of sticky monkeyflower adorn the trail in spring and early summer. After the fifth stream crossing, the trail sticks to the east bank and you soon catch a first glimpse of the upper cascades of the multitiered falls dead ahead, its white noise audible over the whisper of the nearby stream.

At the trail's end, a faint sulfurous odor in the air is juxtaposed against the sweet sight of feathery ribbons of water draped across a travertine outcrop, which forms the lowest tier of the falls. Don't attempt to climb on or around the falls; just enjoy the soothing ambiance of the scene before heading back to the starting point the same way.

Escondido Falls

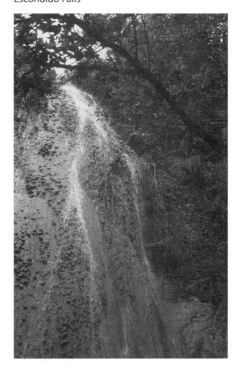

## trip 13  Piuma Overlook

| | |
|---|---|
| **Distance** | 0.6 mile round trip, Out-and-back |
| **Hiking Time** | ½ hour (round trip) |
| **Elevation Gain/Loss** | 150'/150' |
| **Difficulty** | Easy |
| **Trail Use** | Dogs allowed, good for kids |
| **Best Times** | All year |
| **Agency** | SMMC |
| **Optional Map** | USGS 7.5-min *Malibu Beach* |
| **Notes** | Marked trails/obvious routes, easy terrain |

**DIRECTIONS** From Pacific Crest Highway in Malibu, turn north on Las Flores Canyon Road. Proceed 3.4 miles to Rambla Pacifico, and turn right. Go 0.6 miles to Piuma Road and turn left. Now head west on Piuma for about 3 miles, and notice the Piuma roadside overlook on the left. The starting point for the trail (a small parking area on the left side of the road) is 0.25 mile farther, at mile post 2.91.

In a little patch of open space known as the Malibu Canyon Piuma Ridge, high atop the rim of Malibu Canyon, you can take a short hike to a restful spot with a panoramic view of the Pacific Ocean and the Santa Monica Mountains spilling down toward it.

From the trailhead, follow the former roadbed (now a wide trail) that ascends the brushy slope. After only about 0.3 mile, you arrive at a flattish, open area featuring two picnic tables and a virtually unlimited view. Gaze eastward to spot the dramatically tilted sandstone strata on the west flank of Saddle Peak. Look westward into Malibu Creek State Park and spot the Goat Buttes within it. Scan the ocean in the south to as far as the transparency of the air will allow. Those bumps out there in various directions are the Channel Islands, the nearest of which is Santa Catalina Island, about 45 miles away.

## trip 14  West Ridge of Saddle Peak

| | |
|---|---|
| **Distance** | 3.5 miles, Point-to-point |
| **Hiking Time** | 1½ hours |
| **Elevation Gain/Loss** | 350'/1550' |
| **Difficulty** | Moderate |
| **Trail Use** | Dogs allowed, good for kids |
| **Best Times** | October through July |
| **Agency** | NPS |
| **Optional Map** | USGS 7.5-min *Malibu Beach* |
| **Notes** | Marked trails/obvious routes, easy terrain |

**DIRECTIONS** *East End:* From Mulholland Highway, drive south on Stunt Road for 2.9 miles to the start of a connector trail for the Backbone Trail. The trail originates at a small turnout at mile 2.9, and there is a larger parking turnout nearby at mile marker 3.0. *West End:* From Malibu Canyon Road, drive 1.2 miles east on Piuma Road to the Backbone Trail crossing, near mile marker 1.2.

One of the most scenic sections of the Backbone Trail cuts across the northwest flank of Saddle Peak, accomplishing in 3.5 indirect miles what a bird in flight could traverse in about 1.5 miles. Along its winding, scenic course, the trail passes massive sandstone boulders, slices through tangled thickets of chaparral, penetrates secret copses of live oak and bay laurel, and dips to cross a clear-flowing brook in what is appropriately called Dark Canyon. Easy road access on both ends makes this a good point-to-point hike accomplished by either a car-shuttle or a drop-off-and-pick up arrangement.

From Stunt Road, start walking southwest on the Backbone connector trail, up through chaparral. After 0.2 mile you come to a junction with the Backbone Trail. Left leads toward Saddle Peak (Trip 15 below), while our way goes right (west).

Wide-open views to the north are interspersed with shady passages across seasonal rivulets descending from Saddle Peak's boulder-studded heights. At 1.2 miles you traverse a grassy meadow astride a small saddle. Northwest of this meadow a 1942-foot peaklet promises a great view at the expense of a short, leg-scratching climb.

From the saddle you begin a crooked, more-or-less steady descent (1100 feet in 2 miles) down through mostly chaparral—hot going on a sunny afternoon. A cool and pleasant but brief passage across a north-facing slope precedes a final switchbacking plunge down the steep wall of Dark Canyon. There are lots of opportunities to admire Malibu Creek country spread before you—the upthrust Goat Buttes, Brents Mountain, and the green or gold (depending on the season) valleys below. At the bottom, fern-draped Dark Canyon is like a paradise, but the shady passage is a brief one. A final zigzag climb takes you back up into the sunny chaparral, where you come upon Piuma Road.

SANTA MONICA MOUNTAINS

View over marine layer from Saddle Peak

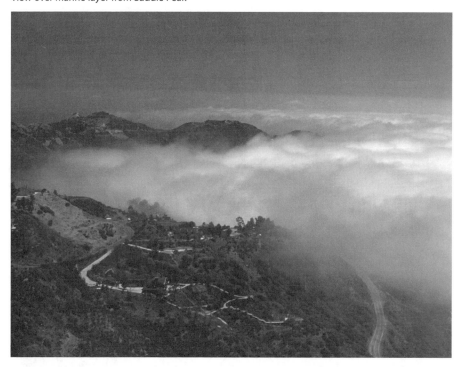

# trip 15  Saddle Peak

| | |
|---|---|
| **Distance** | 3.2 miles round trip, Out-and-back |
| **Hiking Time** | 2 hours (round trip) |
| **Elevation Gain/Loss** | 950'/950' |
| **Difficulty** | Moderate |
| **Trail Use** | Dogs allowed |
| **Best Times** | October through July |
| **Agency** | SMMC |
| **Optional Map** | USGS 7.5-min *Malibu Beach* |
| **Notes** | Marked trails/obvious routes, easy terrain |

see
map on
p. 140

**DIRECTIONS** From Mulholland Highway, drive south on Stunt Road for 2.9 miles to start of a connector trail for the Backbone Trail. The trail originates at a small turnout at mile 2.9, and there is a larger parking turnout nearby at mile marker 3.0.

Saddle Peak's two summits—one topped by antennas and fenced off, the other barren but viewful—soar to an elevation of about 2800 feet. Both preside over a coastline that is only 2.5 miles away. During early morning in spring and early summer, the mountain often stands head and shoulders above a mock ocean of fog that shrouds the coast and sometimes smothers all but the higher ridges of the Santa Monica Mountains. Getting out of bed early to make the trek to the top is worth it to catch the magic of warm sunlight on the pillowy surface of the clouds.

From Stunt Road, start hiking up the Backbone connector trail. Go left after 0.2 mile and proceed uphill though chaparral on a newer stretch of Backbone Trail that at first may seem tedious. By 1.2 miles you reach some blocky sandstone outcrops that lend a spectacular air to the airy views stretching north—assuming you are not still enveloped in fog. Listen for the whoosh of the wings of cliff swallows as they soar and dive among these crags.

At 1.4 miles, turn right (south) on a side trail heading uphill 0.1 mile to a gravel road. Make a left to reach the nearby east (and publicly accessible) summit, or a right to reach the "saddle" of Saddle Peak.

It is also possible to reach Saddle Peak using the Backbone Trail from Saddle Peak Road. This is a slightly shorter, but less scenic approach.

Marine layer from the crest of the Santa Monica Mountains

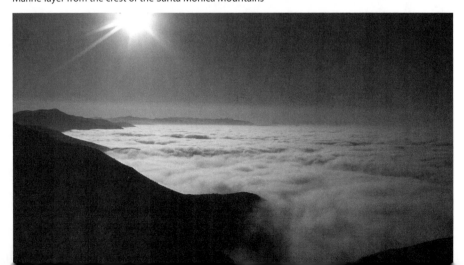

## trip 16   Red Rock Canyon

| | |
|---|---|
| **Distance** | 4.0 miles round trip, Out-and-back |
| **Hiking Time** | 2 hours (round trip) |
| **Elevation Gain/Loss** | 600'/600' |
| **Difficulty** | Moderate |
| **Trail Use** | Suitable for mountain biking, dogs allowed, good for kids |
| **Best Times** | October through June |
| **Agency** | SMMC |
| **Optional Map** | USGS 7.5-min *Malibu Beach* |
| **Notes** | Marked trails/obvious routes, easy terrain |

see map on p. 140

**DIRECTIONS** From Mulholland Highway, drive south on Stunt Road for 1 mile. Turn right into the roadside parking lot on the right, at mile marker 1.0.

Slabs of cavernous sandstone and cobbly conglomerate tilted sharply upward in Red Rock Canyon tell a geologic story of deposition by gentle currents and massive floods, later faulting and folding of the resulting sedimentary rock layers, and ongoing weathering and erosion. The beige and purplish red colors of the rock strata contrast nicely with the greens and grays of oaks, sycamores, and chaparral—altogether making the canyon reminiscent of the cinematic Wild West. This description covers the "back-door" approach to Red Rock Canyon from its top (west) side, ideal for a weekend stroll or mountain bike ride. In addition, hikers (but no dogs or bikes) may want to try a side trip up the slope north of the canyon using the narrow Red Rock Canyon Trail.

From the parking lot on Stunt Road, cross the pavement and pick up the fire road that cuts across a hillside to the north. When you reach a junction in a saddle at 0.7 mile, you're at the head of Red Rock Canyon. Turn right on the crooked road

SANTA MONICA MOUNTAINS

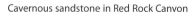

Cavernous sandstone in Red Rock Canyon

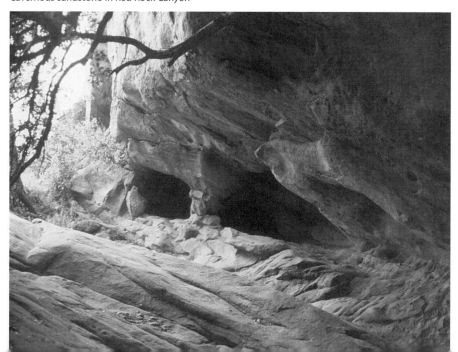

descending into the canyon, enjoying the scenery, which becomes more interesting as the canyon becomes narrower and deeper.

At 1.5 mile, on the left, the 1-mile-long Red Rock Canyon Trail crosses the canyon's seasonal stream, heads abruptly upward along a ridge, and climbs circuitously to the north rim of the canyon. The side trip is worth it if the weather's clear and cool, otherwise probably not. After another 0.5 mile on the canyon road, you come to a picnic site on the grounds of an old Boy Scout camp, and water for drinking. Keep going on the road just a bit farther and you'll discover a spectacular little gorge.

The gorge and picnic site are accessible from the east by car, which pretty much negates the fun of traveling to them on you own power. If you wish to get to the canyon this way, however, take Old Topanga Road 4 miles south from Mulholland Highway, or 2 miles northwest from Topanga Canyon Boulevard, to Red Rock Road. Turn west and drive 0.8 mile to the gorge and a vehicle gate just beyond it.

## trip 17  Calabasas Peak

see map on p. 140

| | |
|---|---|
| **Distance** | 3.6 miles round trip, Out-and-back |
| **Hiking Time** | 2 hours (round trip) |
| **Elevation Gain/Loss** | 1000'/1000' |
| **Difficulty** | Moderate |
| **Trail Use** | Suitable for mountain biking, dogs allowed |
| **Best Times** | October through June |
| **Agency** | SMMC |
| **Optional Map** | USGS 7.5-min *Malibu Beach* |
| **Notes** | Marked trails/obvious routes, easy terrain |

**DIRECTIONS** From Mulholland Highway, drive south on Stunt Road for 1 mile. Turn right into the roadside parking lot on the right, at mile marker 1.0.

The climb to Calabasas Peak should appeal to both exercise buffs and landscape photographers. The non-trivial gain and loss of elevation make a great workout, and the geologic formations passed along the way are some of the most photogenic in the Santa Monica Mountains. In any case, an early or a late start is almost always preferred over a midday excursion. The exercise-minded will find the cool morning air most refreshing. Photographers will appreciate the three-dimensional effect of low-angle sunlight on the rock formations and the long shadows slanting across the shaggy mountainsides.

From the parking lot on Stunt Road, cross the pavement and pick up the fire road that cuts across a hillside to the north. Bear left when you reach a road junction at a saddle (0.7 mile), where you get a glimpse of Red Rock Canyon (see previous trip). Continue north, wending your way past a fascinating collection of tilted sandstone slabs and fins.

At 1.6 miles, just beyond a couple of horseshoe curves in the road, you reach the summit ridge, south of the Calabasas Peak summit. Most of Old Topanga Canyon, to the east, is visible below. The road goes on to traverse the peak's east shoulder, so you leave it (and probably your bike, if you have one) and hop onto a fire break going up toward the peak itself on your left. A low thicket of chaparral guards the rounded summit.

The foreground view, marred at many points around the compass by the encroaching suburbs, may be a bit disappointing. But on clear days, the long views west toward Castro Crest and east to the San Gabriel Mountains are inspiring all the same.

## trip 18  Cold Creek Canyon Preserve

| | |
|---|---|
| **Distance** | 1.8 miles, Point-to-point |
| **Hiking Time** | 2 hours |
| **Elevation Gain/Loss** | 100'/1000' |
| **Difficulty** | Moderate |
| **Trail Use** | Good for kids |
| **Best Times** | All year |
| **Agency** | MRT |
| **Optional Map** | USGS 7.5-min *Malibu Beach* |
| **Notes** | Marked trails/obvious routes, easy terrain |

see map on p. 140

**DIRECTIONS**  Typically the hikes at Cold Creek Canyon Preserve originate at the parking lot on Stunt Road, 1 mile south of Mulholland Highway.

The extravagant lushness of the riparian vegetation growing in Cold Creek Canyon Preserve today is astonishing, especially in view of the fact that 1993's Malibu fire burned virtually everything here to a crisp. Gully-washing El-Nino rains in 1998 sped up the botanical recovery, but also ripped out a large section of the preserve's trail, which took months to repair. While fire and flood have always been part of a regularly recurring cycle in the Santa Monica Mountains, perhaps nowhere else are they expressed more dramatically than here. The preserve lies in a steep, north-facing bowl where retained moisture promotes rampant growth, the underlying rock is weak, and the devil winds of autumn can drive a fire storm upslope in hardly any time

at all. Hopefully your visit to the preserve won't coincide with the recent aftermath of natural disaster.

Cold Creek Canyon is managed by the nonprofit Mountains Restoration Trust, and is not open to the general public. However, docent-led public hikes are offered here nearly every weekend, and it is possible to obtain a permit for hiking on your own from the Mountains Restoration Trust if you decide to join that organization. The guided hikes are listed and described in the quarterly publication *Outdoors, Santa Monica Mountains Recreation Area*, published by the National Park Service, (805) 370-2301, or www.nps.gov/samo. Some of these hikes feature a car shuttle, which allows one-way, downhill travel through the canyon, and

SANTA MONICA MOUNTAINS

Fern glade, Cold Creek Canyon Preserve

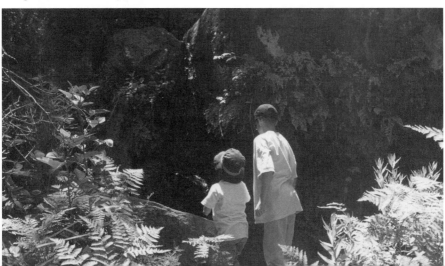

that particular way of exploring the preserve is described here.

The preserve encompasses the former Murphy Ranch, whose owners deeded the property to The Nature Conservancy in 1970. Your starting point, the "upper gate" on the shoulder of upper Stunt Road, is the point where the former access road to the Murphy Ranch began its descent into the canyon. Starting out on this old road (now a trail), you drop 0.4 mile through tall chaparral (including some red shank, which is rare in the Santa Monicas) to reach the canyon bottom, which is graced with sturdy live oak and bay trees. The farther and the lower you go from here, the lusher the canyon becomes.

Presently you pass the remains of an old Dodge pickup hastily abandoned at the end of a dirt road during a 1973 fire. Thereafter, you continue on a narrower trail threading its way through a fairyland of bracken and woodwardia ferns, tules, cattails, Humboldt lilies, and bright green grass thriving on soggy ground. From here on, you are seldom out of earshot of the canyon's delightful little year-round stream.

You'll stop at the site where a 19th Century settler constructed a lean-to between two sandstone outcrops. The settler raised celery (which still grows wild in the canyon) and hauled his crop down to the stage station at Calabasas.

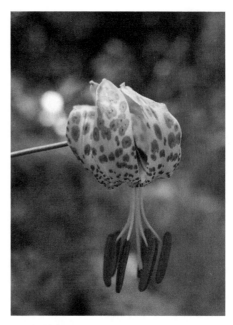

Humboldt lily

After nearly 2 miles of travel, you reach the padlocked "lower gate" on the lower end of Stunt Road, which securely blocks any access into or out of the preserve for those who don't have a key. Hikers who have the energy and wherewithal to travel farther can try linking the Cold Creek Canyon trail into a loop route that would include either Stunt High Trail to the west or the route over Topanga Lookout to the east (see Trip 19).

# trip 19  Topanga Lookout & Stunt High Loop

see map on p. 140

| | |
|---|---|
| **Distance** | 6.5 miles, Loop |
| **Hiking Time** | 3½ hours |
| **Elevation Gain/Loss** | 1800'/1800' |
| **Difficulty** | Moderately strenuous |
| **Trail Use** | Dogs allowed |
| **Best Times** | October through May |
| **Agency** | NPS |
| **Optional Map** | USGS 7.5-min *Malibu Beach* |
| **Notes** | Marked trails/obvious routes, some difficult terrain, possible bushwhacking |

**DIRECTIONS** From Mulholland Highway, drive south on Stunt Road for 1 mile. Turn right into the roadside parking lot on the right, at mile marker 1.0.

This wide-ranging loop has a bit of what feels like genuine mountaineering—a mere class 2.5 or 3 in climber's parlance, but exciting all the same. Save the trip for an exceptionally clear day, as I did, and you'll be rewarded with vistas that must be seen to be believed.

From the parking lot on Stunt Road, cross the pavement and pick up the fire road that cuts across a hillside to the north. Hike uphill to the saddle at the head of Red Rock Canyon, 0.7 mile from Stunt Road. Take neither the road north to Calabasas Peak nor the road east into Red Rock Canyon below. Instead, turn sharply right and climb up a steep bulldozed track. That track soon peters out, but you can continue climbing to a 1766-foot knoll. There you can see what lies ahead: an undulating, brushy, knife-edge ridge, buttressed by tilted sandstone slabs and fins. A narrow, but well-beaten trail up along the ridge testifies to its popularity as a mountaineer's route.

Make your way for a painstaking mile up and over or around the sandstone obstacles and through the brush until you reach the terminus of a fire road. Continue on this for an easy-going 0.4 mile, past a couple of striking columnar rock formations, to the foundation of the long-abandoned Topanga Fire Lookout (2.2 miles). Enjoy the stupefying view, weather permitting. A big section of the San Fernando Valley is visible, along with parts of the L.A.

Basin and Santa Monica Bay. Downtown L.A.'s office towers point the way toward a low spot on the east horizon—San Gorgonio Pass—flanked by Southern California's highest peaks (San Gorgonio and San Jacinto), over 100 miles away.

From the lookout site, walk south on the fire road to Saddle Peak Road (3.1 miles), where there's a better view of Santa Monica Bay and Santa Catalina Island. Over at the intersection of paved roads immediately west, bear right on Stunt Road. Walk easily

Outcrops below Topanga Lookout site

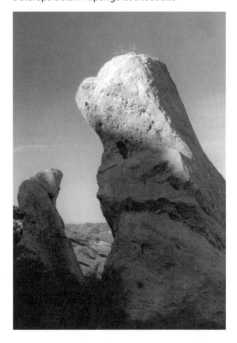

downhill along Stunt Road for a bit over a mile, a not-unpleasant task since the road carries only light traffic and offers nice views throughout.

At a turnout on the right at mile marker 3.0, you'll discover the top end of the Stunt High Trail. Follow the trail's winding course downhill for 0.8 mile through tall chaparral until you hit Stunt Road again. Turn right and walk 0.1 mile east along Stunt Road's left shoulder to the Stunt Ranch entrance road. Follow this for 0.1 mile north, then veer right to continue on the signed Stunt High Trail. Only a mile of walking remains: You wind through more chaparral, go down across a meadow to Cold Creek, and meet an old road paralleling the stream. The final, delightfully shaded stretch goes up along the creek and ends at your starting point, the large turnout at mile 1.0 on Stunt Road.

## trip 20  Hondo Canyon

|  |  |
|---|---|
| **Distance** | 3.5 miles, Point-to-point |
| **Hiking Time** | 2 hours |
| **Elevation Gain/Loss** | 100'/1650' |
| **Difficulty** | Moderate |
| **Trail Use** | Dogs allowed |
| **Best Times** | October through June |
| **Agency** | SMMC |
| **Optional Maps** | USGS 7.5-min *Malibu Beach*, *Topanga* |
| **Notes** | Marked trails/obvious routes, easy terrain |

see map on p. 140

**DIRECTIONS** *West End:* From Mulholland Highway, turn south on Stunt Road. Drive 4.1 miles uphill to the intersection of Saddle Peak Road and Schueren Road. Keep straight there and continue another 0.6 mile east on Saddle Peak Road to reach the trailhead on the left (mile 0.60 on Saddle Peak Road). *East End:* From Topanga Canyon Boulevard, take Old Topanga Canyon Road 0.3 mile northwest to a small turnout, just beyond the bridge over the Old Topanga Canyon stream.

A delightful, remote segment of the Backbone Trail rises between Old Topanga Canyon Road and Saddle Peak Road, zigzagging along slopes densely clothed in chaparral and oaks, and passing near a number of ephemeral waterfalls in Hondo Canyon that contribute a zenlike atmosphere during the rainy season. Assuming you've set up a car shuttle or planned some similar transportation arrangement, you can have the pleasure of following this easygoing stretch of trail in the downhill (west to east) direction.

You start out in dry chaparral at the top on a short connector trail, quickly making a right turn on the segment of Backbone Trail descending into Hondo Canyon. After a few tedious switchbacks, the trail enters a more thickly wooded area consisting not so much of trees, but rather of a rampant growth of tall chaparral. The entire Hondo Canyon drainage was burned in the October 1993 Malibu fire, and has been recovering quickly ever since.

Many more switchbacks take you inexorably downward along the steep south slope of Hondo Canyon, where you encounter Tolkienesque copses of gnarled live oak and fragrant bay laurel. Nearing the bottom of the canyon at about 2 miles, there's a short side path on the left leading to a point where you can view Hondo Canyon's stream tumbling through a little V-shaped gorge.

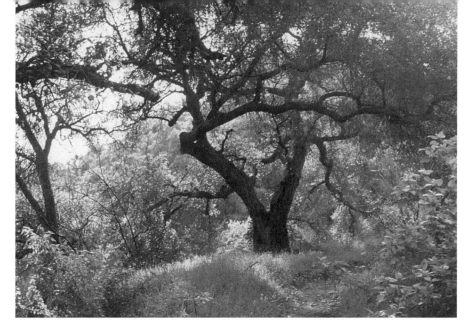

Live oaks in Hondo Canyon

Past this point the trail contours to a saddle, veers right, and descends a grassy slope into a separate lesser ravine, whose bottom is beautifully shaded by majestic live oaks. Water flows in this ravine only after a substantial amount of rain has fallen. A few minutes walk down along the ravine takes you to Old Topanga Canyon's shallow stream and Old Topanga Canyon Road just above it.

# chapter 14

# Santa Monica Mountains: Zuma Canyon

Although it slices only 6 miles inland from the Pacific shoreline near Point Dume, Zuma Canyon harbors one of the deepest gorges in the Santa Monica Mountains. Easily on a par with Malibu and Topanga canyons in scenic wealth, Zuma Canyon holds a further distinction of never having suffered the invasion of a major road.

Ongoing acquisitions of open space in Zuma Canyon and neighboring Trancas Canyon to the west by the National Park Service are serving two goals relevant to the desires of hikers. First, there's public access to lower Zuma Canyon—gateway to the most wild and isolated stretch of canyon bottom in the Santa Monicas. Second, the final uncompleted link of the Backbone Trail is being constructed in the uppermost reaches of Zuma and Trancas canyons. Envisioned more than half a century ago, this 65-mile-long ridgeline trail along the length of the Santa Monica Mountains is finally nearing completion.

In this chapter we visit two hiking routes in lower Zuma Canyon, descend toward upper Zuma Canyon past a couple of waterfalls in Newton Canyon, and ramble through nearby Rocky Oaks Park—a pleasant spot for picnics, wildflower hunting, and birdwatching.

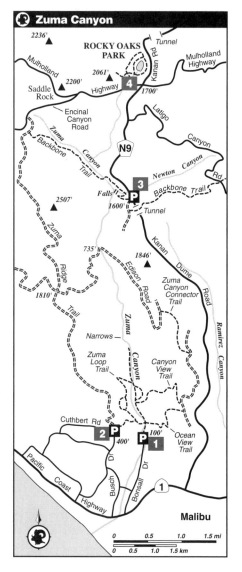

## trip 1  Lower Zuma Canyon

| | |
|---|---|
| **Distance** | 2.8 miles round trip, Out-and-back |
| **Hiking Time** | 1½ hours (round trip) |
| **Elevation Gain/Loss** | 100'/100' |
| **Difficulty** | Easy |
| **Trail Use** | Dogs allowed, good for kids |
| **Best Times** | All year |
| **Agency** | NPS |
| **Optional Map** | USGS 7.5-min *Point Dume* |
| **Notes** | Marked trails/obvious routes, easy terrain |

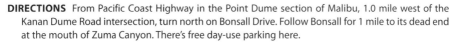

see map on p. 168

**DIRECTIONS**  From Pacific Coast Highway in the Point Dume section of Malibu, 1.0 mile west of the Kanan Dume Road intersection, turn north on Bonsall Drive. Follow Bonsall for 1 mile to its dead end at the mouth of Zuma Canyon. There's free day-use parking here.

The wide mouth of Zuma Canyon offers a small network of riding and hiking trails, and plenty of space to wander along the gravelly bed of the canyon's small creek. For starters, try this easy walk.

From the end of Bonsall Drive, walk past a gate and into the sycamore-dotted flood plain ahead. When you reach trails branching left and right after about 0.2 mile, keep straight and follow along the winter-wet, summer-dry creek, crossing it several times in the next mile. You'll pass statuesque sycamores, tall laurel sumac bushes, and scattered wildflowers in season. This is a promising area for spotting wildlife any-time—squirrels, rabbits, and coyotes are commonly seen, deer and bobcats less so.

After about a mile, the canyon walls close in tighter, oaks appear in greater numbers, and you'll notice a small grove of eucalyptus trees across the creek on a little terrace. A short while later, the trail abruptly ends at a pile of sandstone boulders. During the dry months, surface water may get only this far down the canyon. Usually, however, the water trickles or tumbles past here, disappearing at some point downstream into the porous substrate of the canyon floor. Further travel through the V-shaped canyon ahead is possible only by rock-hopping (Trip 2), so this is a good spot to turn around.

On your return, if you want more exercise, you can follow either the Zuma Loop Trail going up along Zuma Canyon's west slope, or the loop consisting of the Canyon View and Ocean View trails going high up on the canyon's east slope.

**SANTA MONICA MOUNTAINS**

The wilds of Zuma Canyon

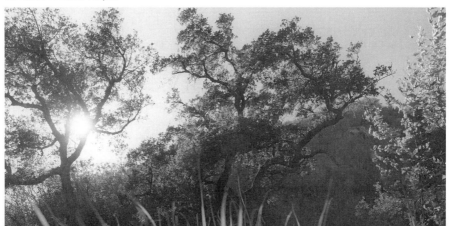

# trip 2  Zuma Canyon & Zuma Ridge Loop

see map on p. 168

| | |
|---|---|
| **Distance** | 8.0 miles, Loop |
| **Hiking Time** | 6 hours |
| **Elevation Gain/Loss** | 1700'/1700' |
| **Difficulty** | Strenuous |
| **Trail Use** | Dogs allowed |
| **Best Times** | October through June |
| **Agency** | NPS |
| **Optional Map** | USGS 7.5-min *Point Dume* |
| **Notes** | Marked trails/obvious routes, difficult terrain, bushwhacking |

**DIRECTIONS** From Pacific Coast Highway in the Point Dume section of Malibu, 1.1 miles west of the Kanan Dume Road intersection, turn north on Busch Drive. Follow Busch 1 mile uphill to where it meets Cuthbert Road. Park in the small lot there.

Squeezed between walls soaring 1500 feet or more, the green, riparian strip along the bottom of Zuma Canyon's mid-section lies undisturbed (save for the crossing of a single, dirt "Edison" road built to give access to electrical towers). Under cover of jungle-like growths of willow, sycamore, oak, and bay, the canyon's small stream cascades over sculpted sandstone boulders and gathers in limpid pools adorned with ferns. These natural treasures yield their secrets begrudgingly, as they should, only to those willing to scramble over boulders, plow through sucking mud and cattails, and thrash through scratchy undergrowth.

Zuma Canyon is passable all the way to the bottom of a 25-foot waterfall just above Newton Canyon. For variety, however, we'll route you part of the way up the canyon, and then back on the Edison powerline road and the Zuma Ridge Trail (a fire road). The roads are shadeless, but offer great vistas of the canyon and the ocean.

Hiking the canyon bottom is least problematical in the fall season before the heavy rains set in. The stream may have shrunk to isolated pools by then, and you'll step mostly on dry rocks with good traction. Winter flooding can render the canyon impassable, but such episodes are rare and short-lived. During spring, the stream flows heartily and there's plenty of greenery and wildflowers; at the same time there's an increased threat of exposure to poison oak

(which is found in fair abundance along the banks) and you're more likely to surprise a rattlesnake. Summer days are usually too oppressively warm and humid for such a difficult hike. Whatever the season, take along plenty of water; the water in the canyon is not potable.

From the Busch Drive parking lot, take the path across the hillside to the east. You lose about 300 feet of elevation as you zigzag down to the flat flood plain at the mouth of Zuma Canyon.

When you reach the bottom, bypass the Zuma Loop Trail and go a little farther to the main Zuma Canyon Trail. Turn left there and walk up along Zuma's creek bed for about a mile. Now you begin a nearly 2-mile stretch of boulder-hopping, 2 or 3 hours worth depending on the conditions. Other than a few rusting pieces of pipeline from an old dam and irrigation system at the lower end, you may find that the canyon is completely litter-free; please keep it that way.

The great variety of rocks that have been washed down the stream or fallen from the canyon walls says a lot about the geologic complexity of the Santa Monicas. You'll scramble over fine-grained siltstones and sandstones, conglomerates that look like poorly mixed aggregate concrete, and volcanic rocks of the sort that make up Saddle Rock (a local landmark near the head of Zuma Canyon) and the Goat Buttes of

Malibu Creek State Park. Some of the larger boulders attain the dimensions of mid-sized trucks, presenting an obstacle course that must be negotiated by moderate hand-and-foot climbing.

About 0.5 mile shy of the dirt road crossing, you'll pass directly under a set of high-voltage transmission lines—so high they're hard to spot. These lines, plus the service road built to give access to the towers, represent the major incursion of civilization into Zuma Canyon. If you can ignore them,

however, it's easy to imagine what all the large canyons in the Santa Monicas were like only a century ago.

From the Edison road crossing, more scrambling and bushwhacking could potentially take you all the way to Kanan Road via Newton Canyon. Going our way, however, you turn left and climb up the twisting service road to the top of the west ridge. From there, the Zuma Ridge Trail, a fire road, takes you back down to the starting point at the end of Busch Drive.

## trip 3 Newton Canyon

|  |  |
|---|---|
| **Distance** | 1.0 mile round trip, Out-and-back |
| **Hiking Time** | 1 hour (round trip) |
| **Elevation Gain/Loss** | 150'/150' |
| **Difficulty** | Easy |
| **Trail Use** | Dogs allowed, good for kids |
| **Best Times** | All year |
| **Agency** | NPS |
| **Optional Map** | USGS 7.5-min *Point Dume* |
| **Notes** | Marked trails/obvious routes, moderate terrain |

**DIRECTIONS** You begin at a large trailhead parking area for the Backbone Trail on the west side of Kanan Dume Road at mile marker 9.5. This is 4.5 miles north of Pacific Coast Highway by way of Kanan Dume Road and 7 miles south of the 101 Freeway by way of Kanan Road and Kanan Dume Road.

Tucked obscurely into an upper tributary of Zuma called Newton Canyon is a pint-sized but charming waterfall accessible by a mere half mile of hiking. Kids will enjoy this little trek, and their parents may feel the same as long as the kids duly observe a couple of safety rules, e.g., watch out for rattlesnakes and don't get too close to precipices.

Start down the uncompleted segment of the Backbone Trail that starts from the north end of the parking lot. Make an easy descent through mature chaparral with an understory of wildflowers and ferns. Very shortly you reach the Newton Canyon stream—which just below this point dribbles some 30 feet down a mossy cliff. Off the Backbone Trail to the left you can get a glimpse of this fall from atop some sandstone outcrops, but

don't step too close to the edge where fallen leaves underfoot may be slippery. To reach the base of the fall, it's safer to continue a bit farther west on the Backbone Trail, take one or another trail going left down the slope to the stream below, and then hike a short distance back upstream.

Going downstream through Newton Canyon's narrow bottom is also fun—a possibly foot-wetting exercise as you hop sandstone boulders and slabs, and dodge the limbs and branches of oaks, sycamores, and bay laurels. After about 250 yards, you reach the top of another dropoff about 50 feet high, just shy of Newton Canyon's confluence with Zuma Canyon. Stay well away from it. This is the end of the line, so back up and return to the starting point the way you came.

## trip 4  Rocky Oaks

see map on p. 168

|  |  |
|---|---|
| **Distance** | 1.0 mile, Loop |
| **Hiking Time** | ½ hour |
| **Elevation Gain/Loss** | 150′/150′ |
| **Difficulty** | Easy |
| **Trail Use** | Suitable for mountain biking, dogs allowed, good for kids |
| **Best Times** | All year |
| **Agency** | NPS |
| **Optional Map** | USGS 7.5-min *Point Dume* |
| **Notes** | Marked trails/obvious routes, easy terrain |

**DIRECTIONS**  Exit the 101 Freeway at Kanan Road in Agoura Hills. Turn south and follow Kanan Road for 5.5 miles to Mulholland Highway. Turn right (west) on Mulholland, and almost immediately turn right again into Rocky Oaks Park.

Diminutive Rocky Oaks Park is typical of the many small properties that have been purchased or earmarked for future acquisition by the National Park Service in the continuing effort to flesh out the Santa Monica Mountains National Recreation Area. The property, a former cattle ranch, was purchased in 1980. Since then it has essentially reverted to a natural state. In the park today, you'll find restrooms, a parking lot, a picnic area, and about 200 acres of wildland consisting of hillsides covered in chaparral and sage scrub, grassy meadows, and (what else?) rocks and oaks.

The trails of Rocky Oaks are open to multiple uses: hiking, mountain biking, and dog-walking. Small kids will perhaps be entertained by the larger-than-life (from their viewpoint) landscape of hills, valleys, and rocky crags.

An easy 1-mile-long loop hike begins across the small stream from the parking lot. Go left and walk 0.2 mile to a four-way intersection, then continue straight ahead up a steep slope to reach an overlook at the top of some wood steps. The cattle pond in the valley below may or may not contain water, depending on recent rains. In the opposite direction is peak 2061 (aka Mitten Mountain), which itself blocks from view the better-known landmark of Saddle Rock. These two crags, as well as the summit you're standing on, consist of the roughly 15-million-year-old Conejo Volcanics rock formation.

The trail continues north, contouring through the tangled growths of chaparral. Dead twigs are accumulating beneath the new growth. In the natural scheme of things, this vegetation sooner or later will burn again, its ashes providing nutrients for the next, almost identical generation of plants.

To complete the 1-mile loop hike, bear right at the next fork, descend to the meadow below, and make your way past the pond back to the parking lot.

# chapter 15

# Santa Monica Mountains: Arroyo Sequit & Sandstone Peak

Toward the western end of the Santa Monica Mountains, the pulse of life slows. Human population is scattered and sparse. People live on little ranches tucked in the canyons, or in modest cottages perched on the hillsides. Some are busy building ostentatious versions of the perfect, hilltop dream house, but those are few and far between. Day-trippers and campers come this way to enjoy the ocean, the fresh coastal breezes, and the picturesque, mostly unspoiled backcountry.

The area depicted on this chapter's map, straddling the Los Angeles-Ventura county line, is dominated by a small stream called Arroyo Sequit. An escarpment stands tall at the northern headwaters of Arroyo Sequit, culminating in a craggy outcrop called Sandstone Peak. At 3111 feet, it's the highest point in the Santa Monicas. The peak, really an outcrop of volcanic rock that looks like sandstone, is one of several similar-looking summits that make up Boney Mountain, which stretches west into Point Mugu State Park (Chapter 16).

Much of this area is protected open space, in big chunks of land like Circle X Ranch and Leo Carrillo State Park, and also more modest-sized parcels, like Arroyo Sequit, and Charmlee parks. Leo Carrillo State Park (formerly Leo Carrillo State Beach), named after the actor, encompasses a mere 6000 feet of ocean frontage, but 2000 acres of interior hillsides and canyons.

Readily accessible from either the Ventura Freeway (U.S. 101) in the north or Pacific Coast Highway in the south, the area is a convenient playground for day hikers, campers, and backpackers. Opportunities for camping here (and also in nearby Point Mugu State Park) help make up for the comparative lack of campsites in the eastern Santa Monicas. Leo Carrillo State Park has two campgrounds: Leo Carrillo (with hot showers), and North Beach. Leo Carrillo Campground has a hiker-biker campground annex.

Generally, hiking is good year round immediately next to the coast where the sea breezes take the heat off the south-facing

Coastline, Leo Carrillo State Park

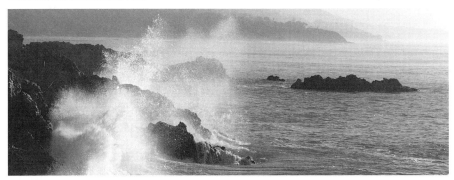

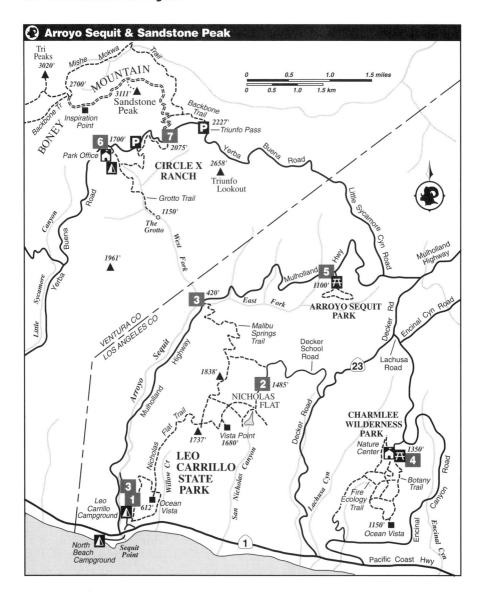

## Arroyo Sequit & Sandstone Peak

slopes. Inland, at places like Circle X Ranch, the temperature can climb to 100 degrees on summer days and drop to well below freezing on calm winter nights.

In addition to hiking, the coastline in and next to Leo Carrillo State Park offers some of the finest beachcombing, surfing, swimming, and sailboarding on the L.A. County coast. At Sequit Point you'll find a jagged stretch of sea bluffs, and rocky pools to explore when the tides are low.

Sequit Point is an especially good vantage for spotting gray whales during their winter migrations. Sometimes they can be seen swimming just beyond the surf line.

The seven trips below encompass many diverse environments and span 3000 feet of elevation change—a world in itself that seems quite disconnected from the multi-millions of people who live within an hour's drive away.

# trip 1  Leo Carrillo Ocean Vista

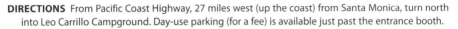

| | |
|---|---|
| **Distance** | 2.0 miles, Loop |
| **Hiking Time** | 1 hour |
| **Elevation Gain/Loss** | 600'/600' |
| **Difficulty** | Moderate |
| **Trail Use** | Good for kids |
| **Best Times** | All year |
| **Agency** | LCSP |
| **Optional Map** | USGS 7.5-min *Triunfo Pass* |
| **Notes** | Marked trails/obvious routes, easy terrain |

see map on p. 174

**DIRECTIONS** From Pacific Coast Highway, 27 miles west (up the coast) from Santa Monica, turn north into Leo Carrillo Campground. Day-use parking (for a fee) is available just past the entrance booth.

For the modest effort of climbing a 612-foot hill, you can enjoy one of the best ocean views available anywhere in the Santa Monica Mountains. If the morning is fog-free and you're ambitious enough, try to make it to the top in time for sunrise. (The sun rises around 7 a.m. in October, November and December, so you don't have to lose much sleep, especially if you're camping nearby.) To the sound of booming surf, you can watch the winter sun's golden beams spill over Palos Verdes and glance off the shimmering ocean surface down below.

The trail begins just beyond the entrance booth. Almost immediately there's a split—go either way to reach the Ocean Vista on the 612-foot hill. The slightly more direct right branch slants across a hillside overlooking the highway, then ducks inland along a slope overlooking the V-shaped ravine of Willow Creek. Near the top, you reverse direction three times and arrive at a four-way junction of trails on a saddle. Turn left and walk the remaining distance to the Ocean Vista.

In addition to the nearby coastline stretching out to Point Dume, you might see

**SANTA MONICA MOUNTAINS**

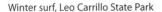

Winter surf, Leo Carrillo State Park

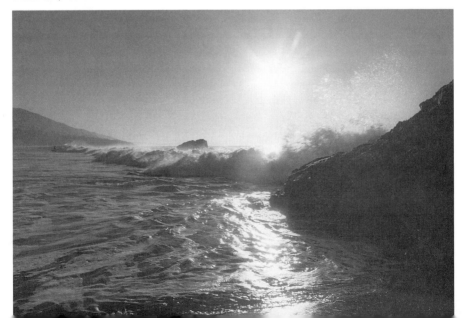

the Palos Verdes peninsula, Santa Catalina Island, and several of the other Channel Islands off Ventura and Santa Barbara. In the north, the toothy crest of Boney Mountain barely peeks over a rounded ridge opposite the Arroyo Sequit. Below, in the west, you'll look down on the sycamore-dotted Leo Carrillo Campground, stretching for almost half a mile along a flat terrace just above Arroyo Sequit's parched bed.

When it's time to go, return to the four-way junction. Take the left branch this time, returning by way of the lower Nicholas Flat Trail.

## trip 2 Nicholas Flat

see map on p. 174

| | |
|---|---|
| **Distance** | 1.5 miles round trip, Out-and-back |
| **Hiking Time** | 1 hour (round trip) |
| **Elevation Gain/Loss** | 100'/100' |
| **Difficulty** | Easy |
| **Trail Use** | Good for kids |
| **Best Times** | All year |
| **Agency** | LCSP |
| **Optional Map** | USGS 7.5-min *Triunfo Pass* |
| **Notes** | Marked trails/obvious routes, easy terrain |

**DIRECTIONS** From Pacific Coast Highway, at a point 25 miles west of Santa Monica, turn north on Decker Road (Highway 23). Continue 2.5 miles north and turn west on Decker School Road. Drive to the roadend, where you will find the Nicholas Flat Trailhead.

Nicholas Flat harbors a small oasis of live oaks and an old cattle pond backed by picturesque sandstone outcrops. During the spring, the grassy meadows above the pond may put on an eye-popping wildflower show. Because so many plant communities converge in this one area—coastal sage scrub, grassland, chaparral, and oak woodland—Nicholas Flat is a good bet for bird- and wildlife-watching too.

From the trailhead, a pleasant, oak-lined path leads south to an intersection just above the pond. Bear right to visit the oak-dotted west shore or the grassy area north of the pond. Amid the oaks you can look for a bedrock *metate* (grinding slick), where the native Americans of the Chumash tribe milled acorns. In wetter times, the pond brims with water, while in drought years it can turn bone-dry by late summer, with gaping cracks up to 2 feet deep in the adobe mud at the bottom.

That's as far as you go for the easy hike as capsulized above. To explore more, you can work your way around the lake to the top of the sandstone outcrops on the south side (watch out for poison oak, though). From there you get a fine view through the gorge of San Nicholas Canyon to the blue ocean below.

A somewhat better view can be had by hiking up to a 1680-foot knob on the ridge to the west (an extra gain and loss of 300 feet, entirely on trail). An excursion farther afield can take you past a 1838-foot high point along the Malibu Springs Trail, and then back to Decker School Road.

Nicholas Flat can also be approached from the Leo Carrillo Campground, a half-day's leisurely hike for the round trip.

## trip 3  Leo Carrillo Traverse

| | |
|---:|:---|
| **Distance** | 5.2 miles, Point-to-point |
| **Hiking Time** | 3 hours |
| **Elevation Gain/Loss** | 1500'/1900' |
| **Difficulty** | Moderately strenuous |
| **Best Times** | October through June |
| **Agency** | LCSP |
| **Optional Map** | USGS 7.5-min *Triunfo Pass* |
| **Notes** | Marked trails/obvious routes, moderate terrain |

see map on p. 174

**DIRECTIONS** *North End:* From Santa Monica, drive 27 miles west (up the coast) from Santa Monica, and turn north on Mulholland Highway. Drive 3.2 miles north on Mulholland to the foot of the Malibu Springs Trail, on the right. *South End:* The route ends at the entrance to Leo Carrillo Campground, just east of the intersection of Pacific Coast Highway and Mulholland Highway.

This one-way hike goes from the confluence of Arroyo Sequit's East and West forks to Leo Carrillo Campground—the hard way. Mulholland Highway is the easy way. You can quickly set up a car shuttle by leaving one car at Leo Carrillo Campground, and taking the other to the starting point at mile 3.2 on Mulholland Highway. (Even if you don't have two cars, you could walk or use a bicycle to cover 3.2 miles of narrow pavement to "close" the loop. Early morning is a good time to try this. Before 7 a.m. there's virtually no traffic on this remote and scenic stretch of Mulholland.)

From the trailhead on Mulholland Highway, an old road bed—now a marked hiking trail—slants up the slope to the south. In essence, you go up and over Arroyo Sequit's east ridge, starting out in oak woodland and chaparral, and ending in coastal sage-scrub vegetation as you approach the ocean. The value of an early-morning start will be apparent as you begin with a bang: 1400 feet of ascent in 2 miles. On the way up, you swing around several hairpin turns, discovering ever-more-impressive vistas of Boney Mountain and the deep crease in the mountains below it—Arroyo Sequit's West Fork. In the north you'll spot the Triunfo Lookout site, now occupied by a huge, boxy structure serving as a passive reflector for microwave transmissions. Down in the val-ley to the east are the big, white "ears" of a satellite tracking station.

Before reaching the top of the ridge, with about 200 vertical feet to go, you pass a trail that forks left and contours eastward. Take it only if you want to extend your hike by circling around to visit Nicholas Flat. This junction also marks the spot where you leave National Park Service land (Malibu Springs open-space area) and enter Leo Carrillo State Park property.

The 1838-foot summit ahead is the highest point on the whole ridge, but you'll have even better ocean views ahead. Drop down to a junction at a saddle (2.4 miles), keep right, and continue south along a brushy ridge overlooking Nicholas Flat. At the next trail junction, where the Nicholas Flat Trail comes in from the left, stay right again. On the saddle just southwest, the Nicholas Flat Trail descends to the right, and a fire break continues south to a 1737-foot knoll. Detour to the top for the best ocean and coastline view of all.

The final, bone-jarring descent to Leo Carrillo Campground features almost 1700 feet of elevation loss in 2.4 miles. A mile from the end, you have a choice: go left down along Willow Creek, or right down the slope overlooking the campground. Both paths are scenic and about equally direct.

**SANTA MONICA MOUNTAINS**

# trip 4  Charmlee Wilderness Park

|              |                           |
|--------------|---------------------------|
| **Distance** | 2.8 miles, Loop |
| **Hiking Time** | 1½ hours |
| **Elevation Gain/Loss** | 500'/500' |
| **Difficulty** | Easy |
| **Trail Use** | Dogs allowed, good for kids |
| **Best Times** | All year |
| **Agency** | CWP |
| **Optional Map** | USGS 7.5-min *Triunfo Pass* |
| **Notes** | Marked trails/obvious routes, easy terrain |

**DIRECTIONS** From Santa Monica, drive 25 miles west on Pacific Coast Highway (Highway 1), turn north on Encinal Canyon Road, and proceed north 4 miles to the park's well-marked entrance. Gates are open 8 a.m. to sunset daily.

Charmlee Wilderness Park (aka Charmlee Natural Area), 590 acres of meadow, oak woodland, sage scrub, and chaparral, was first opened to the public in 1981 as a unit of the Los Angeles County park system. Today the City of Malibu administers the park, which lies on that coastal city's western extremity. Never designed to accommodate a large number of visitors, Charmlee's parking lot is often full on the weekends. A spiderweb of trails totaling 8 miles covers the park, making it a great place to ramble with family and friends for the purpose of wildflower spotting in spring, and ocean watching on any clear day. Here's one option to follow on foot:

From the parking lot, walk on pavement to the nature center (inside, pick up a guide for the Fire Ecology Trail and other interpretive materials). Bear right on a paved road, soon dirt, that bends north up a slope. Make an acute left turn at the top, follow a ridge road past a hilltop water tank (detour and walk around the tank for a good overview of the park and the ocean), and then curve down to a T-intersection. Jog right, then go left on the Fire Ecology Trail. After a few minutes you will be passing under some fire-singed coast live oaks, which are well known for their ability to survive fast-moving wildfires.

Next, go right on the wide trail that winds along the west edge of Charmlee's large, central meadow. Continue all the way to a dry ridge topped by some old eucalyptus trees and a concrete-lined cistern, both relics of cattle-ranching days. From there descend south (stay right at the next junction) to the "Ocean Vista," which really delivers in a big way what its name suggests, especially on clear days. In addition to miles of surf and sand seemingly at your feet, your eyes drink in perhaps a thousand square miles of wind-ruffled ocean.

Circle north from Ocean Vista around the hill with the cistern and then along the east side of the meadow. When you come to the northeast part of the meadow and the dirt road curves west, pick up the hard-to-spot Botany Trail on the right. It winds through mostly chaparral vegetation and takes you to the picnic area just above your starting point.

If it's a spring day and you've kept a tally of wildflowers spotted on the hike, you may be surprised to find your list includes as many as two dozen or more.

# trip 5 Arroyo Sequit Park

| | |
|---|---|
| **Distance** | 1.2 miles, Loop |
| **Hiking Time** | 1 hour |
| **Elevation Gain/Loss** | 150'/150' |
| **Difficulty** | Easy |
| **Trail Use** | Suitable for mountain biking, dogs allowed, good for kids |
| **Best Times** | November through June |
| **Agency** | SMMC |
| **Optional Map** | USGS 7.5-min *Triunfo Pass* |
| **Notes** | Marked trails/obvious routes, easy terrain |

see map on p. 174

**DIRECTIONS** From the 101 Freeway, take the Westlake Boulevard (Highway 23) exit in Thousand Oaks. Turn south on Highway 23, and drive 5 miles south to Mulholland Highway, where you turn right. Watch the roadside mileage markers and drive to mile 5.6 to reach the Arroyo Sequit Park on the left, which has the posted address of 34138 Mulholland Highway. Turn left and park in the small lot, which is open daily 8 a.m. to sunset.

Diminutive Arroyo Sequit Park, a 155-acre former ranch that is now a unit of the Santa Monica Mountains National Recreation Area, is a bit hidden in one of the more remote parts of the mountains between Malibu and Thousand Oaks. This patch of land appears drab and dry at least half the year—but winter rains can transform it instantly into an emerald paradise. Bring the kids here for a little hiking, picnicking, wildflower hunting, or bird watching. It is entirely possible to visit the site on a weekday and see no one else on the trail.

Pass through a gate and walk up the access road into the park. Veer left toward a

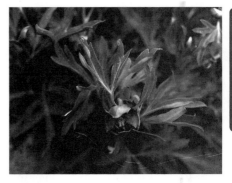

Wild peony

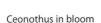

Ceonothus in bloom

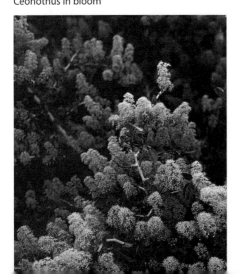

restored barn (used for meetings) and pass a small picnic area shaded by oaks. On the right, you'll see a marked hiking trail slanting up and across a meadow. On that trail, you'll circle to the rim of a little canyon (an upper tributary of the stream called Arroyo Sequit), where you can catch an outstanding view of Boney Mountain, the highest promontory in the Santa Monica range. You then curve back down through more grassland—dotted with spring wildflowers and blooming plants such as wild peony and ceanothus—and loop back to the park entrance.

SANTA MONICA MOUNTAINS

## trip 6  The Grotto

| | |
|---|---|
| **Distance** | 2.6 miles round trip, Out-and-back |
| **Hiking Time** | 1½ hours (round trip) |
| **Elevation Gain/Loss** | 650'/650' |
| **Difficulty** | Moderate |
| **Trail Use** | Dogs allowed, good for kids |
| **Best Times** | All year |
| **Agency** | NPS |
| **Optional Map** | USGS 7.5-min *Triunfo Pass* |
| **Notes** | Marked trails/obvious routes, easy terrain |

see map on p. 174

**DIRECTIONS** From the 101 Freeway, exit at southbound Highway 23 (Westlake Boulevard) in Thousand Oaks. Stay on southbound Highway 23 for 7 miles to reach Mulholland Highway on the right. Take Mulholland 0.4 mile west to Little Sycamore Canyon Road on the right. Then drive 5.5 miles on Little Sycamore Canyon Road (which becomes Yerba Buena Road in a couple of miles when you cross the Ventura County line) to the Circle X Ranch park office on the left.

The 1655-acre Circle X Ranch, formerly run by the Boy Scouts of America but now administered by the National Park Service, is positively riddled with Tom Sawyer-esque hiking paths. The Grotto and Mishe Mokwa (see Trip 7) trails are among the most interesting in the whole Santa Monica Mountain range.

From the park office, start off on a dirt road leading downhill some 100 yards toward a group campground. Walk through or skirt the campsites, and pick up a trail heading south down along a shady, seasonal creek. Keep heading downhill as you pass, in quick succession, two trails coming in from the left. Very shortly afterward, you cross the creek at a point immediately above a 30-foot ledge which becomes a trickling waterfall in winter and spring. You then go uphill, gaining about 50 feet of elevation, and cross an open meadow offering fine views of both Boney Mountain above and Arroyo Sequit's West Fork gorge below. Next you begin a steep descent leading to the bottom of the gorge.

When you come upon an old roadbed at the bottom, stay left, cross the creek, and continue downstream on a narrowing trail along the shaded east bank. Curve left when you reach a grove of fantastically twisted

Live-oak woodland above The Grotto

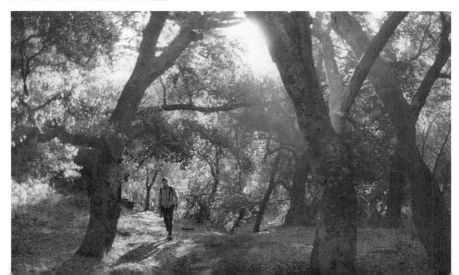

live oaks at the confluence of two stream forks. On the edge of this grove, an overflow pipe coming out of a tank discharges tepid spring water. (From this point on, dogs are prohibited on the "trail," which is actually the streambed itself.) Continue another 200 yards down along the now-lively brook to The Grotto, a narrow, spooky constriction flanked by sheer volcanic-rock walls. If your sense of balance is good and your footwear is appropriate, you can clamber over gray-colored rock ledges and massive boulders fallen from the canyon walls—just as thousands of Boy Scouts have done in the past. At one spot you can peer cautiously into a gloomy cavern, where the subterranean stream is more easily heard than seen. Water marks on the boulders above are evidence that this part of the gorge probably supports a two-tier stream in times of flood.

When you've had your fill of adventuring, return by the same route, uphill almost the whole way.

## trip 7  Sandstone Peak

| | |
|---|---|
| **Distance** | 5.8 miles, Loop |
| **Hiking Time** | 3½ hours |
| **Elevation Gain/Loss** | 1400'/1400' |
| **Difficulty** | Moderately strenuous |
| **Trail Use** | Dogs allowed |
| **Best Times** | October through June |
| **Agency** | NPS |
| **Optional Maps** | USGS 7.5-min *Triunfo Pass, Newbury Park* |
| **Notes** | Marked trails/obvious routes, moderate terrain |

see map on p. 174

**SANTA MONICA MOUNTAINS**

**DIRECTIONS** From the 101 Freeway, exit at southbound Highway 23 (Westlake Boulevard) in Thousand Oaks. Stay on southbound Highway 23 for 7 miles to reach Mulholland Highway on the right. Take Mulholland 0.4 mile west to Little Sycamore Canyon Road on the right. Then drive 4.5 miles on Little Sycamore Canyon Road (which becomes Yerba Buena Road in a couple of miles when you cross the Ventura County line) to a trailhead parking area for the Backbone Trail on the right.

Sandstone Peak is the quintessential destination for peak baggers in the Santa Monica Mountains. The 3111-foot summit can be efficiently climbed from the east via the Backbone Trail in a mere 1.5 miles, but the far more scenic way to go is the looping route outlined below. Take a picnic lunch and plan to make a half day of it. Try to come on a crystalline day in late fall or winter to take best advantage of the skyline views. Or, if it's wildflowers you most enjoy, come in April or May, when the native vegetation blooms best at these middle elevations. In addition to blue-flowering stands of ceanothus, the early-to-mid-spring bloom includes monkey flower, nightshade, Chinese houses, wild peony, wild hyacinth, morning glory, and phacelia. Delicate, orangish Humboldt lilies unfold by June.

Sandstone Peak lies within Circle X Ranch—formerly owned by the Boy Scouts of America, and now a federally managed unit of the Santa Monica Mountains National Recreation Area.

From the trailhead, hike past a gate and up a fire road 0.3 mile to where the marked Mishe Mokwa Trail branches right. On it, right away, you plunge into tough, scratchy chaparral vegetation. The hand-tooled route is delightfully primitive, but requires frequent maintenance so as to keep the chaparral from knitting together across the path. Both your hands and your feet will come into play over the next 40 or 50 minutes as you're forced to scramble a bit over rough-textured outcrops of volcanic rock. You'll make intimate acquaintance with mosses and ferns and several of the more attractive chaparral shrubs: toyon, hollyleaf cherry, manzanita, and red shanks (aka ribbonwood), which is identified by its wispy foliage and perpetually peeling, rust-colored bark. You'll also pass several small bay trees. After about a half hour on the Mishe Mokwa Trail, keep an eye out for an amazing balanced rock that rests precariously on the opposite wall of the canyon that lies just below you.

By 1.7 miles from the start you will have worked you way around to the north flank of Sandstone Peak, where you suddenly come upon a couple of picnic tables and "Split Rock," a fractured volcanic boulder with a gap wide enough to walk through (please do so to maintain the Scouts' tradition). From then on, you continue on an old dirt road that crosses the aforementioned canyon and turns west (upstream). You pass beneath some hefty volcanic outcrops and at 2.8 miles come to a junction with the Backbone Trail. That leg of the Backbone Trail, a narrow path, goes west into Point Mugu State Park. Keep straight (south) on the graded fire road ahead, signed Backbone Trail, and gradually circle east.

A few minutes beyond some water tanks on the right, look for a side path going right. This takes you about 50 yards to the top of an rock outcrop—Inspiration Point. The direction-finder there indicates local features as well as very distant points such as Mount San Antonio, Santa Catalina Island, and San Clemente Island.

Press on with your ascent. At a point just past two closely spaced hairpin turns in the wide Backbone Trail, make your way up a slippery path to Sandstone Peak's windswept top. The plaque on the summit block

honors W. Herbert Allen, a long-time benefactor of the Scouts and Circle X Ranch. To the Scouts this mountain is "Mount Allen," although that name has not, so far, been accepted by cartographers. In any event, the peak's real name is misleading. It, along with Boney Mountain and most of the western crest of the Santa Monicas, consists of beige- and rust-colored volcanic rock, not unlike sandstone when seen from a distance.

On a clear day the view is truly amazing from here, with distant mountain ranges, the hazy L.A. Basin, and the island-dimpled surface of the ocean occupying all 360 degrees of the horizon. To complete the loop, return to the Backbone Trail and resume your travel eastward. One-and-a-half miles of twisting descent will take you back to the trailhead.

Volcanic outcrop on Boney Mountain

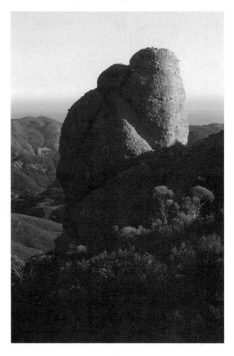

# chapter 16

# Santa Monica Mountains: Point Mugu

**M**ugu, a corruption of the Chumash word *muwu*, meaning beach, lends its name to a rocky promontory jutting into the ocean, a bald peak towering behind it, and one of the larger state parks in California—16,000-acre Point Mugu State Park.

Geographically speaking, the Point Mugu area is the last gasp of the Santa Monica Mountains up the coast from Los Angeles. Geologists, however, say that the underpinnings of these mountains really extend as far west as the Channel Islands off Santa Barbara. The intervening low area, occupied by the flat, silty Oxnard Plain and part of the continental shelf offshore, is a structurally huge syncline, or downfold of crustal rocks. Paleontological evidence has shown that for a long period ending 1 or 2 million years ago the islands were linked to the mainland by an isthmus. This ancient feature is named the Cabrillo Peninsula, after the 16th Century explorer Juan Rodriguez Cabrillo, who was buried on the westernmost island, San Miguel.

Point Mugu State Park lies entirely outside Los Angeles County's boundary, but it's an integral and important part of the Santa Monica Mountains National Recreation Area so it merits a chapter in this book. Recreational opportunities here are superb. Almost half the park's area comprises the Boney Mountain State Wilderness—remote, wild, and open to hikers and equestrians only.

The two principal park entrances—both off Pacific Coast Highway—are Big Sycamore Canyon and the Ray Miller Trailhead at La Jolla Canyon. Big Sycamore Canyon, in particular, is one of the favored areas on the California coast for overwintering Monarch butterflies.

Abutting the north end of the park, next to suburban Newbury Park, is the Rancho Sierra Vista/Satwiwa natural area and cultural park, managed by the National Park Service. In addition to serving as a northern trailhead for the state park (easily accessible from the Ventura Freeway), Rancho Sierra Vista features the Satwiwa Native American Indian Culture Center, where park rangers or Native American hosts offer interpretive programs on the weekends.

With about 100 miles of trails lacing the Point Mugu area, it's possible to devise more than a dozen loop trips significantly different from one another. Six routes are included in this chapter, on trails ranging from paved service roads and graded fire roads to primitive pathways suitable for hikers only. These specific routes are not available for use by mountain bicyclists, because they include portions of "single-track" trail, which (for the purposes of state park rules) are reserved for hikers and equestrians.

Camping opportunities in the Point Mugu area are plentiful. There are developed campgrounds at Thornhill Broome Beach and Sycamore Canyon (hot showers at the latter). Backpackers can pitch a tent at La Jolla Valley Walk-in Camp, a 2.5-mile hike by the shortest route. Organizations can reserve group-camping facilities at the Danielson and Sycamore Multi-use areas.

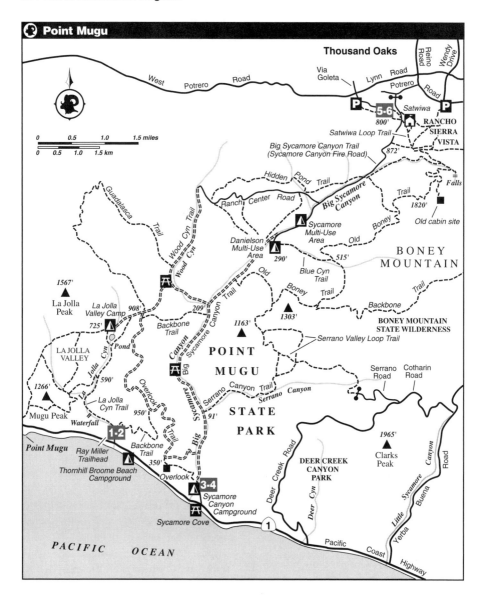

## trip 1  La Jolla Falls

| | |
|---|---|
| **Distance** | 1.8 miles round trip, Out-and-back |
| **Hiking Time** | 1 hour (round trip) |
| **Elevation Gain/Loss** | 250'/250' |
| **Difficulty** | Easy |
| **Trail Use** | Good for kids |
| **Best Times** | December through June |
| **Agency** | PMSP |
| **Optional Map** | USGS 7.5-min *Point Mugu* |
| **Notes** | Marked trails/obvious routes, easy terrain |

see map on p. 184

**DIRECTIONS** From Santa Monica, drive west (up the coast) on Pacific Coast Highway for 34 miles to the Ray Miller Trailhead, on the right, in Point Mugu State Park.

The modest 15-foot-tall cascade in La Jolla Canyon is a pleasant destination for an introductory exploration of Point Mugu State Park. Just be sure to come after recent rains have been sufficient to enliven the flow of water through the canyon.

From the Ray Miller Trailhead, follow the wide La Jolla Canyon Trail north. Your route initially follows a dirt road used to haul stone for the construction of Pacific Coast Highway in the 1920s. After about 0.7 mile, the trail passes the quarry site and starts climbing. With a small amount of huffing and puffing, you arrive at the falls. Willows and a native species of walnut tree grace the canyon hereabouts. They're handy if you're looking for some shade.

Beyond the falls, the trail continues sharply uphill toward La Jolla Valley (covered in Trip 2 below)—but you simply turn back at this point, assuming your only destination is the falls.

## trip 2  La Jolla Valley & Mugu Peak

| | |
|---|---|
| **Distance** | 10.8 miles, Loop |
| **Hiking Time** | 5½ hours |
| **Elevation Gain/Loss** | 1950'/1950' |
| **Difficulty** | Moderately strenuous |
| **Trail Use** | Suitable for backpacking |
| **Best Times** | October through June |
| **Agency** | PMSP |
| **Optional Map** | USGS 7.5-min *Point Mugu* |
| **Notes** | Marked trails/obvious routes, easy terrain |

see map on p. 184

**DIRECTIONS** From Santa Monica, drive west (up the coast) on Pacific Coast Highway for 34 miles to the Ray Miller Trailhead, on the right, in Point Mugu State Park.

Lazily curving up the rumpled slopes of the western Santa Monica Mountains, the Ray Miller Trail takes in sweeping views of the Point Mugu coastline and the distant Channel Islands. This is the westernmost link in the nearly completed Backbone Trail, which skims along the crest of the Santa Monicas for some 65 miles. The Ray Miller Trail offers a well-graded and scenic approach to the rounded ridge that divides

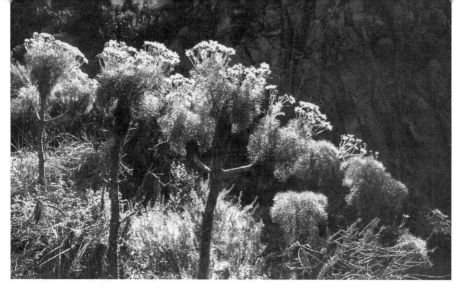

Giant coreopsis, Point Mugu State Park

the two largest canyons in Point Mugu State Park: La Jolla and Big Sycamore canyons.

The Ray Miller Trail is just the start of the big loop we're suggesting here: a comprehensive trek through the western quadrant of Point Mugu State Park. If this is too big a chunk to bite off for a single day, there are short cuts, as this chapter's map suggests. You could also extend your trip by staying overnight at La Jolla Valley Walk-in Camp. For that, you must register with a park ranger first.

Start hiking at the Ray Miller Trailhead. Two trails diverge from the parking lot there. The wide one going up along the dry canyon bottom ahead is the La Jolla Canyon Trail—your return route. To begin, take the narrower Ray Miller (aka Backbone) Trail to your right. It doggedly climbs 2.4 miles to a junction with the Overlook Trail, a wide fire road. This is the major ascent along the loop—better to get it over with at the beginning. Ever-widening views of the ocean and fine, springtime wildflower displays keep your mind off the effort.

Turn left when you reach the Overlook Trail, and wend your way around several bumps on the undulating ridge. You arrive at a saddle (4.5 miles from the start), where five trails diverge. Take the trail to the left (west) that descends into the green- or flaxen-colored (depending on the season) La Jolla Valley.

The valley is managed by the state park as a natural preserve to protect the native bunchgrasses that flourish there. Because so much of California's coast ranges have been biologically disturbed by grazing for more than a century, opportunistic, non-native grasses have taken over just about everywhere. The authentic California "tallgrass prairie" in parts of La Jolla Valley is a notable exception.

The La Jolla Valley Walk-in Camp ahead has piped water, restrooms, and oak-shaded picnic tables. Just south of there, beside a trail leading directly back to the Ray Miller Trailhead, you'll find a tule-fringed pond, seasonally dry in some years. Look for chocolate lilies on the slopes around it.

From the camp, continue west in the direction of a military radar installation on Laguna Peak. Stay right where marked trails diverge to the left, circling the perimeter of the La Jolla Valley grassland, and rising sharply on the Chumash Trail to a saddle (6.7 miles) on the northwest shoulder of the Mugu Peak ridge. At that saddle you'll have a great view of the Pacific Ocean. The popping noises you may hear below are from a military shooting range, near Pacific Coast Highway. Up the coast lies the Point Mugu Naval Air Station.

From the saddle, Chumash Trail descends sharply to Pacific Coast Highway. You veer left on the Mugu Peak Trail, and contour south and east around the south flank of Mugu Peak. You arrive (7.7 miles) at another saddle just east of Mugu's 1266-foot summit. Five minutes of climbing on a steep path puts you on top, where there's a dizzying view of the east-west-oriented coastline. You can look down upon The Great Sand Dune (coastal dunes) and Pacific Coast Highway, where it barely squeezes past some coastal bluffs. On warm days there's a desertlike feel to this rocky and sparsely vegetated mountain, oddly juxtaposed with the sights and sounds of the surf below.

Return to the saddle east of the peak and continue descending to a junction in a wooded recess of La Jolla Canyon. Turn right, proceed east along a hillside, and then hook up with the La Jolla Canyon Trail (9.7 miles), where you turn right.

There's an exciting stretch down through a rock-walled section of La Jolla Canyon, where you'll see magnificent springtime displays of giant coreopsis. This plant is quite common in the Channel Islands, but is found only in scattered coastal locales from far western Los Angeles County to San Luis Obispo County. Some coreopsis plants have forked stems towering as high as 10 feet, head and shoulders above the surrounding scrub. The massed, yellow, daisylike flowers are an unforgettable sight in March and April.

Descending toward the canyon's mouth, you'll pass a little grove of native walnut trees and the small, seasonal La Jolla Canyon waterfall. After a final descent, you'll join an old dirt road that leads straightway to your starting point, the Ray Miller Trailhead.

La Jolla Canyon, Point Mugu State Park

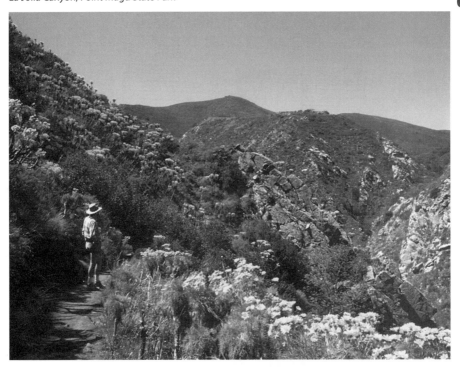

## trip 3  Overlook Loop

see map on p. 184

| | |
|---|---|
| **Distance** | 2.6 miles, Loop |
| **Hiking Time** | 1½ hours |
| **Elevation Gain/Loss** | 350'/350' |
| **Difficulty** | Easy |
| **Trail Use** | Good for kids |
| **Best Times** | All year |
| **Agency** | PMSP |
| **Optional Map** | USGS 7.5-min *Point Mugu* |
| **Notes** | Marked trails/obvious routes, easy terrain |

**DIRECTIONS** From Santa Monica, drive west (up the coast) on Pacific Coast Highway for 32 miles to Sycamore Canyon Campground, on the right, in Point Mugu State Park. There's a day-use parking lot here.

The Overlook above Sycamore Canyon Campground offers an almost straight-down view of white, foamy surf and turquoise-tinted shallows. When the tide and surf conditions are just right, and the water's glassy, you can watch the swells reflect off the shore and head back out to sea, producing an ever-changing interference pattern on the surface of the water.

This is an easy loop trip, unlike the much longer one that hikers and mountain bikers often take by linking the whole,

Indian paintbrush

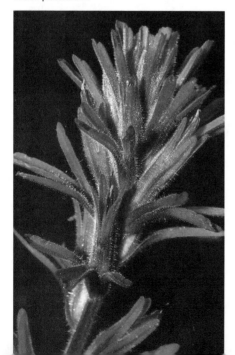

ridge-running Overlook Trail with trails in Wood and Big Sycamore canyons. This more leisurely approach will give you time to pay closer attention to the wildflowers and wildlife. Deer frequent these slopes in the early morning and evening.

From the day-use parking lot at Sycamore Canyon Campground, head north through the campground and past a vehicle gate. Just past that gate start up the Scenic Trail on the left. You curve up a hillside and arrive after about 15 minutes at a saddle overlooking the ocean. Walk down to a little flat below for a better view. Nestled against the cliff below is a sloping blanket of sand called The Great Sand Dune. Prevailing sea breezes from the west and south keep it in place.

When it's time to go, pick up the fire road that curves down the high ridge to the north—the Overlook Trail. Follow its winding course downhill to Big Sycamore Canyon, turn right, and walk back to the campground.

## trip 4  Serrano & Big Sycamore Loop

| | |
|---|---|
| **Distance** | 9.8 miles, Loop |
| **Hiking Time** | 4½ hours |
| **Elevation Gain/Loss** | 1250'/1250' |
| **Difficulty** | Moderately strenuous |
| **Best Times** | October through July |
| **Agency** | PMSP |
| **Optional Maps** | USGS 7.5-min *Point Mugu, Triunfo Pass* |
| **Notes** | Marked trails/obvious routes, easy terrain |

see
map on
p. 184

**DIRECTIONS** From Santa Monica, drive west (up the coast) on Pacific Coast Highway for 32 miles to Syca-more Canyon Campground, on the right, in Point Mugu State Park. There's a day-use parking lot here.

There's something nice about this hike in just about any season. October through December can bring warm, dry winds and fall color—muted yellows and oranges—to the sycamores. During the rainy season, mostly December through March, runoff cascades through the canyon bottoms, and the grasslands come to life. March, April and May are great for wildflowers—even as the grass bleaches to white and gold. June and July are warm, but tolerable under the shade of the spreading oaks in Serrano Canyon, where delicate, orange Humboldt lilies sway in the breeze.

Two caveats: Bring all the water you'll need, and watch out for poison oak, especially in Serrano Canyon. From the day-use parking lot, head north through Sycamore Campground, past the vehicle gate, and up along the wide dirt road (Big Sycamore Canyon Trail) through park-like Big Sycamore Canyon. Proceed to a major fork in the canyon, 1.5 miles from Pacific Coast Highway, and bear right on the Serrano Canyon Trail. After a rather dry, open stretch you enter the steep-walled canyon.

Serrano Canyon is a real treasure—narrow, private, filled with thickets of dark live oaks, pale sycamores, pungent bay laurels, and a green carpet of wild blackberry, ferns, and poison oak. The stream carves its way in a couple of spots through bedrock and gathers in shallow pools.

At 2.9 miles, the Serrano Canyon Trail leaves the canyon, bearing left up a ravine and onto a grassy slope. Stay left at the next three intersections, ignoring the Serrano Valley Loop Trail, which loops around the valley. You gain elevation through chaparral and reach a gap in the ridge above you. At this gap (4.5 miles) you can look down upon a slice of Big Sycamore Canyon. You're now on the far west shoulder of Boney Mountain; eastward the ridge undulates toward its high point at Sandstone Peak. Follow the trail for another 0.4 mile, up along the ridge and then down a little to meet the Old Boney Trail. Swing left there and go sharply downhill for 1.2 miles to Big Sycamore Canyon Trail.

Four pleasant, easy miles remain in Big Sycamore Canyon. The park's brochure boasts of the canyon as being "the finest example of a sycamore savanna in the State Park System." It's true enough. Some of the gangly sycamores soar to heights of about 80 feet. Look for deer, bobcats, and coyotes in the grass, and owls and hawks nesting in the trees. If it's fall or early winter, you may see masses of Monarch butterflies in some of the trees.

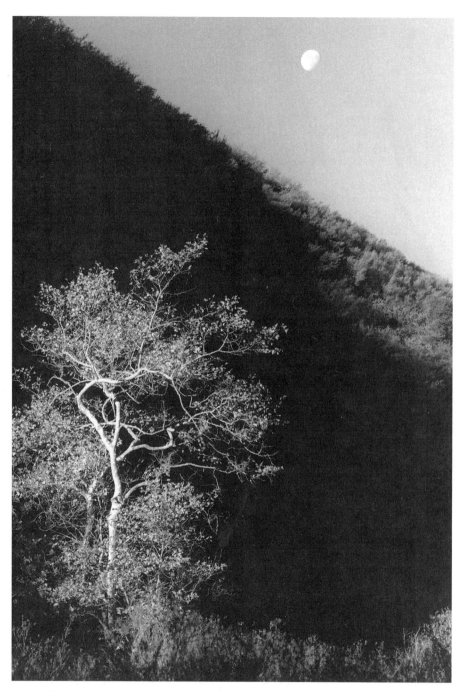

Serrano Canyon sycamores in late afternoon

## **trip 5**  Sycamore Canyon Waterfall

see map on p. 184

| | |
|---|---|
| **Distance** | 3.4 miles round trip, Out-and-back |
| **Hiking Time** | 2 hours (round trip) |
| **Elevation Gain/Loss** | 350'/350' |
| **Difficulty** | Moderate |
| **Trail Use** | Good for kids |
| **Best Times** | December through June |
| **Agency** | NPS |
| **Optional Map** | USGS 7.5-min *Newbury Park* |
| **Notes** | Marked trails/obvious routes, easy terrain |

**DIRECTIONS**  Exit Highway 101 at Lynn Road in Thousand Oaks, and turn south. Drive 5.6 miles on Lynn Road to the Rancho Sierra Vista/Satwiwa Park entrance on the left. Continue past a gate (open daylight hours) and arrive, after a half mile, at a large trailhead parking area.

Point Mugu State Park's Big Sycamore Canyon is famous for its miles-long promenade of magnificent California sycamore trees. Higher up and farther inland, hidden in that same drainage, you can find an intimate little waterfall. The falls deliver a melodious whisper most of the year—but try to visit them in the aftermath of recent rainfall, when they play at a larger volume.

From the trailhead, head southeast on an unpaved service road to the paved Big Sycamore Canyon Trail, 0.2 mile away. Jog briefly right, then veer left on the Satwiwa Loop Trail, bypassing the Satwiwa Native American Culture Center and a Chumash Indian demonstration village (worth a visit on the return leg of your hike). Following signs to the waterfall, aim southeast across a gorgeous meadow, more or less toward the toothy ridgeline called Boney Mountain. You pick up the Old Boney Trail (an old roadbed), which climbs to a small crest (1.0 mile) and then starts descending into the upper reaches of Big Sycamore Canyon. You're now crossing from Rancho Sierra Vista Park into Point Mugu State Park.

At the bottom of the grade, Old Boney Trail swings across the Big Sycamore stream (1.5 miles), and then strikes uphill. That's where you leave Old Boney Trail and turn left onto the narrow, rough Waterfall Trail. You work your way 0.2 mile upstream to the cascades, which lie in a north-facing grotto almost perpetually shaded from the direct rays of the sun. The falling and flowing water around you is framed by a wild and tangled assortment of oak and sycamore limbs overhead. Given that you've spent only an hour walking in to this spot from the edge of the suburbs, the beauty, serenity, and splendid isolation of the place is a bit hard to believe. Don't get too carried away—rattlesnakes seem to like this cozy corner as well.

Big Sycamore Canyon, Point Mugu State Park

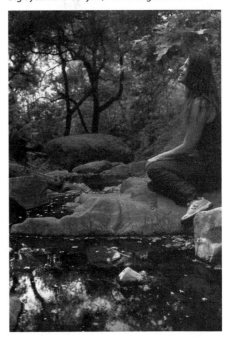

SANTA MONICA MOUNTAINS

# trip 6  Old Boney Loop

see
map on
p. 184

|  |  |
|---|---|
| **Distance** | 10.3 miles, Loop |
| **Hiking Time** | 5 hours |
| **Elevation Gain/Loss** | 2000'/2000' |
| **Difficulty** | Moderately strenuous |
| **Best Times** | November through June |
| **Agency** | PMSP |
| **Optional Maps** | USGS 7.5-min *Newbury Park, Triunfo Pass* |
| **Notes** | Marked trails/obvious routes, easy terrain |

**DIRECTIONS**  Exit Highway 101 at Lynn Road in Thousand Oaks, and turn south. Drive 5.6 miles on Lynn Road to the Rancho Sierra Vista/Satwiwa Park entrance on the left. Continue past a gate (open daylight hours) and arrive, after a half mile, at a large trailhead parking area.

This hike takes you through the heart of the Boney Mountain State Wilderness, which encompasses nearly all the Point Mugu State Park lands east of the Big Sycamore Canyon Trail. As in wilderness areas under federal management (those in the Angeles National Forest and elsewhere), policy here prohibits travel by any mechanical conveyance—even bicycles. Old roads exist from the ranching days, but they are not maintained or improved anymore, except to allow for the passage of hikers and horses.

Boney Mountain, which is the top part of a mass of volcanic rock that solidified roughly 15 million years ago and was later uplifted to its present dominant position, overshadows the area. You'll pass beneath its craggy heights while hiking the Old Boney Trail during the latter part of this trip.

You enter the state park the back way, from Rancho Sierra Vista/Satwiwa park. From the trailhead, head southeast on an unpaved service road to the paved Big Sycamore Canyon Trail, 0.2 mile away. Bear right and follow the pavement, passing into Point Mugu State Park and arriving at an 872-foot summit with a water tank on the right (0.6 mile). You can now look down on Big Sycamore Canyon and the ribbon of pavement you'll be following for the next 2.5 miles. Walking this paved service road is not unpleasant at all, but if you tire of

it there are dirt paths that parallel it from time to time.

Just before the road's end at a ranger residence (3.1 miles), turn left into the Danielson Multi-use Area, one of two such facilities in the park that cater to organized groups of campers, backpackers, and equestrians. The Danielson facility lies on the grounds of the former Danielson Ranch, which was incorporated into Point Mugu State Park in 1973. There are restrooms, and a beautiful, oak-shaded barbecue pit and patio, which is great for a picnic if it's not occupied. Top off your water bottles here with enough to last the rest of the trip.

Now the harder part begins. Head east on the Blue Canyon Trail, under an oak- and sycamore-canopy, until you reach an intersection with the Old Boney Trail (4.1 miles). Make a sharp left there and trudge uphill through hot, dry chaparral to an open ridge. You'll follow the undulating ridge for a while, under the gaze of Boney Mountain's crags, then climb in earnest to another, higher ridge (5.8 miles).

You're going against the grain of the land now, and it feels like it. There's a steep descent of about 200 feet and then another climb of about 550 feet to an 1820-foot summit (6.8 miles). En route you pass a trail leading down to Big Sycamore Canyon; stay right. On a clear day all this labor is offset by the tremendous view of the Oxnard

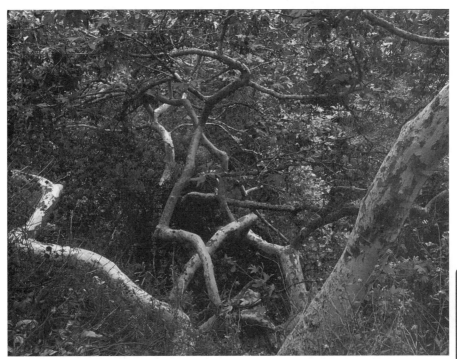

Big Sycamore Canyon sycamores

Plain, the Channel Islands, the far-off ridges of the Los Padres National Forest, and the discontinuous urban sprawl of Ventura County before you.

Beyond the 1820-foot summit, the Old Boney Trail pitches steeply downward, heading toward the uppermost reaches of Big Sycamore Canyon. On the way down, don't miss the side trail on the right, which leads to the "Old Cabin Site," which consists of a foundation and a rock chimney. Nearby is a beautiful monument to Richard E. Danielson made of rock and wrought-iron. Danielson and his family donated a part interest in the lands, which were acquired to expand the state park and create the Rancho Sierra Vista/Satwiwa park.

By 8.5 miles, you'll be swinging around a hairpin turn that wraps around upper Big Sycamore Canyon's stream. At that turn, a side path (Waterfall Trail—see Trip 5 above) goes east to some cascades. Don't miss that little detour if the water's flowing decently.

Back on the Old Boney Trail, continue west 0.2 mile, uphill to where you hook up with the Satwiwa Loop Trail. Follow it northwest toward the Satwiwa Native American interpretive center,which is just west of the paved Big Sycamore Canyon Trail and your starting point.

# chapter 17

# Angeles Forest: Piru Creek

Although relatively unknown among hikers, Piru Creek and its tributaries offer a rugged wilderness experience barely one hour's drive away from the San Fernando Valley and Santa Clarita Valley suburbs. Los Padres National Forest and Angeles National Forest share administrative responsibilities for the area, which lies west of Interstate 5 along the Los Angeles-Ventura county line. The area, which has few roads and trails, is being managed primarily for its value as watershed and wildlife habitat.

In 1992 the gargantuan (220,000-acre) Sespe Wilderness was carved out of lands lying mostly west of Piru Creek. This wilderness area includes the Sespe Condor Sanctuary (closed to all recreational use), where California condors raised in captive breeding programs have been released into the wild. While you're out exploring the places described below, keep an eye on the skies. Spotting a soaring condor is possible; spotting a golden eagle or a turkey vulture is somewhat probable; spotting common raptors such as red-tailed hawks is virtually certain.

Since the first edition of this book was published in 1991, access to the remote wild section of Piru Creek (aka Piru Gorge) has been made more difficult by the closure of Blue Point Campground at the north end of Lake Piru, and the closure (to vehicles) of the paved road around Lake Piru's west shoreline. Trail maintenance has generally been suspended as well, which will make any journey into the remote section of Piru Creek and its Agua Blanca tributary a true wilderness experience.

We begin with a civilized dayhike up a slope not far from Interstate 5—the Oak Flat Trail. The other two trips are best done as overnight backpacks. Fire regulations apply; you'll need a fire permit from Los Padres National Forest in order to operate a camp stove.

All trips in this chapter require a National Forest Adventure Pass ($5 per day, $30 per year) for trailhead parking.

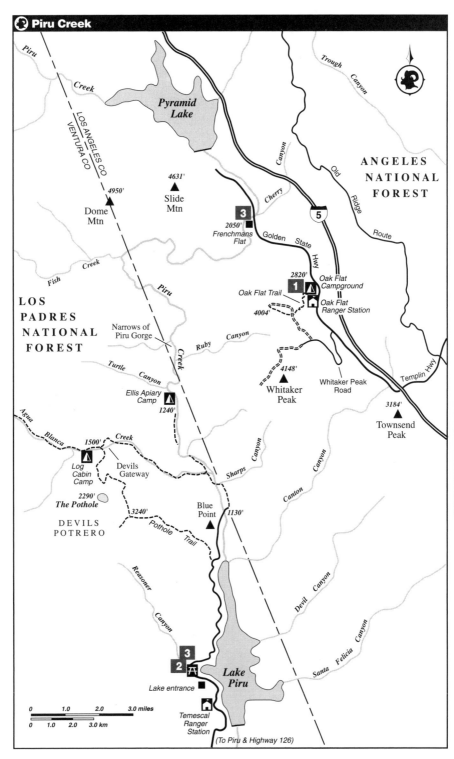

Piru

Creek

LOS ANGELES CO
VENTURA CO

Pyramid
Lake

*4631'*
▲
Slide
Mtn

*4950'*
▲
Dome
Mtn

**ANGELES
NATIONAL
FOREST**

Trough

Canyon

Canyon

Cherry

Old

Ridge

Route

**3**
*2050'* ■
Frenchmans
Flat

Golden    State    Hwy

**5**

Fish    Creek

Piru

**LOS
PADRES
NATIONAL
FOREST**

Narrows of
Piru Gorge

Ruby    Canyon

*2820'*
Oak Flat Trail **1** 🏕
*4004'*

Oak Flat
Campground

Oak Flat
Ranger Station

Turtle    Canyon

Creek

Ellis Apiary
Camp  🏕
*1240'*

*4148'*
▲
**Whitaker
Peak**

Whitaker Peak
Road

Templin Hwy

*3184'*
▲
Townsend
Peak

Agua

Blanca

*1500'*
🏕
Log
Cabin
Camp

Creek

Devils
Gateway

*2290'*
**The Pothole**

**DEVILS
POTRERO**

Sharps    Canyon

Canton    Canyon

Canyon

*3240'*

Pothole    Trail

Blue
Point
▲    *1130'*

Reasoner

Canyon

Devil    Canyon

**3**
**2** 🏕

Lake entrance ■

Temescal
Ranger
Station

*Lake
Piru*

Santa    Felicia    Canyon

0    1.0    2.0    3.0 miles
0    1.0    2.0    3.0 km

(To Piru & Highway 126)

## trip 1 Oak Flat Trail

| | |
|---|---|
| **Distance** | 2.8 miles round trip, Out-and-back |
| **Hiking Time** | 1½ hours (round trip) |
| **Elevation Gain/Loss** | 950'/950' |
| **Difficulty** | Moderate |
| **Trail Use** | Good for kids |
| **Best Times** | All year |
| **Agency** | ANF/SCMRD |
| **Optional Map** | USGS 7.5-min *Whitaker Peak* |
| **Notes** | Marked trails/obvious routes, easy terrain |

see map on p. 195

**DIRECTIONS** Exit I-5 at Templin Highway, about 45 miles northwest of central Los Angeles. Pick up the frontage road on the west side of I-5 (old Highway 99, formerly the main highway) and drive an additional 3 miles northwest to the Oak Flat Campground entrance. Turn left and continue 0.3 mile to a parking area next to the Oak Flat Ranger Station, just short of the Verdugo Oaks Boy Scout camp.

The Oak Flat Trail, the only developed trail along the Interstate 5 corridor through the Angeles National Forest, offers ever-widening vistas of fault-tortured canyon country, and a close look on the way up at some interesting outcrops of breccia—a sedimentary rock resembling conglomerate in appearance, except that the imbedded stones are sharp, not rounded.

The signed Oak Flat Trail begins on the left side of the big, grassy area just inside Camp Verdugo Oaks. Switchbacks take you under a shady canopy of valley oaks and live oaks. Soon, however, you'll climb to scrub-covered slopes exposed to the morning and midday sun.

After surmounting a final set of steeply inclined switchback segments, you reach the Whitaker Spur Road (1.4 miles). From there you can look west into the gorge of Piru Creek, and, if it's clear, farther west into the remote Los Padres country where Cobblestone Mountain, White Mountain, and a half dozen other summits over 5000 feet raise their shaggy heads. In the foreground is a breccia outcrop with a window

Cavernous sedimentary rock above Oak Flat Trail

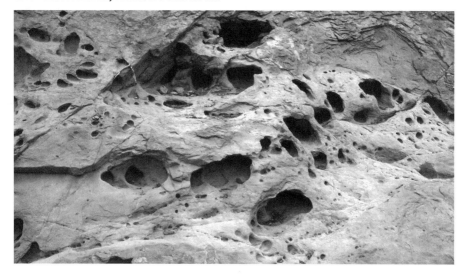

in it. Turning north and east, you'll be able to trace the long hogbacks of Liebre and Sawmill mountains and the gashed face of Redrock Mountain (in the area covered by Chapter 18).

At this point you're standing just east of the San Gabriel Fault, whose trace is not obvious here. The fault continues southeast and east about 70 miles into the San Gabriel Mountains, where it parallels the West and East forks of the San Gabriel River, roughly dividing the so called "Front Range" of the San Gabriels from the "High Country."

You'll return down the same trail. In the meantime, you may want to try following the Whitaker Spur Road 0.7 mile west to a 4004-foot summit offering a nice view of Pyramid Lake to the north. You can also go 0.4 mile south on the same road to see a large outcrop of pock-marked breccia.

## trip 2  Agua Blanca Trail

| | |
|---|---|
| **Distance** | 20 miles round trip (including paved road), Out-and-back |
| **Hiking Time** | 10 hours (round trip) |
| **Elevation Gain/Loss** | 500'/500' |
| **Difficulty** | Moderately strenuous |
| **Trail Use** | Suitable for backpacking, dogs allowed |
| **Best Times** | November through May |
| **Agency** | LPNF/OD |
| **Recommended Map** | USGS 7.5-min *Cobblestone Mtn.* |
| **Notes** | Navigation required, moderate terrain, bushwhacking |

see map on p. 195

**DIRECTIONS** Exit Interstate 5 at westbound Highway 126 (just north of Santa Clarita). Drive 11 miles west to the town of Piru and follow the signs north to Lake Piru. There's a substantial charge for entry and day use of the recreational area at the end of the road. The area above Lake Piru is seldom visited and is mostly out of range of cell-phone signals, so it is imperative to contact Los Padres National Forest (805-646-4348) for the latest information on possible flood conditions, wilderness area rules, and logistics.

In previous editions of this book, the trail following Agua Blanca Creek was linked to the Pothole Trail in the form of a loop hike. That was when hikers had access by car to Blue Point and the former Blue Point Campground nearby. Then, the Pothole Trail became severely overgrown, and the paved service road along the west side of Lake Piru was closed to autos. So today's strategy for reaching the wild and beautiful Agua Blanca Creek is to hike a tedious 6 miles of service road from the Lake Piru Recreation Area to where it ends at Piru Creek. The remainder of the hike takes you up upstream along Piru Creek and then west into its tributary, Agua Blanca Creek. Clever travelers should consider the use of a bicycle for those initial 6 miles and final 6 miles!

From the end of the paved service road, cross Piru Creek and pass through the grounds of the defunct Blue Point Campground. Head north on an old dirt road up along the wide floodplain of Piru Creek. After a mile, swing left at the mouth of the canyon of Agua Blanca Creek. This is in an area called Kesters, a private inholding of property within the national forest. Follow the trail that goes into the canyon—the Agua Blanca Trail. The trail (or at least remnants of it) stays mostly along the steep, shaded south wall of the canyon, but it also fords the creek several times down on the narrow flood plain. At these crossings, you can admire (during times of good flow in winter and spring, at least) the extraordinary transparency of the water.

The going is easier at first, then more difficult as you approach the sheer-walled Devils Gateway. The trail detours around the Gateway by rising some 250 feet up and around the north wall, but as an option you can wade through the 20-foot-wide Gateway itself—in water that's likely to be waist-deep or more during the spring.

Your destination (if you care to press on that far), just beyond Devils Gateway, is the unmaintained Log Cabin trail camp. It is 4 miles from the roadend and a total of 10 miles from Lake Piru's entrance.

## trip 3  Piru Creek

see map on p. 195

| | |
|---|---|
| **Distance** | 21 miles, Point-to-point |
| **Hiking Time** | 14 hours |
| **Elevation Gain/Loss** | 400'/1300' |
| **Difficulty** | Strenuous |
| **Trail Use** | Suitable for backpacking, dogs allowed |
| **Best Times** | October through June |
| **Agency** | LPNF/OD |
| **Recommended Maps** | USGS 7.5-min *Whitaker Peak, Cobblestone Mtn.* |
| **Notes** | Navigation required, moderate terrain, bushwhacking |

**DIRECTIONS  North End:** From Interstate 5, take the Templin Highway exit and drive up the west-side frontage road (old Highway 99) to a point 2 miles past Oak Flat Campground's entrance. There you'll find Frenchmans Flat, a large, dirt parking area on the left. **South End:** Exit Interstate 5 at westbound Highway 126 (just north of Santa Clarita). Drive 11 miles west to the town of Piru and follow the signs north to Lake Piru. There's a substantial charge for day use of the recreational area at the end of the road. The area is seldom visited and mostly out of range of cell-phone signals, so it is imperative to contact Los Padres National Forest (805-646-4348) for the latest information on possible flood conditions, wilderness area rules, and logistics.

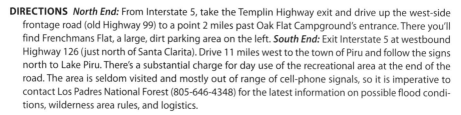

Experienced hikers/backpackers can mount a 2-day expedition down Piru Creek, which involves almost no true climbing but rather many miles of riverbank walking and foot-wetting creek crossings. If the water in the creek is flowing too fast, you will want to postpone your trip.

The unmaintained Ellis Apiary trail camp, on an oak-shaded bench on the west bank of Piru Creek, is a pleasant place to spend the night. The water in Piru Creek can be quite murky, so either bring all the drinking water you'll need or use a water filter.

From Frenchmans Flat, work your way down the cottonwood- and willow-fringed banks, crossing whenever necessary. (Anglers by the score park at Frenchmans Flat and then hike down along Piru Creek in search of trout fishing holes, so there may be plenty of human company initially.) The stream slips over water-worn boulders, some the size of cars, and collects in silt-bottomed pools. You should resign yourself right away to walking in squishy boots. Once you get used to it, the interludes of wading will feel refreshing.

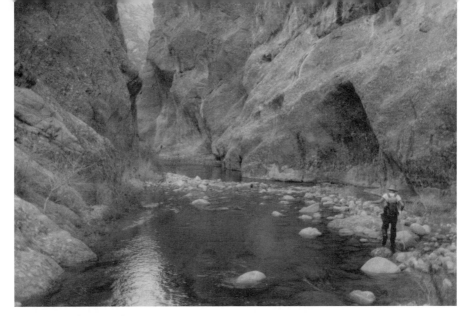

The Narrows of Piru Creek

The seamed and shattered walls down the length of the gorge ahead, up to 500 feet high, disclose at least five distinct changes in the bedrock as you travel downstream. These rocks reflect a variety of ages, from older than 600 million years (Precambrian metamorphic rocks) to tens of millions of years old (Eocene sedimentary rocks). Several faults cross the route, including the northernmost end of the San Gabriel Fault. If you care to keep apprised of your progress down the canyon, be sure to keep updating your position on a topographic map. The Fish Creek confluence at 5.2 miles into the hike is a major milestone; there you change your general direction of travel from west to south.

The most interesting part of the canyon is an otherworldly passage just north of the confluence of Ruby Canyon (9.5–10 miles). There you make your way between gro-tesquely sculpted conglomerate-rock walls, wading most of the time.

South of that narrow section the canyon widens considerably and you sometimes have the luxury of walking on flat, sandy terraces on either side of the creek. After passing Ellis Apiary (11.5 miles), you can follow a remnant of an old trail on the canyon's west side for some distance before being forced back into the rocky bed of the creek. At 13.2 miles, you pick up traces of an old road that will take you to former parking and picnic area opposite the defunct Blue Point Campground (elevation 1130 feet), some 15 miles from Frenchmans Flat. You're now 6 miles away by paved road, closed to vehicle traffic, from where you can reliably reach a parked automobile: the entrance to Lake Piru. Perhaps you have planted a second car there earlier, or someone can meet you at that finish point.

# chapter 18

# Angeles Forest:
# Liebre Mountain & Fish Canyon

I made my first acquaintance with Angeles National Forest as a child, while riding in the family car north of L.A. on Highway 99 (yesteryear's version of Interstate 5). The signs said "National Forest," but my obvious question (probably voiced by millions before and since) was simply "Where are the trees?"

There are trees aplenty, if you know where to look for them—high on the ridges, down in the canyons, tucked away on north-facing slopes. If you take the poetic name of the chaparral—*elfin forest*—literally, there's plenty of that along Interstate 5 as well. In fact, 78 percent of the entire Angeles National Forest is covered by either chaparral or sage-scrub vegetation.

The predominance of chaparral is particularly true in the area mapped for this chapter. It is part of a triangular-shaped region bounded by the south edge of Antelope Valley on the north, Interstate 5 on the southwest, and Antelope Valley Freeway on the southeast. In a geologic sense this triangle is simply an extension of the San Gabriel Mountains, though you don't usually find that name associated with it on maps.

In earlier editions of this book there were eight trips in this triangular area. Now it's down to only two worth including in this present edition. This is because over the years road access has been increasingly restricted, and cost-cutting measures have resulted in the virtual abandonment of most trails in the area, save for the Pacific Crest Trail. Even several roadside National Forest campgrounds have been abandoned and obliterated in recent years.

A few hardy adventurers continue to explore the rugged and forbidding interior spaces around Red Rock Mountain and Cienaga Canyon on the sketchiest of trails. Previous editions of this book may be of help if you wish to do some further research on the old, disused trails.

All trips below require a National Forest Adventure Pass ($5 per day, $30 per year) for trailhead parking.

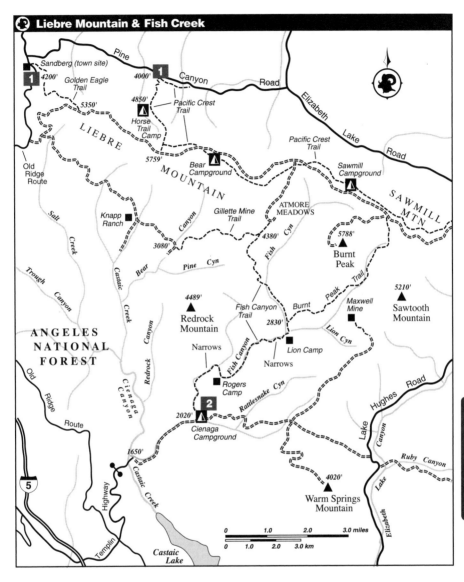

**Liebre Mountain & Fish Creek**

Sandberg (town site)
4200'
Golden Eagle Trail
5350'
Pine
4000'
Canyon
Road
Elizabeth
Lake
4850'
Pacific Crest Trail
Horse Trail Camp
LIEBRE
Pacific Crest Trail
Sawmill Campground
Old Ridge Route
5759'
MOUNTAIN
Bear Campground
SAWMILL MTN
Salt
Creek
Knapp Ranch
Canyon
Gillette Mine Trail
ATMORE MEADOWS
Fish Cyn
5788'
Burnt Peak
3080'
Bear
Pine Cyn
4380'
Trough
Canyon
Castaic
Creek
4489'
Redrock Mountain
Fish Canyon Trail
Burnt
2830'
Peak Trail
Lion Cyn
Maxwell Mine
5210'
Sawtooth Mountain
ANGELES NATIONAL FOREST
Redrock Canyon
Narrows
Narrows
Lion Camp
Cienaga Canyon
Rogers Camp
Rattlesnake Cyn
Hughes
Road
Old
Ridge
Route
2020'
Cienaga Campground
1650'
Lake Canyon
Ruby Canyon
Highway
5
Castaic Creek
4020'
Warm Springs Mountain
Elizabeth Lake
Templin
Castaic Lake

0    1.0    2.0    3.0 miles
0    1.0    2.0    3.0 km

## trip 1 Liebre Mountain

| | |
|---|---|
| **Distance** | 9.0 miles, Point-to-point |
| **Hiking Time** | 5 hours |
| **Elevation Gain/Loss** | 2100'/1900' |
| **Difficulty** | Moderately strenuous |
| **Trail Use** | Suitable for backpacking, dogs allowed |
| **Best Times** | October through June |
| **Agency** | ANF/SCMRD |
| **Recommended Map** | USGS 7.5-min *Liebre Mtn.* |
| **Notes** | Navigation required, easy terrain |

see map on p. 201

**DIRECTIONS** *East End:* From central Los Angeles, drive northwest on Interstate 5 about 65 miles to the Highway 138 exit. After 4 miles on 138, turn right on Old Ridge Route (County Route N2). Go 2.2 miles south, turn left (east) on Pine Canyon Road, and go 4.2 miles to mile marker 13.5, where the Pacific Crest Trail crosses Pine Canyon Road. Park off the pavement in the dirt area to the south. *West End:* From the Old Ridge Route/Pine Canyon Road intersection, drive 0.5 mile south on Old Ridge Route to the defunct townsite of Sandberg. Park next to the historic plaque.

The cool, forested north slopes of Liebre Mountain rear up in stark contrast to the wide, brown Antelope Valley at their feet. The San Andreas Fault, which lies along Liebre Mountain's north base, is responsible for this juxtaposition. Vertical movements have occurred along the fault, as well as the more familiar horizontal movements.

Black oak with mistletoe, Liebre Mountain

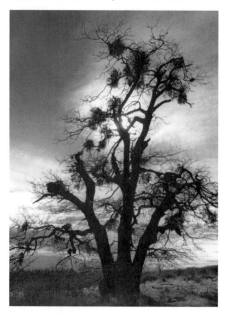

Atop Liebre Mountain's sparsely wooded, mile-high crest you can gaze north to the rolling Tehachapis and the southern Sierra, west toward the Sespe country and the highest (8000+ feet) summits of Los Padres National Forest, and south and southeast over much of Angeles National Forest. Seemingly at your feet is the flat, arid floor of the Mojave Desert, stretching to a hazy vanishing point on the eastern horizon.

This is a shuttle trip requiring two cars. (If you have a single car, you can elect to walk—or send the fastest runner of your group—down the 5 miles of pavement between the two points to close the loop.)

Just south (uphill) of Pine Creek Road, you'll find the Pacific Crest Trail. Go right and begin a leisurely switchback ascent through red-barked manzanitas, wispy gray pines, and deciduous black oaks. Patches of Great Basin sagebrush remind you that the high desert is not far away.

The mix of mountain-desert vegetation is soon enhanced by many large California buckeye shrubs. Leafless and gray until about April, buckeye becomes one of California's most handsome blooming plants by June, showing off myriad sprays of white blossoms. Botanically, this slope resembles much of central California's Coast Ranges and the lower Sierra foothills. Here on Liebre Mountain, both buckeye and gray pine are very close to their southern geographical limits.

Nearly 2 miles up, the trail becomes steeper amidst closely spaced pines. On a little flat to the right, you'll discover a wilderness campsite, with a picnic table, for hikers on the PCT. There's no water, but the breeze soughing through the long, thin pine needles overhead sets a peaceful mood, and the desert air, whether warm or cool, feels nice on the skin.

Past the campsite, you continue over the broad top of a 4923-foot peaklet and descend to a wooded saddle. From there the trail switchbacks up through bigcone Douglas-fir and joins an old road bed. You enter a grassy clearing dotted with black oaks (5400′)—a good place to admire the view of the Antelope Valley while catching your breath.

Ahead another half hour (3.5 miles from the start), you arrive at a junction where the PCT veers east toward Sawmill Mountain. Keep straight and walk up to Liebre Mountain Truck Trail (5759′), which is open to motor traffic when road conditions allow. Turn right and follow this road west along the oak-dotted crestline. An overgrown, abandoned segment of the PCT lies right and then left of the road. Originally PCT travelers were to have used this alignment, passing near Quail Lake, to reach the Tehachapis. Later the PCT was rerouted on the path you followed up the hill.

At mile 6.6, exactly where the topo map indicates a campground (non-existent now), take the narrow, unmarked trail that forks right. This point is 0.3 mile short of a 5345-foot peaklet labeled "Sandberg" on the topo map, where the road bends left and starts descending quickly toward Old Ridge Route. Use by hikers and mountain bikers keeps this abandoned section of the PCT in fairly good shape. It is referred to by some as the "Golden Eagle Trail."

As you descend through the chaparral you'll spot the weathered concrete ribbon of Old Ridge Route winding like a snake down below. This venerable roadway was a key (and dreaded) link in the original "Valley Route" linking Los Angeles with the Central Valley and points north. Paved with a narrow ribbon of concrete in 1919, the Ridge Route between Castaic and Gorman featured 642 turns in 38 miles, the equivalent of 97 complete circles! Widening and additional asphalt paving in the 1920s eliminated about one-third of the turns. The road was virtually abandoned in 1933 when a new bypass (U.S. 99) opened to the west. Today a third-generation Ridge Route—eight-lane Interstate 5—carries virtually 100 percent of the through traffic.

The trail ends on Old Ridge Route's shoulder, near the defunct townsite of Sandberg, which was a popular stopover on the old highway.

The Old Ridge Route

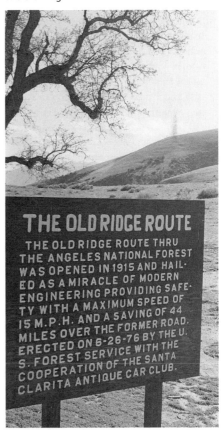

ANGELES FOREST

## trip 2  Fish Canyon Narrows

see map on p. 201

| | |
|---|---|
| **Distance** | 4.4 miles round trip, Out-and-back |
| **Hiking Time** | 3½ hours (round trip) |
| **Elevation Gain/Loss** | 400'/400' |
| **Difficulty** | Moderately strenuous |
| **Trail Use** | Suitable for backpacking, dogs allowed |
| **Best Times** | October through June |
| **Agency** | ANF/SCMRD |
| **Recommended Maps** | USGS 7.5-min *Whitaker Peak, Liebre Mtn.* |
| **Notes** | Navigation required, moderate terrain, bushwhacking |

**DIRECTIONS** From Castaic (on the northernmost fringe of Santa Clarita) exit Interstate 5 at Lake Hughes Road. Drive east and north on Lake Hughes Road for 13.2 miles to the unpaved, gated Forest Service Road on the left, next to the Warm Springs Rehabilitation Center. If the gate is open, drive west on this road for 7 miles to the defunct Cienaga Campground.

For many years, easy access to the trailhead from the west (Templin Highway) has been blocked by a formidable gate and no-trespassing signs. Lately, access has only been possible by way of a dirt road from the east, originating at Lake Hughes Road. Check with the Forest Service (661-296-9710) first to see if this dirt road is open to cars. If not, you might be able to mountain-bike-ride the 7 miles in to the start of the hike.

In the trenchlike confines of Fish Canyon, aridity and moisture stand side by side, separated by a matter of a few yards. Mountain mahogany, manzanita, and other drought-resistant chaparral shrubs cling to the walls, while a shallow stream gurgles merrily past a line of oaks, sycamores, willows, and cottonwoods. It's almost as if a little slice of the Pacific Northwest were transplanted to Southern California. Around the time of winter solstice, sunbeams fail to reach the innermost confines of the canyon and frost can linger on the creeping blackberry vines till midmorning.

From old Cienaga Campground begin hiking north up the main Fish Canyon on an old road bed, closed to motor traffic. (Take care not to head east up Fish Canyon's east fork.) The oak-shaded roadbed takes you 1.0 mile to a sharp bend to the right, where a narrow section of Fish Canyon begins. On the right, you can examine an old mining prospect, called the Pianobox, named for a piano that was once hauled in there.

The narrow section ahead is flanked by towering walls made of a strange, battered-looking, gray- and tan-colored rock. They're part of a 15-mile-wide formation of Precambrian gneiss (metamorphosed granite) covering most of Redrock Mountain, Sawmill Mountain, Fish Canyon, and upper Elizabeth Lake Canyon.

Only the merest pretense of a trail threads through the narrows, but the going is usually fairly easy along flat benches to either side of the creek. You'll cross the shallow creek perhaps two dozen times in the next mile.

After four sharp bends in the canyon, you arrive at unmaintained Rogers Camp (2.2 miles), perched atop a grassy, oak-shaded bench on the right—opposite an old mining tunnel bored in the north wall. The campsite was used by Scouts in the past. More opportunities for establishing a trail camp can be found a few hundred yards ahead, where the canyon widens.

Rogers Camp is a good turnaround point for a first hike or backpack into Fish Canyon. Intrepid explorers can press on through an upper narrow section of Fish Canyon, and perhaps trace the unmaintained upper Fish Canyon and Burnt Peak trails, which climb the slopes of mile-high Liebre Mountain and Sawmill Mountain.

# chapter 19

# Angeles Forest:
# Tujunga Canyons

Rising starkly behind the San Fernando and La Crescenta valley communities of Sylmar, San Fernando, Sunland and Tujunga, the westernmost ridges of the main San Gabriels have a lean and hungry look—at least from a distance. As seen at closer range—as along Big Tujunga Canyon Road—that impression is certainly reinforced. Canyon walls, some soaring a half mile in height, bear scraggly growths of brush and widely scattered trees. Sharply cut ravines, filled with accumulated rock rubble, appear to sweep down from the rounded ridgelines above. There's an almost palpable sense of violent events past and future. Fires, floods, and landslides keep material on these slopes moving downward even as fault movements heave the whole mountain mass upward.

This dramatic if unforgiving landscape has a gentler, mostly hidden side too. That's what you'll discover off the main roads and especially on the trails. Here you'll find mile-high peaks (including Mount Lukens, highest point within L.A.'s city limits), one of the more picturesque waterfalls in the county (in Trail Canyon), riparian glens, and pocket forests of oaks and conifers.

Three large drainage systems penetrate the area. Pacoima Canyon, on the north, stretches east to Mount Gleason and drains the south slopes of the mile-high Santa Clara Divide. Little Tujunga Canyon, along with its biggest tributary, Gold Creek, drains the rolling foothill country between two prominent ridges—Mendenhall and Yerba Buena. Big Tujunga Canyon, the largest of the three, penetrates deep into the High Country of the San Gabriels (Chapter 22). Big Tujunga Canyon Road threads the lower reaches of this canyon, permitting almost instant access to the canyon's lower trails by San Fernando Valley residents.

All trips below require a National Forest Adventure Pass ($5 per day, $30 per year) for trailhead parking.

The Station Fire, which burned about 160,000 acres of the San Gabriel Mountains from August through October 2009, profoundly affected both of the Tujunga canyons. Riparian vegetation in the canyon and ravine bottoms of this area will likely return quickly. Most of the native oaks, which are typically veterans of past fires, will send out new leaves right way and will likely fully recover in a few years. Chaparral on the canyon slopes always experiences regrowth; it is hoped that this assemblage of native vegetation won't be replaced by too many nonnative, weedy plants. Most of the trails in this chapter will be closed for an undetermined amount of time, so it is wise to contact Angeles National Forest, (626) 574-5200, www.fs.fed.us/r5/angeles, for the latest information.

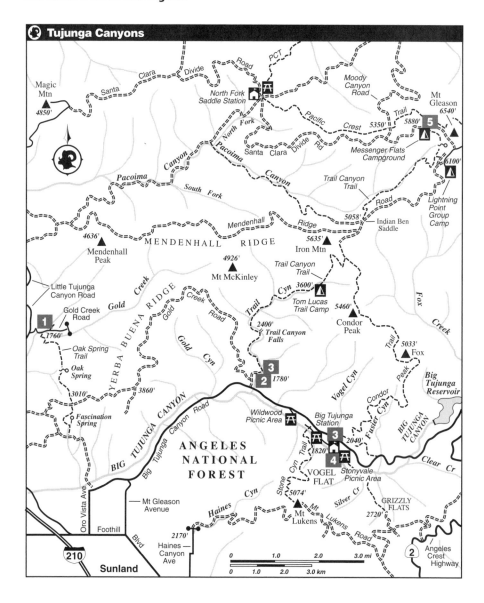

**Tujunga Canyons**

# trip 1  Yerba Buena Ridge

| | |
|---|---|
| **Distance** | 4.6 miles round trip, Out-and-back |
| **Hiking Time** | 3 hours (round trip) |
| **Elevation Gain/Loss** | 1400'/1400' |
| **Difficulty** | Moderately strenuous |
| **Trail Use** | Suitable for backpacking, dogs allowed |
| **Best Times** | October through May |
| **Agency** | ANF/LARD |
| **Recommended Map** | USGS 7.5-min *Sunland* |
| **Notes** | Navigation required, moderate terrain, bushwhacking |

see map on p. 206

**DIRECTIONS** Exit Interstate 210 at Foothill Boulevard in Lake View Terrace. Turn toward the north side of the freeway and immediately turn left on Osborne Street. After a mile Osborne Street becomes Little Tujunga Canyon Road. At about 4 miles from I-210, turn right on Gold Creek Road. Continue 1 mile to the trailhead for the Oak Spring Trail on the right.

The Oak Spring Trail, right on the western border of Angeles National Forest, provides a quick escape from the teeming, aging suburban "foothill" and San Fernando Valley communities down below. The area traversed by the trail was burned in the 2009 Station Fire, and could be closed to the public for an unknown amount of time. When access is allowed again, the growth of pioneering shrubs may be rapid, and you could face challenges associated with encroaching vegetation.

From the trailhead on Gold Creek Road, the Oak Spring Trail strikes steadily uphill. It switches back seven times, crosses a hillside, goes over a saddle, and then drops into a grassy bowl containing Oak Spring (1.4 miles). The spring itself lies hidden beneath a cluster of live oaks. From there, the trail contours south for a while, and resumes climbing up ceanothus-smothered slopes that can become waves of white blossoms during the late winter or early spring.

After 2.3 miles of general ascent, you reach the wide, graded fire road following the crest of Yerba Buena Ridge. A rim-of-the-world view of La Crescenta and San Fernando valleys unfolds there—and (as an option) you can enhance that view by walking higher on the fire road. Otherwise, simply turn around and retrace your earlier footsteps.

ANGELES FOREST

# trip 2  Trail Canyon Falls

| | |
|---|---|
| **Distance** | 3.0 miles round trip, Out-and-back |
| **Hiking Time** | 1½ hours (round trip) |
| **Elevation Gain/Loss** | 700'/700' |
| **Difficulty** | Moderate |
| **Trail Use** | Dogs allowed |
| **Best Times** | December through May |
| **Agency** | ANF/LARD |
| **Optional Map** | USGS 7.5-min *Sunland* |
| **Notes** | Marked trails/obvious routes, moderate terrain |

see map on p. 206

**DIRECTIONS**  To reach the trailhead from the foothill community of Sunland take either Oro Vista Avenue or Mount Gleason Avenue north to Big Tujunga Canyon Road and turn right. Some 5 miles up the canyon (mile 2.0 according to highway mile markers), look for a Forest Service fire road on the left. Drive 0.2 mile uphill to a fork, go right, and descend 0.2 mile to an oak-shaded parking area on the right, just above Trail Canyon's melodious creek.

When soaking rains come, Trail Canyon's normally indolent flow becomes a lively torrent. After tumbling through miles of rock-bound constrictions and sliding across many gently inclined declivities, the water comes to the lip of a real precipice. There the bubbly mixture momentarily attains weightlessness during a free-fall of about 30 feet. If you can manage to ignore the vastly smaller scale of this spectacle, you might easily imagine yourself in Yosemite Valley during spring runoff.

Trail Canyon Falls

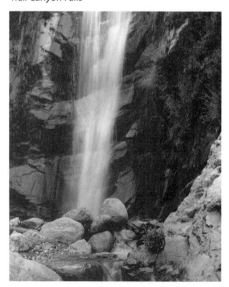

The falls in Trail Canyon are fairly easy to approach, except during the most intense flooding, when the several fords you must cross on the way may be dangerously deep. Sturdy footwear may be helpful at some of the deeper crossings in high water.

From the trailhead, continue up remnants of the same road on foot, passing a few cabins and fording the creek for the first time. The now-very-deteriorated road goes on to follow an east tributary for a while, doubles back, contours around a ridge, and drops into Trail Canyon again (0.6 mile). The old road ends there, and you continue up-canyon on a footpath. The path clings to the banks for 0.5 mile, crossing the stream several times, and then climbs the west wall to avoid a narrow, alder-choked section of the canyon. The falls come into view as you round a sharp bend about 1.5 miles from the parking area.

Although many people have obviously done so, it's difficult and dangerous to slide down from the trail to the base of the falls. The falls can also be reached by bushwhacking up the canyon from the point where the trail begins its ascent of the west wall; this is fun scrambling during low water, hazardous during high water.

Trail Canyon was swept by the 2009 Station Fire; the canyon trail will be closed for an indefinite amount of time.

# trip 3  Condor Peak & Trail Canyon

|  |  |
|---|---|
| **Distance** | 14.0 miles, Point-to-point |
| **Hiking Time** | 10 hours |
| **Elevation Gain/Loss** | 4260'/4520' |
| **Difficulty** | Strenuous |
| **Trail Use** | Suitable for backpacking, dogs allowed |
| **Best Times** | October through May |
| **Agency** | ANF/LARD |
| **Required Maps** | USGS 7.5-min *Condor Peak, Sunland* |
| **Notes** | Navigation required, moderate terrain, bushwhacking |

see map on p. 206

**DIRECTIONS** *East End:* From the foothill community of Sunland take either Oro Vista Avenue or Mount Gleason Avenue north to Big Tujunga Canyon Road and turn right. Some 7 miles up the canyon (mile 4.3 according to highway mile markers) on the left, park in a turnout opposite the entrance to Big Tujunga Station and Vogel Flat. *West End:* About 5 miles up Big Tujunga Canyon from Sunland (mile 2.0 according to highway mile markers), look for a Forest Service fire road on the left. Drive 0.2 mile uphill to a fork, go right, and descend 0.2 mile to an oak-shaded parking area on the right, just above Trail Canyon's melodious creek.

This all-day trip has a little of everything: long, winding passages across fragrant chaparral-clothed slopes, outstanding views from the open summit of Condor Peak, and a soothing, foot-wetting descent along Trail Canyon's delightful stream. The elevation gains and losses, however, are punishing to all but well-conditioned hikers and back-packers. The first half of the route (Condor Peak Trail) is infrequently maintained, sometimes eroded, and often overgrown, so lug soles and long pants or gaiters are recommended. An early start, ideally before sunrise, is advised too. That way you can be off the lower, south-facing slopes before midday's heat.

Ceonothus, Condor Peak Trail

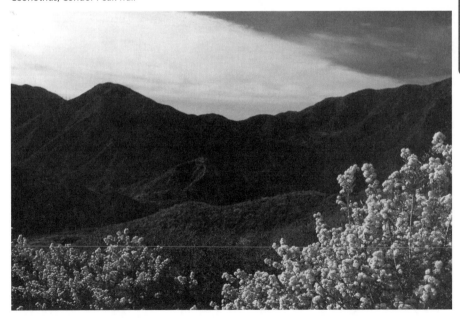

ANGELES FOREST

A five-minute car shuttle will connect together the start and end points. (Alternatively you can take only one car and have someone in your party sprint 3 miles along Big Tujunga Canyon Road to close the loop.)

Start off by walking east on the north shoulder of Big Tujunga Canyon Road to the mile 4.5 marker, where you will find the Condor Peak Trail going up a gully.

About 0.5 mile up the trail, a lateral of the Condor Peak Trail comes in from the right. This 1-mile-long trail was constructed in 1980 after rock slides had closed a section of Big Tujunga Canyon Road. Stay left at the trail junction and continue winding steadily uphill along the ridge between Vogel and Fusier canyons. In March, thousands of white-flowering ceanothus shrubs burst into bloom on these slopes, suffusing the air with a sublime perfume. A few coniferous trees, the survivors of past fires, rise above the ubiquitous blanket of chaparral.

After 2.0 miles the trail bends around several gullies draining into Fusier Canyon. The biggest gully you cross (3.2 miles) is a cool, ferny oasis with surface water present until at least April or May. At 5.5 miles (4600'), the Condor Peak Trail joins an old fire break coming down from Fox Peak—one of several bumps on the ridge running northwest toward Condor Peak. Follow the fire break up and over the undulating ridge 1.2 miles more to a point just below the east brow of Condor Peak. Leave the trail and scramble 300 feet up the slope on sandy soil and over fractured granite (watch for loose rocks). On the windswept summit plateau, there are two small peaklets, each containing a climbers' register hidden in a cairn.

A pleasant, but dry camp could be made here on the summit plateau or on any neighboring ridge, if the weather is calm. Wind-sheltered campsites lie about 3 miles ahead at Tom Lucas Trail Camp in upper Trail Canyon.

From Condor Peak, the Pacific Ocean sprawls more than a quarter of the way around the compass. To the south, barely clearing the broad profile of Mount Lukens, Santa Catalina Island floats in serene splendor on the hazy blue horizon. To the west, over the San Fernando Valley and through the low gap of Santa Susana Pass, rises Santa Cruz Island, the biggest and tallest of the Channel Islands, about 90 miles away.

If time allows, consider scrambling 0.8 mile down the ridge west of Condor Peak to a 5250-foot knob. From there you can peer almost straight down on upper Trail Canyon, threaded by a dark-green line of riparian vegetation.

After soaking in the view, retrace your way back to the Condor Peak Trail and continue going north on the old fire break. At 8.3 miles, you come to a 4840-foot saddle at the head of Trail Canyon and the intersection of the Trail Canyon Trail. Make a sharp left and zigzag steeply down the scrubby slopes to a dry, sloping bench. At 9.7 miles you reach the line of willow and bay trees making up Big Cienaga, the source of Trail Canyon's almost-perennial stream. Down-canyon another 0.3 mile, on a small, grassy flat surrounded by oaks and jungle-like riparian vegetation, is cozy Tom Lucas Trail Camp, sometimes occupied by Scouts or other groups.

The last 4 miles along the trench-like confines of the canyon are thoroughly delightful if you don't mind occasional rocky stretches and foot-wetting fords. On clear afternoons, warm sunlight filters through the alders, casting flitting shadows amid the crystalline pools and stream-side boulders. The soothing music of water flowing over stone assuages the weariness almost every hiker feels at this point.

The Condor Peak/Trail Canyon area was almost completely burned in the 2009 Station Fire. With the anticipated reopening of the trails (at some indefinite future date) the route could showcase for a number of years impressive displays of fire-following wildflowers.

# trip 4  Mount Lukens & Grizzly Flats Loop

see map on p. 206

| | |
|---|---|
| **Distance** | 12.2 miles, Loop |
| **Hiking Time** | 8 hours |
| **Elevation Gain/Loss** | 3400'/3400' |
| **Difficulty** | Strenuous |
| **Trail Use** | Suitable for backpacking, dogs allowed |
| **Best Times** | October through May |
| **Agency** | ANF/LARD |
| **Recommended Map** | USGS 7.5-min *Condor Peak* |
| **Notes** | Navigation required, easy terrain |

**DIRECTIONS** From the foothill community of Sunland take either Oro Vista Avenue or Mount Gleason Avenue north to Big Tujunga Canyon Road and turn right. Some 7 miles up the canyon (mile 4.3 according to highway mile markers) take the road to the right which leads to Big Tujunga Station and Vogel Flat. Drive to the bottom of the hill, turn right, and park at the Vogel Flat parking lot, open from 8 a.m. to 6 p.m. (The parking lot at Stonyvale Picnic Area stays open longer—6 a.m. to 10 p.m.—so consider parking there if you think you may finish the hike late.)

This all-day adventure lets you walk on the wild side of the Tujunga canyon and peak country. After a grueling climb up the north slope from Big Tujunga Canyon, you circle back by way of a long, gradually descending route that passes through secluded Grizzly Flats. The hike feels best on a cool day, but beware of periods following heavy rain: the trip begins and ends with crossings of Big Tujunga creek, which can be hazardous in high water. If you're in doubt, call the Forest Service to check on flood conditions.

On foot, head west down a narrow, paved road (private, but with public easement) through the cabin community of Stonyvale. When the pavement ends after 0.7 mile, continue on dirt for another quarter mile or so. Choose a safe place to ford Big Tujunga creek, wade across, and find the Stone Canyon Trail on the far bank. From afar you can spot this trail going straight up the sloping terrace just left (east) of Stone Canyon's wide, boulder-filled mouth. Settle into a pace that will

Northwest panorama, Mount Lukens

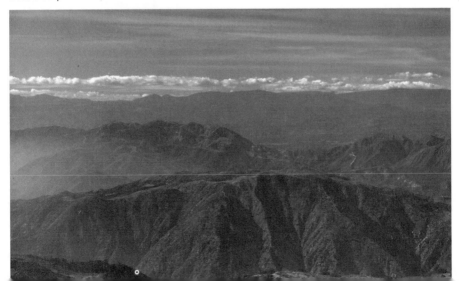

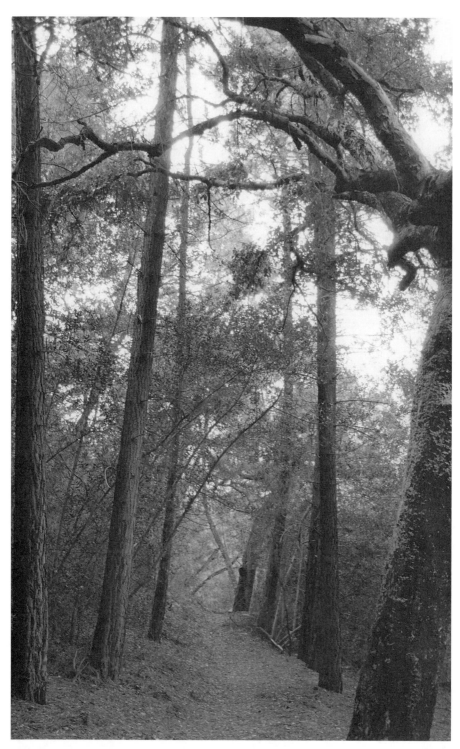

Trail below Grizzly Flats

allow you to persevere over the next 3 miles and 3200 feet of vertical ascent.

From the vantage point of the first switchback, you can look down on the thousands of storm-tossed granitic boulders filling Stone Canyon from wall to wall. Although the boulders are frozen in place, you can almost sense their movement over geologic time. Indeed, floods continue to reshape this canyon and many others in the San Gabriels during every major deluge.

Ahead, you turn along precipitous, chaparral-covered slopes. At or near ground level, a profusion of ferns, mosses, and herbaceous plants forms its own pygmy understory.

The dizzying view encompasses a long, obviously linear stretch of Big Tujunga Canyon. This segment of the canyon is underlain by the San Gabriel Fault and its offshoot, the Sierra Madre Fault. The latter fault splits from the former near Vogel Flat and continues southeast past Grizzly Flat, following a course roughly coincident with the final leg of our loop hike. According to current understanding, the San Gabriel Fault is presently inactive and not likely to be the cause of major movement or earthquakes in the near future. The depth of Big Tujunga Canyon and the steepness of its walls are due primarily to stream cutting following uplift of the whole mountain range.

Between 1.8 and 2.6 miles (from the start), the trail hovers above an unnamed canyon to the east, nearly equal in drainage to Stone Canyon, but very steep and narrow. Down below you can often hear, and barely glimpse, an inaccessible waterfall. Long and short switchback segments take you rapidly higher to a steep, bulldozed track leading to the bald summit ridge of Mount Lukens. Go 0.5 mile farther (connecting with Mount Lukens Road along the way) to reach the highest point on the ridge (4.2 miles), which is occupied by several antenna structures. Technically the summit lies within the city limit of Los Angeles, and is the highest point in any incorporated city in the county.

Glendale almost claims this honor, as its corporate limit reaches within 300 yards of the summit. Both cities encompass parts of the Angeles National Forest, of course. The view can be fabulous on a clear day.

The remaining two-thirds of the hike is almost entirely downhill—a little monotonous, but mostly easy on the knees. Follow Mount Lukens Road southeast down the main ridge, keeping left at the next two road junctions. At 7.2 miles you begin dropping toward a saddle. At the four-way junction there (9.0 miles), choose the road to the far left and continue on a zigzag course past beautiful oaks and bay laurels to Grizzly Flats (10.0 miles), where a terrace of planted pines slopes down to a ravine called Vasquez Creek. The leftmost of several diverging roads on the flat leads to a water tank. Behind that you'll find a maintained remnant of the old Dark Canyon Trail from Angeles Crest Highway to Big Tujunga Canyon—roughly the escape route used by the outlaw Tiburcio Vasquez and his unsuccessful pursuers during a hot chase over a century ago.

From the water tank, follow the trail down to a creek bedecked with woodwardia fern and wild strawberry. You then descend moderately through oak forest, descend sharply down a ridge overlooking the pit-like gorge of Silver Creek, and finally reach a wildflower-dotted bench along Big Tujunga creek. Wild fruit trees and eucalyptus there silently speak of former homesteads. Head downstream, crossing the creek five times in the next mile, to reach Stonyvale Picnic Area, a quarter mile upstream from your car at Vogel Flat.

The 2009 Station Fire swept through most of the area described in this trip, and heavily damaged visitor facilities and homes at Vogel Flat. While the vegetation will largely recover in the next several years, parts of this looping route may be out of commission due to washouts or other conditions deemed dangerous by the Forest Service.

ANGELES FOREST

**trip 5**  # Messenger Flats

see map on p. 206

| | |
|---|---|
| **Distance** | 3.3 miles, Loop |
| **Hiking Time** | 2 hours |
| **Elevation Gain/Loss** | 800'/800' |
| **Difficulty** | Moderate |
| **Trail Use** | Dogs allowed, good for kids |
| **Best Times** | March through November |
| **Agency** | ANF/SCMRD |
| **Optional Map** | USGS 7.5-min *Acton* |
| **Notes** | Marked trails/obvious routes, easy terrain |

**DIRECTIONS**  Exit the Antelope Valley Freeway (Highway 14) at Angeles Forest Highway, 5 miles south of Palmdale. Follow Angeles Forest Highway south into the San Gabriel Mountains. After about 10 miles of uphill driving, you reach Mill Creek summit. Turn right (west) there on Mount Gleason Road (aka Santa Clara Divide Road). After another 10 miles on this mostly paved, but narrow national-forest roadway, you'll arrive at the trailhead, Messenger Flats Campground.

Tucked amid a lovely grove of pines on the remote north ridge of the San Gabriel Mountains is pint-size Messenger Flats Campground, an Angeles National Forest facility available on a first-come, first-served basis. The Pacific Crest Trail (PCT), the 2650-mile "gorilla" of all hiking trails in the West, passes right through, and you can use a section of it to piece together a viewful 3.3-mile hike overlooking the vast Mojave Desert, which lies to the north.

Note that Messenger Flats Campground is seasonally closed due to snow at some

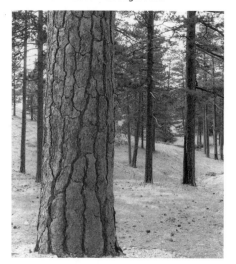

Ponderosa forest at Messenger Flats

point during the winter season. Also, if you are interested in mountain biking in this area, be aware that you must stay on any of the numerous forest roadways in the area. The PCT is off-limits to all mechanized transport, including bicycles.

The PCT parallels Santa Clara Divide Road at a point 20 yards north of the campground entrance. Go left (west) and follow the trail as it veers away from the road and starts to descend along steep, north-facing slopes. This is a narrow, rough-cut, seldom traveled section of the PCT. Conifers and oaks provide welcome shade at frequent intervals. Far below is Soledad Canyon, the broad, east-west gash separating the main block of the San Gabriel Mountains from outlying ranges to the northwest. In the hills beyond Soledad Canyon, the tilted sedimentary slabs known as the Vasquez Rocks glow a bright beige amid the otherwise muted gray-green and brown land.

After 1.5 miles, the PCT dips into a shady ravine and crosses Moody Canyon Road. Leave the trail and follow the road 0.2 mile uphill to Santa Clara Divide Road. Turn left there and return to Messenger Flats, uphill all the way.

The 2009 Station Fire burned through Messenger Flats, so check with the Forest Service to determine whether the campground and trails are accessible.

# chapter 20

# Angeles Forest:
# Arroyo Seco & Front Range

**D**espite regular invasions by smoggy air (mostly at lower elevations), Angeles National Forest's Arroyo Seco drainage can be a hiker's and backpacker's paradise. In this chapter we'll cover a host of trail trips featuring fantastic views from high ridges, passages through lush forests, and visits to sparkling waterfalls and mirror-like pools. The same can be said for the broader, so-called Front Range of the San Gabriels—the sharply rising massif closest to L.A. and Pasadena—covered in this chapter and the next chapter.

Although hardly qualifying as wilderness by bureaucratic standards (there are too many roads through it), much of the Arroyo Seco area has the look and the feel of wilderness. Most of the fire roads that were carved into the mountainsides decades ago are now blocked to unauthorized vehicle traffic. Once off the pavement, travelers must get around on their own power, much as people did during the so-called Great Hiking Era of the early 1900s. Then, the Front Range and "High Country" beyond were regarded as a local frontier for weekend exploration and recreation. Scenic trails were constructed, and dozens of trailside camps and hostelries sprang up to serve the needs of overnight guests. The road-building era that followed in the late 1930s and '40s ended that idyllic chapter of the mountains' history.

There's a renewed interest in rambling the mountains of the Front Range today, with the focus on day hiking. Volunteers have teamed up with the Forest Service to refurbish the old trails and construct new ones. Several of the old resorts have been replaced by trail camps that are popular on weekends among youth groups and backpackers.

A clear advantage of the Front Range trails is that many of them can be reached so quickly and easily from the metropolitan basin below. Down in the canyon recesses, a hiker can quickly forget the sights and sounds of the city, hardly aware that his or her peaceful, uncrowded world lies only a few miles from the edge of one of the world's largest cities.

Most of the trips below require a National Forest Adventure Pass ($5 per day, $30 per year) for trailhead parking.

Note: The Station Fire, which swept through about 160,000 acres of the San Gabriel Mountains from August through October 2009, profoundly affected nearly all of the trips in this chapter. Riparian vegetation in the canyon and ravine bottoms of this area will likely return quickly. The fate of coniferous trees, which stood at higher elevations, is less certain. Most of the native oaks, which are typically grizzled veterans of past fires, will send out new leaves right way and will likely fully recover in a few years. The chaparral zones will probably recover quickly as well. Most of the trails in this chapter will need extensive repair; they'll be closed for an undetermined amount of time. Contact Angeles National Forest, (626) 574-5200, www.fs.fed.us/r5/angeles, for the latest information.

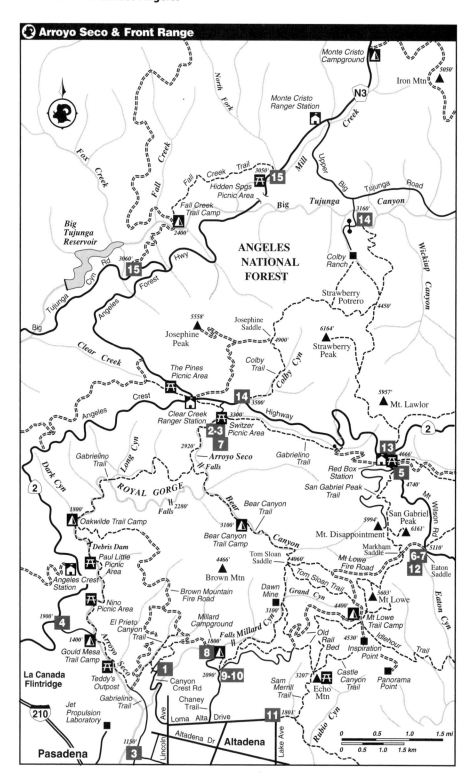

**Arroyo Seco & Front Range**

## trip 1  El Prieto Loop

| | |
|---|---|
| **Distance** | 2.4 miles, Loop |
| **Hiking Time** | 1½ hours |
| **Elevation Gain/Loss** | 600'/600' |
| **Difficulty** | Moderate |
| **Trail Use** | Dogs allowed, good for kids |
| **Best Times** | All year |
| **Agency** | ANF/LARD |
| **Optional Map** | USGS 7.5-min *Pasadena* |
| **Notes** | Marked trails/obvious routes, moderate terrain |

see map on p. 216

**DIRECTIONS**  Exit Interstate 210 at Lincoln Avenue in Pasadena. Go north on Lincoln for 1.9 miles, and turn left on Canyon Crest Road. Wind uphill for 1.1 miles to Cloverhill Road. Turn left, go two short blocks, and turn right (north) on El Prieto Road. Park on the street at or near the north end of El Prieto Road.

The quiet, shady interior of El Prieto Canyon seems impossibly remote given its stone's-throw proximity to the edge of an Altadena subdivision. Majestic live oaks flank the canyon's stream, casting dense pools of shade, particularly in the fall and winter. A few willows and sycamores are here, too, lending highlights of warm, autumn color. El Prieto Canyon Trail, which crookedly navigates the canyon bottom, is a delight in any season, though.

From the north end of El Prieto Road, squeeze around a steel-bar fence, go up past a water tank, and continue on the steeply rising dirt road. At 0.4 mile, you hit pavement next to a rustic house on the right. Just beyond, find the narrow trail on the left that descends sharply into the shady bottom of El Prieto Canyon.

Right down below, you reach a fork in the trail. Stay right and begin a side trip (highly recommended, and an integral part of this hike's mileage) up the canyon bottom a half mile to the Lower Brown Mountain Fire Road (a popular mountain bike route). On that out-and-back stretch, you work your way around or over several check dams that help control erosion during times of flood. That means that some of the cascades here aren't exactly natural, but they're beautiful all the same.

Back at the fork, turn right and continue to make your way downstream, past more check dams, enjoying more gorgeous wooded scenery. After about 0.7 mile on this leg of the hike, look for the trail on the left bank that slants steeply uphill to the subdivision above. Follow it and you'll emerge on El Prieto Road at a point 100 feet north of Cloverhill Road, near where you have parked your car.

El Prieto Canyon Trail is also accessible via the lowermost end of Lower Brown Mountain Fire Road, near the Gabrielino Trail through the Arroyo Seco canyon. That approach to it is much longer.

Note: Much of El Prieto Canyon was burned in the 2009 Station Fire. Recovery of the natural landscape will likely start with the riparian vegetation in the very bottom of the canyon, which benefits from a year-round supply of water.

**ANGELES FOREST**

## trip 2  Switzer Falls

see
map on
p. 216

| | |
|---|---|
| **Distance** | 3.6 miles round trip, Out-and-back |
| **Hiking Time** | 2 hours (round trip) |
| **Elevation Gain/Loss** | 700'/700' |
| **Difficulty** | Moderate |
| **Trail Use** | Suitable for backpacking, dogs allowed, good for kids |
| **Best Times** | All year |
| **Agency** | ANF/LARD |
| **Optional Map** | USGS 7.5-min *Condor Peak* |
| **Notes** | Marked trails/obvious routes, moderate terrain |

**DIRECTIONS** Exit Interstate 210 at Angeles Crest Highway in La Cañada-Flintridge. Drive 10 miles north to the turnoff for Switzer Picnic Area on the right (mile-marker 34.2). Drive 0.5 mile down the paved access road to the parking lot next to the picnic area. (If the access road happens to be closed and gated, you can park at the top and walk down into the picnic area—250 feet of elevation loss in a half mile.)

Amid a precarious setting of crumbling rock walls, the waters of the upper Arroyo Seco slide some 50 feet down a steep incline known as Switzer Falls. Normally a modest dribble, but occasionally an exuberant cascade, the falls are tantalizingly secretive—they can be approached at close range only by some foolhardy scrambling over unstable or slippery rock (definitely not recommended—many people have been seriously hurt this way). Our route takes you by trail around the main falls and down to a lesser cascade in the canyon below.

From the far end of Switzer Picnic Area, pick up the signed Gabrielino Trail. Make your way past outlying picnic tables, and then down along the alder-shaded stream. Soon nothing but the clear-flowing stream and rustling leaves disturb the silence. Remnants of an old paved road are occasionally

Lower falls below Switzer's

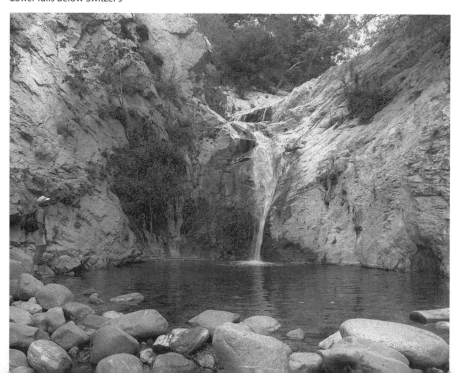

underfoot. In a couple of spots you ford the stream by boulder-hopping—no problem except after heavy rain.

One mile down the canyon you come upon the foundation remnants of Switzer's Camp. Established in 1884, the camp became the San Gabriels' premier wilderness resort in the early 1900s, patronized by Hollywood celebrities as well as anyone who had the gumption to hike or ride a burro up the tortuous Arroyo Seco trail from Pasadena. After the completion of Angeles Crest Highway as far as Red Box in 1934, and then a severe flood in the 1938, the resort lost its appeal. It was finally razed in the late 1950s.

Below Switzer's Camp the stream slides 50 feet over Switzer Falls—but don't go that way. Instead, cross the stream and continue on the Gabrielino Trail as it edges along the canyon's right (west) wall. To the left are glimpses of the falls, a dark pit below them, and the crumbled foundation of a miniature stone chapel (a part of the resort) that perched on a ledge above the falls. Continue 0.2 mile to a trail junction. Take the left fork (the trail to Bear Canyon) and descend to the canyon bottom (1.5 miles). There's a severe, unfenced dropoff on the left on the way down, so watch your step and that of your kids.

Leave the trail there and walk along the banks, or rock hop through the stream itself, 0.2 mile up-canyon. You'll come upon a dark, shallow pool, fed by a 15-foot-high cascade just below the main Switzer Falls. This is a peaceful and secluded spot for a picnic. Signs here warn against climbing farther up the canyon, and that is advice well-taken.

Note: Reconstruction of certain trails in this area (in the aftermath of the 2009 Station Fire) could take several years.

## trip 3  Down the Arroyo Seco

see map on p. 216

| | |
|---|---|
| **Distance** | 9.6 miles, Point-to-point |
| **Hiking Time** | 5 hours |
| **Elevation Gain/Loss** | 450'/2600' |
| **Difficulty** | Moderately strenuous |
| **Trail Use** | Suitable for backpacking, suitable for mountain biking |
| **Best Times** | October through June |
| **Agency** | ANF/LARD |
| **Optional Maps** | USGS 7.5-min *Condor Peak, Pasadena* |
| **Notes** | Marked trails/obvious routes, easy terrain |

**ANGELES FOREST**

**DIRECTIONS** *North End:* Exit Interstate 210 at Angeles Crest Highway in La Cañada-Flintridge. Drive 10 miles north to the turnoff for Switzer Picnic Area on the right (mile-marker 34.2). Continue 0.5 mile down the paved access road to the parking lot next to the picnic area. (If the access road happens to be closed and gated, you can park at the top and walk down into the picnic area—250 feet of elevation loss in a half mile.) *South End:* From Interstate 210 in Pasadena, exit Windsor Avenue and go north 1 mile to where Windsor meets Ventura Street. A large parking are on the left serves as the trailhead for the Gabrielino Trail.

The Spanish colonists who christened Arroyo Seco ("dry creek") evidently observed only its lower end—a hot, boulder-strewn wash emptying into the Los Angeles River. Upstream, inside the confines of the San Gabriels, Arroyo Seco is a scenic treasure—all the more astounding when you consider that its exquisite sylvan glens and sparkling brook lie just 12–15 miles from L.A.'s city center. If you haven't yet been freed from the notion that Los Angeles is nothing but a seething megalopolis, walk down the canyon of the Arroyo Seco. You'll be convinced otherwise.

A botanist's and wildflower seeker's dream, the canyon features generous growths of canyon live oak, western sycamore, California bay, white alder, bigleaf maple, bigcone Douglas-fir, and arroyo willow. A quick census one spring day (in a dry year, no less) yielded for me the following blooming plants: golden yarrow, prickly phlox, western wallflower, Indian pink, live-forever, wild pea, deerweed, bush lupine, Spanish broom, baby-blue-eyes, yerba santa, phacelia, chia, black sage, bush poppy, California buckwheat, shooting star, western clematis, Indian paintbrush, sticky monkey flower, scarlet bugler, and purple nightshade.

You'll be traveling the westernmost leg of the Gabrielino Trail, one of four routes in Angeles National Forest specially designated as "National Recreation Trails." The Arroyo Seco stretch of the Gabrielino Trail receives considerable use—and also a lot of much-needed maintenance—by mountain-bike club members. The upper and middle portions, which are in places narrow with steep drops to one side, are challenging

Arroyo Seco above Pasadena

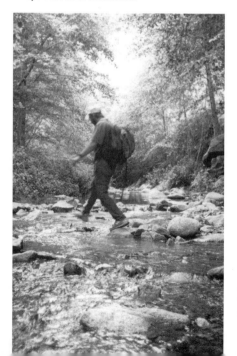

even for expert riders, although not at all hard for hikers. The lower end consists of remnants of an old road built as far up the canyon as the Oak Wilde resort (now Oak-wilde Campground) in the 1920s.

Several rest stops and picnic sites line the trail's lower half, making this a great route for a leisurely saunter. Most of these stops are located on the sites of early tourist camps or cabins erected in the early 1900s. Virtually all the structures were either destroyed by flooding in 1938 or removed through condemnation proceedings (based on water and flood-control needs) in the '20s, '30s, and '40s.

Some kind of car-shuttle or drop-off-and-pick-up transportation arrangement is obviously required for this long one-way hike or backpack trip. Carry along whatever drinking water you'll need for the duration of the trip; there may be piped water at one or another of the rest stops along the way, but don't count on it. Pleasantly shaded Oakwilde Campground near the midpoint is the best place to stay if you're backpacking the route.

From the west end of the Switzer Picnic Area, start hiking on the signed Gabrielino Trail. Make your way past outlying picnic tables, and then down along the alder-shaded stream. Soon nothing but the clear-flowing stream and rustling leaves disturb the silence. Remnants of an old paved road are occasionally underfoot. In a couple of spots you ford the stream by boulder-hopping—no problem except after heavy rain.

One mile down the canyon you come upon the foundation remnants of Switzer's Camp, a former resort, now occupied by a trail campground. Walk down to a fork in the trail 0.2 mile beyond the trail camp. You will probably hear, if not clearly see, the 50-foot cascade known as Switzer Falls, to the east. Our way continues on the right fork (Gabrielino Trail), which now begins a mile-long traverse through chaparral. This less-than-perfectly-scenic stretch avoids a narrow, twisting trench called Royal Gorge, through which the Arroyo Seco stream tumbles and sometimes abruptly drops.

At 2.3 miles (from the start) the trail joins a shady tributary of Long Canyon, and later Long Canyon itself, replete with a trickling stream. Alongside the trail you'll discover at least five kinds of ferns, plus mosses, poison oak, and Humboldt lilies (in bloom during early summer).

At 3.4 miles, the waters of Long Canyon swish down through a sculpted grotto to join Arroyo Seco. The trail descends to Arroyo Seco canyon's narrow floor and stays there, crossing and recrossing many times over the next few miles. The stretch from Long Canyon to Oakwilde Campground (4.5 miles) is perhaps the most gorgeous of all, flanked by soaring walls and dappled with shade cast by the ever-present alders. Bigleaf maples put on a great show here in November, their bright yellow leaves boldly contrasting with the earthy greens, grays, and browns of the canyon's dimly lit bottom.

Beyond Oakwilde Campground the canyon widens a bit and the trail assumes a more gentle gradient. There's a sharp climb at 5.3 miles—to bypass the large Brown Canyon Debris Dam—then a long trek out to the mouth of the canyon with no further significant climbing. Toward the end, the trail becomes a dirt road, and finally a paved service road, complete with bridged crossings of the Arroyo Seco (purists can follow a narrow, equestrian trail alongside). During the last couple of miles you're likely to run into lots of cyclists, joggers, parents pushing strollers, and even skateboarders.

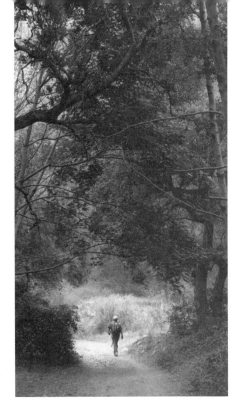

Gabrielino Trail, Arroyo Seco, before the Station Fire

Note: The 2009 Station Fire swept nearly the entire area described in this trip, taking out campground and picnic facilities, and thoroughly incinerating most of the vegetation. The trails also suffered serious damage. The demand for the use of the lower and middle portions of the Gabrielino Trail will likely lead to their rehabilitation at an earlier date. The upper end of trail, which clings to steeper slopes, will likely be out of service longer. Springtime displays of fire-following wildflowers could be spectacular for several years after the Station Fire, especially in wet years.

# trip 4  Royal Gorge

| | |
|---|---|
| **Distance** | 12.4 miles round trip, Out-and-back |
| **Hiking Time** | 8 hours (round trip) |
| **Elevation Gain/Loss** | 1600'/1600' |
| **Difficulty** | Strenuous |
| **Trail Use** | Suitable for backpacking, dogs allowed |
| **Best Times** | October through July |
| **Agency** | ANF/LARD |
| **Recommended Maps** | USGS 7.5-min *Pasadena, Condor Peak* |
| **Notes** | Navigation required, moderate terrain, bushwhacking |

see map on p. 216

**DIRECTIONS**  Exit Interstate 210 at Angeles Crest Highway in La Cañada-Flintridge. Drive 2 miles north to a trailhead parking area on the right, at mile 26.4.

Easy trail hiking, then moderate boulder-hopping, and finally some knee-deep wading will take you deep into the sublime hideaway of the Royal Gorge, the narrow, rock-walled section of Arroyo Seco that has repelled trail builders for over a century. There you'll come upon a small waterfall and a deep, dark, swimmable pool whose setting suggests to me the name "Royal Pool" or perhaps "King's Bathtub."

From the parking area, step around the locked gate and descend 1 mile on a paved service road to reach the Gabrielino Trail, just upstream from Gould Mesa Campground. Follow the Gabrielino Trail upstream (north) past Oakwilde Trail Camp (3.6 miles) to the point where the Gabrielino Trail leaves Arroyo Seco and starts going up Long Canyon (4.7 miles). Abandon the trail at this point and start boulder-hopping up the main stream to the right—this is Royal Gorge. (Note: Forget about reaching the Royal Pool if the first couple of creek crossings are difficult; that would indicate that the water level was extraordinarily high.)

After following the stream around several horseshoe bends, you enter (at about 6.0 miles) a section of the gorge where the sheer walls pinch in tight. Clamber over some boulders and wade through a couple of pools to reach the Royal Pool ahead. Fed by water that slides about 8 feet down a 45-degree incline, then 10 feet more almost vertically, the rock-bound pool measures about 50 feet long, 30 feet wide, and 10 feet deep at the middle.

Don't try climbing around the falls to reach the upper gorge. The south wall may look "do-able," but it consists of horrendously loose, battered Precambrian metamorphic rock (it looks its age).

It is possible to approach the upper lip of the falls from the upstream side (an hour's walk and boulder-hop from the Bear Canyon Trail), but there's no safe way to descend from there—even by sliding over the precipice into the pool. A small rock ledge juts from the base of the falls near the pool's surface. Anyone using the falls as a water slide would probably experience a very hard (possibly fatal) landing.

Note: The 2009 Station Fire burned through the section of the Arroyo Seco described in this trip. Check with the Forest Service to ascertain if the Gabrielino Trail is open.

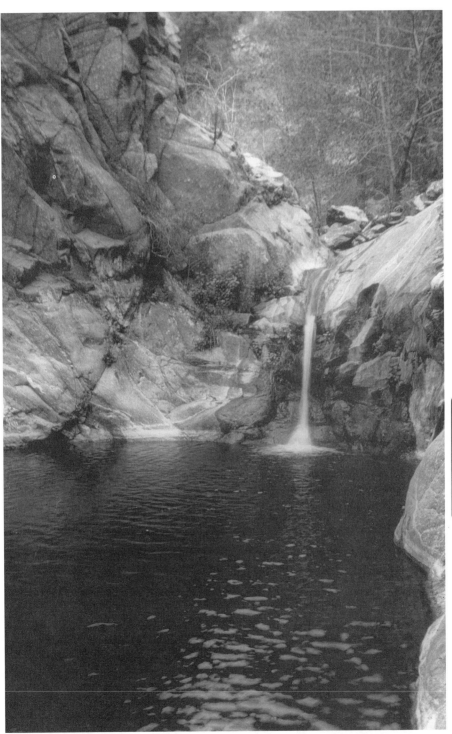

Royal Pool in Royal Gorge

see map on p. 216

## trip 5 San Gabriel Peak

| | |
|---|---|
| **Distance** | 4.2 miles round trip, Out-and-back |
| **Hiking Time** | 2½ hours (round trip) |
| **Elevation Gain/Loss** | 1450'/1450' |
| **Difficulty** | Moderate |
| **Trail Use** | Dogs allowed, good for kids |
| **Best Times** | All year |
| **Agency** | ANF/LARD |
| **Optional Maps** | USGS 7.5-min *Chilao Flat, Mt. Wilson* |
| **Notes** | Marked trails/obvious routes, easy terrain |

**DIRECTIONS** Exit Interstate 210 at Angeles Crest Highway in La Cañada-Flintridge. Drive 13.5 miles north and east to Red Box Station and the intersection of Mount Wilson Road. Turn right on Mount Wilson Road and proceed just 0.4 mile to a turnout at the gated Mount Disappointment service road on the right. This is also the trailhead for the San Gabriel Peak Trail.

The San Gabriel Peak Trail, built by JPL (Jet Propulsion Laboratory) Hiking Club volunteers in 1987–88, bypasses a less-interesting, paved service road to Mount Disappointment used by hikers in the past.

Disappointment was the name given to the peak in 1875 by surveyors who were trying to establish a triangulation point on the area's highest promontory. After a laborious struggle through brush, they discovered they'd reached a false summit. San Gabriel Peak, 100 feet higher, lay beyond.

Today's Mount Disappointment is a disappointing shadow of its former self. The U.S. Army blasted off its top in the 1950s, installed a Nike missile base, and built a service road to the top. Currently the flat-tened summit serves as an antenna site. San Gabriel Peak's summit is not so abused, and makes a fine destination for a high-country hike anytime.

From the trailhead, the San Gabriel Peak Trail wastes no time in zigzagging straight up the steep, oak- and conifer-shaded slopes to the west. Starting at about 0.5 mile, the trail comes abreast of and parallels for a while a stretch of the service road. It then resumes switchbacking, offering occasional conifer-framed views of the Mount Wilson and West Fork (San Gabriel River) country to the east. You come up alongside the service road again at about 1.5 miles. Soon afterward, the trail switchbacks up and joins the service road.

Bigcone Douglas-firs, San Gabriel Peak Trail

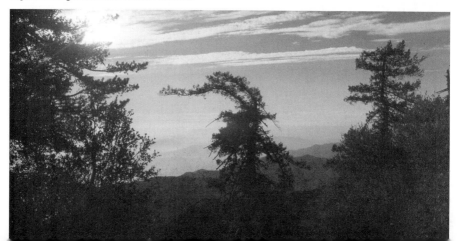

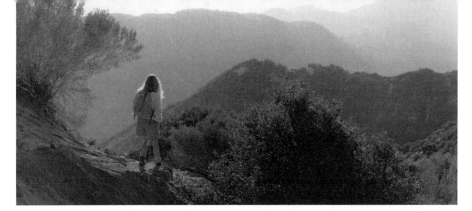

Descending San Gabriel Peak

You can turn north on the service road for a side trip to Mount Disappointment, if you like. Our route to San Gabriel Peak, however, continues southeast over the broad saddle between Mount Disappointment and San Gabriel Peak. You come to a trail junction: the right branch goes south, dropping to Markham Saddle. Take the left branch, going east up San Gabriel Peak's flank, gaining 400 feet in about 0.4 mile. The view from the top is panoramic, but not quite so impressive as that from Mount Lowe, which is about a mile closer to the great L.A. Basin below.

San Gabriel Peak can also be climbed by way of Eaton Saddle and Markham Saddle—a shorter and slightly easier but less scenic approach through the chaparral.

Note: Although San Gabriel Peak was near the 2009 Station Fire perimeter, the entire route described here was within the burn zone.

## trip 6  Mount Lowe

| | |
|---|---|
| **Distance** | 3.2 miles round trip, Out-and-back |
| **Hiking Time** | 1½ hours (round trip) |
| **Elevation Gain/Loss** | 500'/500' |
| **Difficulty** | Moderate |
| **Trail Use** | Dogs allowed |
| **Best Times** | All year |
| **Agency** | ANF/LARD |
| **Optional Maps** | USGS 7.5-min *Mt. Wilson* |
| **Notes** | Marked trails/obvious routes, easy terrain |

see map on p. 216

ANGELES FOREST

**DIRECTIONS** Exit Interstate 210 at Angeles Crest Highway in La Cañada-Flintridge. Drive 13.5 miles north and east to Red Box Station and the intersection of Mount Wilson Road. Turn right on Mount Wilson Road and proceed 2.4 miles to a roadside parking area at Eaton Saddle.

Late in the year, when the smog lightens but temperatures still hover within a moderate register, come up to Mount Lowe to toast the setting sun. You can sit on an old bench, pour the champagne, and watch Old Sol sink into Santa Monica Bay.

From Eaton Saddle, walk past the gate on the west side and proceed up the dirt road (Mount Lowe Fire Road) that carves its way under the precipitous south face of San Gabriel Peak. As you approach a short tunnel (0.3 mile) dating from 1942, look for the remnants of a former cliff-hanging trail to the left of the tunnel's east entrance. At Markham Saddle (0.5 mile) the fire road starts to descend slightly—don't continue on the road. Instead, find the Mount Lowe Trail on the left (south). You contour southwest

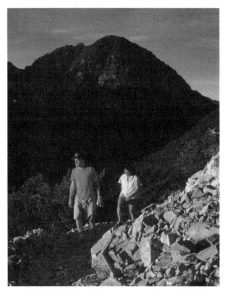

Mount Lowe Trail

above the fire road about 0.6 mile, and then start climbing across the east flank of Mount Lowe without much change of direction.

At 1.3 miles, make a sharp right turn. Proceed 0.2 mile uphill, then go left on a short spur trail to Mount Lowe's barren summit. Mount Lowe was the proposed upper terminus for Professor Thaddeus Lowe's famed scenic railway (see Trip 11 in this chapter). Funding ran out, however, and tracks were never laid higher than Ye Alpine Tavern (later named Mount Lowe Tavern), 1200 feet below. During the railway's heyday in the early 1900s, thousands disembarked at the tavern and tramped Mount Lowe's east- and west-side trails for world-class views of the basin and the surrounding mountains. Some reminders of that era remain on the summit of Mount Lowe and along some of the trails: volunteers have repainted, relettered, and returned to their proper places some the many sighting tubes that helped the early tourists familiarize themselves with the surrounding geography.

Note: The 2009 Station Fire licked its way around the slopes of Mount Lowe, burning nearly all of the vegetation and damaging the trails. Access to the peak, as described here, may be unavailable for some time to come.

## trip 7 Bear Canyon

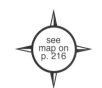

see map on p. 216

| | |
|---|---|
| **Distance** | 7.5 miles, Point-to-point |
| **Hiking Time** | 4 hours |
| **Elevation Gain/Loss** | 1000'/2800' |
| **Difficulty** | Moderately strenuous |
| **Trail Use** | Suitable for backpacking, dogs allowed |
| **Best Times** | All year |
| **Agency** | ANF/LARD |
| **Recommended Maps** | USGS 7.5-min *Mt. Wilson, Pasadena, Condor Peak* |
| **Notes** | Navigation required, moderate terrain |

**DIRECTIONS** *East End:* Exit Interstate 210 at Angeles Crest Highway in La Cañada-Flintridge. Drive 13.5 miles north and east to Red Box Station and the intersection of Mount Wilson Road. Turn right on Mount Wilson Road and proceed 2.4 miles to a roadside parking area at Eaton Saddle. *West End:* From a point on Angeles Crest Highway 10 miles north of La Cañada-Flintridge (3.5 miles west of Mount Wilson Road) turn south and descend into Switzer Picnic Area.

**B**ear Canyon, as secluded and beautiful as any small canyon in the Front Range country, enjoys the added benefit of good trail access from two sides. Graced by a sparkling rivulet of water, and shaded by beautiful sycamore, alder, bigcone Douglas-fir, bigleaf maple, and bay trees, the canyon's innermost confines are scarcely disturbed at all by the little-improved remains of the historic Tom Sloan Trail—built in 1923 to serve the needs of hikers traveling between Mount Lowe Tavern and Switzer's Camp. The stretch through the canyon is a special delight in November, when the leaves of the maples turn crispy yellow, and you scuff through leaf litter so thick it's hard to recognize the path. The one-way hike suggested here adds some driving logistics, it but makes the hiking/backpacking part a lot easier than hoofing it in both directions.

From the start at Eaton Saddle, take the Mount Lowe Fire Road west to Markham Saddle (0.5 mile). Continue southwest and west without leaving the fire road until you reach a 180-degree bend to the left (1.8 miles) atop the long west ridge coming down from Mount Lowe's summit. Leave the road there and continue, on trail now, westward along the same ridge. Here and there along the way you can look south over Millard Canyon and across the often hazy lowlands to Palos Verdes and Santa Catalina Island. Upper Bear Canyon lies to the north, its rugged, chaparral-clad slopes hardly suggesting the beauty that exists down along the hidden stream. After a few downhill

switchbacks, you arrive at Tom Sloan Saddle (2.8 miles), where several trails meet: a trail coming up from Dawn Mine, the east leg of the Tom Sloan Trail from the Mount Lowe Tavern site, and the west leg of the Tom Sloan Trail (aka the Bear Canyon Trail) coming up from Bear Canyon. In addition, there's a ridgetop fire break, sometimes followed by hikers, leading west to the summit of Brown Mountain.

From Tom Sloan Saddle, you go north, descending switchbacks through chaparral until you reach Bear Canyon's stream (3.5 miles). There you'll discover the remains of a small, stone shed and cabin foundations hidden amid the poison oak and wild blackberry vines.

The trail deteriorates as you turn downcanyon, and progress slows. From time to time, boulder-hopping may become the way to travel until you reach Bear Canyon Trail Camp, 4.2 miles, on an oak-shaded terrace to the left. Beyond here the pathway becomes easier to follow. A section of trail carved precariously into a sheer wall on the right (mile 5.4) heralds your arrival at Bear Creek's confluence with Arroyo Seco. From there on the path is wide and obvious, and you'll be climbing for almost all of the remaining 2 miles. You follow Arroyo Seco upstream past some sparkling mini-falls

Bigleaf maples, Bear Canyon

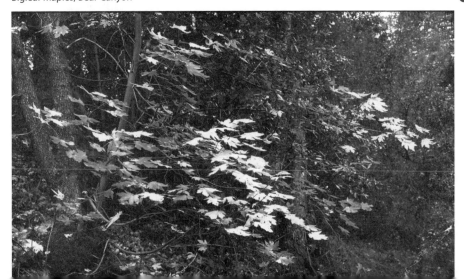

and rock-bound pools. A half mile later you start an ascent up the slope to the left, and soon thereafter join the Gabrielino Trail. You pass Switzer Falls, skirt Switzer's Camp, and finally arrive at Switzer Picnic Area. (If the access road to the picnic area is gated at the top, you'll need to hike an additional 0.5 mile, 250 feet elevation gain, to reach Angeles Crest Highway.)

Note: The 2009 Station Fire burned most of the area traversed in the foregoing trip. The west end of the trip, in particular, involves trails in steep and unstable terrain that may be closed for years to come.

## trip 8  Millard Canyon Falls

see map on p. 216

| | |
|---|---|
| **Distance** | 1.4 miles round trip, Out-and-back |
| **Hiking Time** | 1 hour (round trip) |
| **Elevation Gain/Loss** | 300'/300' |
| **Difficulty** | Moderate |
| **Trail Use** | Dogs allowed, good for kids |
| **Best Times** | All year |
| **Agency** | ANF/LARD |
| **Optional Map** | USGS 7.5-min *Pasadena* |
| **Notes** | Marked trails/obvious routes, moderate terrain |

**DIRECTIONS**  Exit Interstate 210 at Lincoln Avenue in Pasadena. Go north on Lincoln for 1.8 miles, and turn right on Canyon Crest Road. Proceed 0.6 mile east to Chaney Trail (a paved road) on the left. Drive past a sturdy gate, typically open 6 a.m. to 10 p.m., go up and over Sunset Ridge, and then down to the road's end into a large parking lot alongside the Millard Canyon stream.

During heavy rains, Millard Canyon's modest watershed gathers enough runoff to stage a real spectacle near its lower end—Millard Canyon Falls. Even in the dry season, when the water dribbles over the rock by way of several serpentine paths, the steep-walled grotto containing the falls is pleasantly cool, and worth a visit.

From the parking lot, hike upstream, past a vehicle gate, and through Millard Campground (a walk-in facility). Continue up the canyon, boulder-hopping from time to time, beneath oaks and alders, until you reach the falls. Part of the falling water is blocked from view by several large boulders wedged like chockstones high above. It's difficult to take a photograph that does justice to this cool, dark or sun-dappled, pleasant place.

Although much of Millard Canyon was burned in the 2009 Station Fire, it is possible that the streamside access to Millard Canyon Falls will not be seriously curtailed. Check with the Forest Service to be sure.

## trip 9  Dawn Mine Loop

| | |
|---|---|
| **Distance** | 5.6 miles, Loop |
| **Hiking Time** | 3½ hours |
| **Elevation Gain/Loss** | 1600'/1600' |
| **Difficulty** | Moderately strenuous |
| **Trail Use** | Suitable for backpacking, dogs allowed |
| **Best Times** | October through June |
| **Agency** | ANF/LARD |
| **Optional Map** | USGS 7.5-min *Pasadena* |
| **Notes** | Marked trails/obvious routes, moderate terrain |

see map on p. 216

**DIRECTIONS** Exit Interstate 210 at Lincoln Avenue in Pasadena. Go north on Lincoln for 1.8 miles, and turn right on Canyon Crest Road. Proceed 0.6 mile east to Chaney Trail (a paved road) on the left. Drive past a sturdy gate, typically open 6 a.m. to 10 p.m., and proceed sharply uphill to the road crest at Sunset Ridge, where there's parking space by the roadside.

**M**illard Canyon's happily splashing stream, presided over by oaks, alders, maples, and bigcone Douglas-firs, is the main attraction on this hike. But you can also do a little snooping around the site of the Dawn Mine, one of the more promising gold prospects in the San Gabriels, worked intermittently from 1895 until the early 1950s.

An early start is emphatically recommended. That way you'll take advantage of shade during the climbing phase of the hike, and you'll be assured of finding a place to park your car at the trailhead (which is as popular with mountain bikers as with hikers).

Start by walking east on the gated, paved Sunset Ridge fire road. After about 100 yards, you pass a foot trail on the left leading down to Millard Campground. Continue another 300 yards to a second foot trail on the left (Sunset Ridge Trail). Take it. On it you contour north and east along Millard Canyon's south wall, passing above a sometimes-vociferous 50-foot waterfall. You begin climbing in earnest at about 0.7 mile and soon reach a trail fork. The left branch (your return route) goes down 100 yards past a private cabin

ANGELES FOREST

Dawn Mine ruins

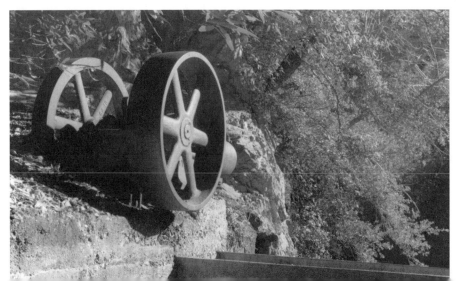

to the canyon bottom. You go right, uphill. Switchbacks long and short take you farther up along the pleasantly shaded canyon wall to an intersection with Sunset Ridge fire road (2.3 miles), just below a rocky knob called Cape of Good Hope.

Turn left on the fire road, and walk past Cape of Good Hope. The trail to Echo Mountain, intersecting on the right, and the fire road ahead are both part of the original Mount Lowe Railway bed (see Trip 11 in this chapter)—now a self-guiding historical trail. Continue your ascent on the fire road/railway bed to post #4 on the left (2.8 miles). There you'll find a trail descending to Dawn Mine in Millard Canyon. This is a reworked but primitive version of the mule path once used to haul ore from the mine to the railway above. On the way down you may encounter a dicey passage or two across loose talus.

After reaching the gloomy canyon bottom (3.4 miles), the trail goes upstream along the east bank for about 100 yards to the long-abandoned Dawn Mine, perched on the west-side slope. The gaping entrance to the lower shaft may seem inviting to explore, but it could collapse without warning.

From the mine, head down-canyon past crystalline mini-pools, the flotsam and jetsam of the mining days, and storm-tossed boulders. Much of the original trail in the canyon has been washed away, but a new generation of hikers has beaten down a pretty good semblance of a path. About a half mile below the mine a wider area of the canyon, with a high and dry terrace on the right, could be used as a wilderness campsite for backpackers.

After swinging around an abrupt bend to the right, the canyon becomes dark and gloomy once again. After another 0.5 mile you'll come to the aforementioned exit trail climbing up to the left. Pass the private cabin and hook up with the Sunset Ridge Trail, which will take you back to the Sunset Ridge fire road and your car.

Note: The 2009 Station Fire thoroughly incinerated upper Millard Canyon, and swept away portions of the Sunset Ridge Trail. It is unknown when the route described here will be available for hiking again.

## trip 10  Upper Millard Canyon

| | |
|---|---|
| **Distance** | 10.6 miles, Loop |
| **Hiking Time** | 6 hours |
| **Elevation Gain/Loss** | 2700'/2700' |
| **Difficulty** | Strenuous |
| **Trail Use** | Suitable for backpacking, dogs allowed |
| **Best Times** | October through May |
| **Agency** | ANF/LARD |
| **Recommended Maps** | USGS 7.5-min *Pasadena, Mt. Wilson* |
| **Notes** | Navigation required, moderate terrain |

**DIRECTIONS** Exit Interstate 210 at Lincoln Avenue in Pasadena. Go north on Lincoln for 1.8 miles, and turn right on Canyon Crest Road. Proceed 0.6 mile east to Chaney Trail (a paved road) on the left. Drive past a sturdy gate, typically open 6 a.m. to 10 p.m., and proceed sharply uphill to the road crest at Sunset Ridge, where there's parking space by the roadside.

**O**n this longer version of the Dawn Mine loop described just above, you'll climb all the way to Tom Sloan Saddle at the head of Millard Canyon, and then take the east leg of the historic Tom Sloan Trail down toward Mount Lowe Trail Camp (the site of the historic Mount Lowe Tavern). If this is your first visit to the area, it's better to travel around the loop in a clockwise direction as we describe here, returning via the Mount Lowe Railway bed.

Begin by walking up the Sunset Ridge fire road and veering left onto the Sunset Ridge Trail after 400 yards. Bear left at 1.0 mile (where the Sunset Ridge Trail climbs right), descend to Millard Canyon's stream, and work your way up along the banks to Dawn Mine (2.4 miles).

Continue upstream another 0.2 mile to a confluence where a large tributary, Grand Canyon, branches east. On the left you should find a narrow switchback trail going up the shady ravine heading north. You cross the ravine five times and negotiate several switchbacks before arriving at Tom Sloan Saddle (3.6 miles) atop the high ridge shared by Brown Mountain and Mount Lowe. Of the many paths that converge there, take the one farthest right—you will see its trace slanting across the chaparral-covered north wall of Grand Canyon. Reworked in 1988-89, this 1923 trail retains much of the charm of the original. Just wide enough for hikers, it climbs on a constant, moderate grade, chiseling across rock faces, ducking beneath oaks, tunneling through tall chaparral. South across Grand Canyon, you'll spot the old railway bed cutting across the opposing canyon wall.

When you reach the Mount Lowe Fire Road (5.2 miles), turn right and walk about a quarter mile. You may hear voices from Mount Lowe Trail Camp, 150 feet below, on the right. Find a good place to cut down the slope—you'll save almost a half mile of road-walking this way. Year-round water is available at the trail camp, but it must be filtered or purified.

From the trail camp it's downhill virtually all the way back. Follow the fire road/old railway bed 2.6 miles west and south, down past a couple of hairpin turns, to Cape of Good Hope, where the pavement begins. Just past the Cape, use the Sunset Ridge Trail to return to the starting point. Alternatively you can walk down the paved Sunset Ridge fire road, which is slightly shorter, but sun-exposed and a lot less scenic.

Note: The 2009 Station Fire thoroughly incinerated upper Millard Canyon, and swept away portions of the Sunset Ridge Trail. It is unknown when the route described here will be available for hiking again.

**trip 11**  ## Mount Lowe Railway

see map on p. 216

|  |  |
|---|---|
| **Distance** | 11.4 miles, Loop |
| **Hiking Time** | 6 hours |
| **Elevation Gain/Loss** | 2800'/2800' |
| **Difficulty** | Moderately strenuous |
| **Trail Use** | Suitable for backpacking, dogs allowed |
| **Best Times** | October through May |
| **Agency** | ANF/LARD |
| **Optional Maps** | USGS 7.5-mi *Mt. Wilson, Pasadena* |
| **Notes** | Marked trails/obvious routes, easy terrain |

**DIRECTIONS** Exit Interstate 210 at Lake Avenue in Pasadena. Drive north on Lake Avenue for 3.6 miles to where the street bends left and becomes Loma Alta Drive. Find the any curbside parking space nearest this intersection.

An engineering marvel when built in the 1890s, the Mount Lowe Railway has had a checkered past full of both glory and destruction. Before its final abandonment in the mid-1930s, the line carried over 3 million passengers—virtually all of them tourists. Unheard of by most Southland residents today, the railway was for many years the most popular outdoor attraction in Southern California.

Today hikers are taking a new interest in the old road bed; the Rails-to-Trails Conservancy (which promotes the conversion of abandoned rail corridors into recreation trails) ranked the Mount Lowe Railway as one of the nation's 12 most scenic and historically significant recycled rail lines.

The line consisted of three stages, of which almost nothing remains today. Passengers rode a trolley from Altadena into lower Rubio Canyon, then boarded a steeply inclined cable railway which took them 1300 feet higher to Echo Mountain, where two hotels, a number of small tourist attractions, and an observatory stood. At Echo Mountain, non-acrophobic passengers hopped onto the third phase, a mountain trolley that climbed another 1200 vertical feet along airy slopes to the end of the line—Ye Alpine Tavern (later Mount Lowe Tavern, on whose ruins stands today's Mount Lowe Trail Camp).

The Forest Service and volunteers have put together a self-guiding trail, featuring ten markers fashioned from railroad rails, along the route of the mountain trolley. The middle portion of the old railway bed can be reached by hiking either the paved road or the trail coming up from the Chaney Trail above Millard Canyon. The more direct, easier, and more exciting way to reach Station 1 at Echo Mountain, however, is to go by way of the Sam Merrill Trail from Altadena.

The Sam Merrill Trailhead lies on the grounds of the long-demolished Cobb Estate, at the north end of Lake Avenue in Altadena. Walk east past the stone pillars at the entrance and continue 150 yards on a narrow, blacktop driveway. The driveway bends left, but you keep walking straight (east). Soon you come to a water fountain on the rim of Las Flores Canyon and a sign indicating the start of the Sam Merrill Trail.

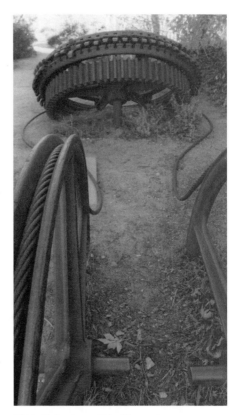

Old bullwheel atop Echo Mountain

This trail goes left over the top of a small debris dam and begins a switchback ascent of Las Flores Canyon's precipitous east wall, while another trail (the Altadena Crest equestrian trail) veers to the right, down the canyon.

Inspired by the fabulous views (assuming you're doing this early on one of L.A.'s clear winter days), the 2.5 miles of steady ascent on the Sam Merrill Trail may seem to go rather quickly. Turn right at the top of the trail and walk south over to Echo Mountain, which is more like the shoulder of a ridge. There you'll find a historical plaque and some picnic tables near a grove of incense cedars and bigleaf maples. Poke around and you'll find many foundation ruins and piles of concrete rubble. An old "bullwheel" and cables for the incline railway were thoughtfully left behind after the Forest Service cleared away what remained of the buildings here in the 1950s and '60s. After visiting Echo Mountain, you'll go north on the signed Echo Mountain Trail, where you'll walk over railroad ties still imbedded in the ground.

Here's a log of the stops along the self-guiding rail bed tour (numbers in parentheses refer to hiking mileage starting from Echo Mountain.):

**Station 1 (0.0) Echo Mountain**. This was known as the White City during its brief heyday in the late 1890s, but most of its tourist facilities were destroyed by fire or windstorms in the first decade of the 1900s. The mountain remained a transfer point for passengers until the mid-1930s.

**Station 2 (0.5) View of Circular Bridge**. You can't see it from here, but passengers at this point first noticed the 400-foot-diameter circular bridge (Station 6) jutting from the slope above. As you walk on ahead, you'll notice the many concrete footings that supported trestles bridging the side ravines of Las Flores Canyon.

**Station 3 (0.8) Cape of Good Hope**. You're now at the junction of the Echo Mountain Trail and Sunset Ridge fire road. The tracks swung in a 200-degree arc around the rocky promontory just west—Cape of Good Hope. (Walk around the Cape, if you like, to get a feel for the experience.) North of this dizzying passage, riders were treated

to the longest stretch of straight track— only 225 feet long. The entire original line from Echo Mountain to Ye Alpine Tavern had 127 curves and 114 straight sections. [Note: plenty of mountain bikers use this section of the old railroad grade. They mostly arrive by way of the Sunset Ridge fire road.]

**Station 4 (1.0) Dawn Station/Devil's Slide**. Dawn Mine lies below in Millard Canyon. Gold-bearing ore, packed up by mules from the canyon bottom, was loaded onto the train here. Ahead lay a treacherous stretch of crumbling granite, the Devil's Slide, which was eventually bridged by a trestle. (The current fire road has been shored up with much new concrete, and cement-lined spillways seem to do a good job of carrying away flood debris.)

**Station 5 (1.2) Horseshoe Curve**. Just beyond this station, Horseshoe Curve enabled the railway to gain elevation above Millard Canyon. The grade just beyond Horseshoe Curve was 7 percent—steepest on the mountain segment of the line.

**Station 6 (1.6) Circular Bridge**. An engineering accomplishment of worldwide fame, the Circular Bridge carried startled passengers into midair over the upper walls of Las Flores Canyon. Look for the concrete supports of this bridge down along the chaparral-covered slopes to the right.

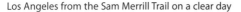

Los Angeles from the Sam Merrill Trail on a clear day

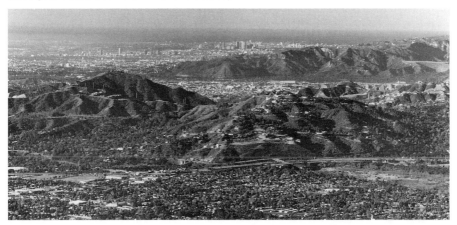

**Station 7 (2.0) Horseshoe Curve Overview**. Passengers here looked down on Horseshoe Curve, and could also see all three levels of steep, twisting track climbing the east wall of Millard Canyon.

**Station 8 (2.4) Granite Gate**. A narrow slot carefully blasted out of solid granite on a sheer north-facing slope, Granite Gate took 8 months to cut. Look for the electric wire support dangling from the rock above.

**Station 9 (3.4) Ye Alpine Tavern**. The tavern, which later became a fancy hotel, was located at Crystal Springs, the source that still provides water (which now requires purification) for backpackers staying overnight at today's Mount Lowe Trail Camp. The rails never got farther than here, although it was hoped they would one day reach the summit of Mount Lowe, 1200 feet higher.

**Station 10 (3.9) Inspiration Point**. From Ye Alpine Tavern, tourists could saunter over to Inspiration Point along part of the never-finished rail extension to Mount Lowe. Sighting tubes (still in place there) helped visitors locate places of interest below.

Inspiration Point is the last station on the self-guiding trail. The fastest and easiest way to return is by way of the Castle Canyon Trail, which descends directly below Inspiration Point. After 2 miles you'll arrive back on the old railway grade just north of Echo Mountain. Retrace your steps on the Sam Merrill Trail.

Note: Only the uppermost (northernmost) portions of the foregoing trip were affected by the 2009 Station Fire. Check with the Forest Service to determine if the entire loop is open.

## trip 12  Inspiration Point

see map on p. 216

| | |
|---|---|
| **Distance** | 6.0 miles, Loop |
| **Hiking Time** | 3½ hours |
| **Elevation Gain/Loss** | 1500'/1500' |
| **Difficulty** | Moderately strenuous |
| **Trail Use** | Suitable for backpacking, dogs allowed |
| **Best Times** | October through June |
| **Agency** | ANF/LARD |
| **Optional Map** | USGS 7.5-min *Mt. Wilson* |
| **Notes** | Marked trails/obvious routes, easy terrain |

**DIRECTIONS** Exit Interstate 210 at Angeles Crest Highway in La Cañada-Flintridge. Drive 13.5 miles north and east to Red Box Station and the intersection of Mount Wilson Road. Turn right on Mount Wilson Road and proceed 2.4 miles to a roadside parking area at Eaton Saddle.

This trip rambles down to Inspiration Point the back way—via Mount Lowe. It's a down-and-up route, so save most of your energy for the trip back. On the way down and later back, you'll have a chance to use both the east and west trails on the slopes of Mount Lowe. These were among the best-used trails during the era of the railway, and both were brought back into service in the late 1980s.

From Eaton Saddle, walk past the gate on the west side and proceed up the dirt road (Mount Lowe Fire Road) that carves its way under the precipitous south face of San Gabriel Peak. As you approach a short tunnel (0.3 mile) dating from 1942, look for the remnants of a former cliff-hanging trail to the left of the tunnel's east entrance. At Markham Saddle (0.5 mile) the fire road starts to descend slightly—don't continue

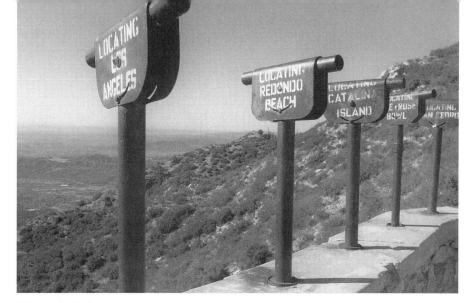

At Inspiration Point

on the road. Instead, find the Mount Lowe Trail on the left (south). You contour southwest above the fire road for about 0.6 mile, and then start climbing across the east flank of Mount Lowe without much change of direction.

At 1.3 miles, there's a trail junction. Go either way (straight for the east trail, sharply right for the west trail), but plan to use the other trail on your return. Either way you'll end up descending to meet the Mount Lowe Fire Road at a point above Mount Lowe Trail Camp. Go south on the fire road to Inspiration Point, where the view is truly inspiring whenever the marine inversion layer lies low across the L.A. Basin—a fairly common occurrence early in the day. On very clear days the ocean horizon can be seen *behind* the gap at Two Harbors on Santa Catalina Island, and San Clemente Island sprawls indistinctly just left of the leftmost tip of Santa Catalina.

If you're interested in side trips, you can climb the 4714-foot peaklet just west of Inspiration Point. Or you can travel 1 mile southeast on the flat fire road going out to Panorama Point—the ridge overlooking Eaton Canyon. Starting around 1915, tourists could traverse this stretch on board a mule-pushed (not drawn, so passengers could avoid dust) observation car that rolled along narrow-gauge rails. This O. M. & M. (One Man and a Mule) Railroad became a popular side attraction for Mount Lowe Tavern guests and day-trippers.

Today's fire road out toward Panorama Point curls south and ends at a concrete water tank, where views of the L.A. Basin are probably more fantastic than from any other land-based vantage point. On a clear night, the view of millions of lights almost a mile of elevation lower is surreal. From this close-in point, less than 2 beeline miles from the edge of the city, the soft droning of a hundred thousand engines, accented now and again by an accelerating motorcycle or unmuffled car, floats upward on the updrafts.

Return the way you came, except in circling Mount Lowe.

Nearly the entire area covered by the foregoing trip was burned in the 2009 Station Fire. That approach may be closed for repairs for possibly years to come. Access to Inspiration Point and Panorama Point may be possible at a much earlier time using routes approaching from the south—Trip 11 in this chapter being one example.

## trip 13 Strawberry Peak

see
map on
p. 216

| | |
|---|---|
| **Distance** | 6.6 miles round trip, Out-and-back |
| **Hiking Time** | 4 hours (round trip) |
| **Elevation Gain/Loss** | 1900'/1900' |
| **Difficulty** | Moderately strenuous |
| **Trail Use** | Suitable for backpacking, dogs allowed |
| **Best Times** | October through June |
| **Agency** | ANF/LARD |
| **Recommended Map** | USGS 7.5-min *Chilao Flat* |
| **Notes** | Navigation required, moderate terrain |

**DIRECTIONS** Exit Interstate 210 at Angeles Crest Highway in La Cañada-Flintridge. Drive 13.5 miles north and east to Red Box Station (at the intersection of Mount Wilson Road). Park in either the ranger station or picnic-ground lots.

Strawberry Peak's 6164-foot summit beats by a smidgen 6161-foot San Gabriel Peak, thus claiming the honor of being the highest peak in the Front Range. Although its profile appears rounded as seen from most places, in reality its flanks fall away sharply on three sides, leaving only one relatively easy route to the top.

In March 1909, Strawberry Peak garnered national attention when a gas balloon and gondola carrying six passengers over Tournament Park in Pasadena was swept by violent gusts into storm clouds over the San Gabriel Mountains. After being tossed to as high as 14,000 feet, the balloon descended in white-out conditions and crash-landed just below Strawberry's snow-covered summit—its gondola coming to rest just 10 feet from a vertical precipice. Nearly three days later, a telephone call from Switzer's Camp brought news to the world below that the riders had survived.

On this hike you'll climb Strawberry by way of the fastest and easiest way—first by trail, then on a well-beaten but sometimes steep path along an old fire break. You'll be traveling mostly along hot, south-facing slopes and open ridges exposed to the sun, so an early-morning start is best.

The starting point, Red Box Gap, is named for a red box of fire-fighting tools placed there around 1908. The gap, or saddle, divides the Arroyo Seco from the West Fork of the San Gabriel River. Today, of course, it's an important crossroads for mountain-going auto traffic.

From Red Box, walk east along the left shoulder of Angeles Crest Highway 0.1 mile to an abandoned fire road slanting left up the hillside. Continue up the eroded bed of that road for 0.6 mile to reach a trail on the left. From there, a switchbacking trail through chaparral takes you northwest to a saddle due south of Mount Lawlor's summit.

When you reach a saddle on the northwest shoulder of Mount Lawlor (2.2 miles from Red Box) and the trail starts to descend north, leave the maintained trail and start climbing along the overgrown fire break slanting left along an undulating, chaparral-covered ridge. Work your way north and finally west to Strawberry's shaggy-looking summit—rocky and slippery going in places.

Scattered Coulter pines and bigcone Douglas-firs struggle for existence near the summit, their wind-blown limbs swept back in gestures that seem defiant. The view from the top is panoramic, but not so exciting as from peaks such as Mount Lowe or Mount Lukens. On the other hand, Strawberry often basks in clean air while the basin-bordering ramparts are wreathed in smoggy air.

The foregoing trip was affected by the 2009 Station Fire. Check with the Forest Service to determine if the route is open.

## trip 14  Colby Canyon to Big Tujunga

| | |
|---|---|
| **Distance** | 8.4 miles, Point-to-point |
| **Hiking Time** | 5½ hours |
| **Elevation Gain/Loss** | 1700'/2040' |
| **Difficulty** | Moderately strenuous |
| **Trail Use** | Suitable for backpacking, dogs allowed |
| **Best Times** | October through May |
| **Agency** | ANF/LARD |
| **Recommended Maps** | USGS 7.5-min *Condor Peak, Chilao Flat* |
| **Notes** | Navigation required, moderate terrain, bushwhacking |

see map on p. 216

**DIRECTIONS** *South End:* Exit Interstate 210 at Angeles Crest Highway in La Cañada-Flintridge. Drive 9.8 miles north to an unpaved turnout on the left at mile marker 34.5. *North End:* From Clear Creek Station, 9.1 miles north of Interstate 210 via Angeles Crest Highway, turn north on Angeles Forest Highway. Proceed 8.4 miles and turn right on Upper Big Tujunga Road. Continue 1.2 miles and turn right on the dead-end road to Colby Camp. Descend on narrow and sharply twisting pavement to a large unpaved lot along Big Tujunga Canyon's creek.

A newer bypass of the old Colby Trail through Colby Ranch allows hikers to swing by Strawberry Peak and descend all the way to the bank of Big Tujunga Canyon's creek. (Formerly, the trail ended inside the ranch property—now a private Methodist camp.) For the most part you'll be following a route hewn over the mountains in the 1890s by pioneer Delos Colby. The trail connected Switzer's Camp in the Arroyo Seco with Colby's ranch in Coldwater Canyon, a tributary of Big Tujunga. Around the turn of the century, the ranch catered to hikers, hunters, and fishermen independent and determined enough to travel beyond the fancy resorts of the Arroyo Seco and Mount Lowe areas.

The highlight of the trip is Strawberry Potrero, a series of gentle depressions tucked under the granite cliffs and talus of Strawberry Peak's sheer north flank. Beyond Strawberry Potrero, the route tends to be less maintained and possibly overgrown and sketchy. It would be wise to contact the Forest Service before attempting this trip for up-to-date information.

From the turnout on Angeles Crest Highway, head up the Colby Trail. In the first half mile you'll be charmed by the woodsy atmosphere and (in season at least) the brook trickling down the narrow canyon bottom. All too soon you're struggling up slopes thickly grown with chaparral and punctuated by the giant white plumes of blooming yuccas. The well-graded but at times rock-strewn trail zigzags expeditiously to Josephine Saddle, 2.0 miles. There you meet an old fire road going west toward Josephine Peak, and a sketchy footpath going northeast, gently uphill, left of the boulder-backed ridge leading to Strawberry Peak. Follow the footpath. Almost immediately you'll notice the well-worn climbers' route to Strawberry's summit veering right; our route follows the trail contouring ahead.

For 2 more miles the trail stays close to the 5000-foot contour, bending around several precipitous gullies that often serve as chutes for rockfall. Unlike Strawberry Peak's wind-beaten, nearly barren top (unseen more than 1000 feet above), oaks, pines, and bigcone Douglas-firs cling tenaciously to this level of the mountain—wherever the soil is stable enough to retain moisture. Clusters of prickly phlox and Indian paintbrush brighten the muted tones of earth and forest.

Following a moderate descent, you arrive (4.6 miles) at the westernmost clearing of Strawberry Potrero (the Spanish word *potrero* means pasture), a sandy basin

ANGELES FOREST

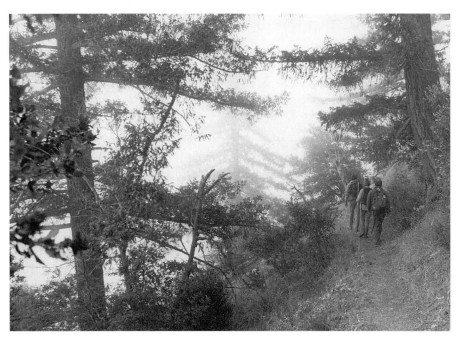

Colby Trail north of Josephine Saddle

ringed by live oaks and Coulter pines. The sheer, granite cliffs and talus of Strawberry Peak's north face preside over this superb camping/picnic spot. There's a picnic table and flat, sandy spaces for pitching tents. Depending on the season, water might be obtained from runoff or snowmelt on the slopes above.

A trail (Colby's original route) continues north down to Colby Ranch. Our way, however, contours east along the base of the talus slope, passes through a second clearing, and descends through a shady ravine to a third, open basin—this one a true meadow filled with sedges and grasses.

At the next trail junction, 5.6 miles from the start, go left (north). When you come to the next fork, 0.2 mile farther, keep right (northeast) to follow the newer trail down to Big Tujunga.

At 6.6 miles the trail comes to the nose of a ridge offering a view of cars in the unpaved lot at the trail's end, 1000 feet below but almost 2 miles away via the trail. Two steep firebreaks diverge here, one to the northwest, the other to the northeast. Our route follows the latter. Slip and slide down, losing about 150 feet, and find the continuation of the trail going left (northwest) along an oak-bowered slope. Gentle switchbacks take you from there to Big Tujunga Canyon.

Note: The entire area covered by the Colby Canyon to Big Tujunga traverse was swept by the 2009 Station Fire. Check with the Forest Service to determine if the route is open.

# trip 15  Fall Creek Trail

| | |
|---|---|
| **Distance** | 5.5 miles, Point-to-point |
| **Hiking Time** | 2½ hours |
| **Elevation Gain/Loss** | 1600'/1600' |
| **Difficulty** | Moderate |
| **Trail Use** | Dogs allowed |
| **Best Times** | October through June |
| **Agency** | ANF/LARD |
| **Optional Map** | USGS 7.5-min *Condor Peak* |
| **Notes** | Marked trails/obvious routes, easy terrain, possible bushwhacking |

see map on p. 216

**DIRECTIONS** *East End:* From Clear Creek Station, 9.1 miles north of Interstate 210 via Angeles Crest Highway, turn north on Angeles Forest Highway. You come to the intersection of Big Tujunga Canyon Road after 3.8 miles. Continue north on Angeles Forest Highway for another 3 miles to reach Hidden Springs Picnic Area, just beyond a tunnel. *West End:* The hike ends at a turnout on Big Tujunga Canyon Road, 0.7 mile west of Angeles Forest Highway.

**F**all Creek Trail threads the steep, north wall of Big Tujunga Canyon and offers unique vistas of Big Tujunga's dramatic "Narrows" section below. Big Tujunga Canyon drains much of the western end of the San Gabriel Mountains, and was the site, a century ago, of the shooting of one of the last of California's native grizzly bears.

The Fall Creek Trail offers fine vistas of the looming "skyline" to the south, consisting of Josephine and Strawberry peaks. The hike is best as a one-way trek—down into Big Tujunga Canyon, and back up the other side. Be aware, however, that flood conditions could render Big Tujunga's creek unsafe to ford. Also, the trail traverses thick growths of chaparral, which in fairly short order could knit together across the trail, rendering it difficult to trace.

Both end-points of the hike lie on virtually the same elevation contour, so it makes little difference which way you go. Mornings,

Springtime chaparral along Fall Creek Trail

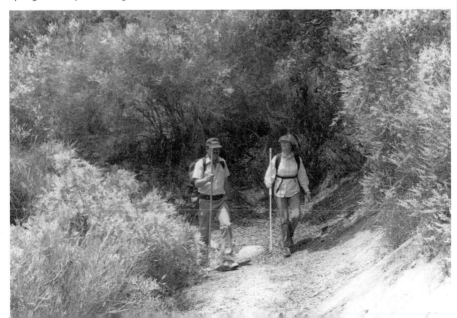

ANGELES FOREST

you may prefer going west to keep the sun out of your eyes; afternoons, going east is probably better. Assuming you go from east to west, you start at Hidden Springs Picnic Area. The trail doesn't begin exactly there, but rather from the road shoulder about 300 yards north. It goes up along a small canyon (North Fork Mill Creek) a short distance and then veers left along a brushy hillside. After gaining roughly 800 feet in 1 mile, the trail levels, contours for another mile, and then begins dropping steadily into Big Tujunga Canyon.

You're almost never out of sight or sound of the curling ribbons of asphalt and traffic below, but at least the trail smells of wilderness and wild chaparral. The sun-warmed slopes reek of pungent yerba santa and sage. While you're descending, enjoy the view up the V-shaped gash of Big Tujunga's Narrows to the east.

At 3.5 miles, the footpath you're on ends at a junction of dirt roads. The left branch leads 200 yards east to Fall Creek Trail Camp (a former work camp—tables, stoves, and ornamental plantings gone wild), while the middle branch (our route) descends to the gravelly floor of Big Tujunga Canyon.

After fording the normally shallow creek, continue west on the fire road that crookedly ascends Big Tujunga Canyon's steep south wall. On the way up, look across the canyon to see water shooting (or dribbling) down a moss-covered ledge in Fall Creek.

Note: The Fall Creek traverse was swept by the flames of the 2009 Station Fire. The chaparral landscape will likely return within a few years, but trail damage has resulted and may take some time to be repaired. Check with the Forest Service to determine if the route is open.

# chapter 21

# Angeles Forest:
# Mount Wilson & Front Range

In the lush and shady recesses of Big Santa Anita Canyon, Eaton Canyon, and other drainages at the foot of Mount Wilson, you can easily lose all sight and sense of the hundreds of square miles of dense metropolis lying just over a single ridge. With very easy access, by city street or mountain road and then by trail, these are perfect spots to discover the San Gabriel Mountains' beguiling charms.

The flattish, rambling summit of Mount Wilson, a sort of centerpiece for the area covered in this section, is hardly notable for its elevation of about 5700 feet. But its long history of use, dating back to 1864, has made it a major node in the trail network of the San Gabriels. Today the drive to Mount Wilson is an easy one—half an hour at best from I-210 at La Cañada. You can play tourist by visiting Skyline Park (open 10 a.m. to 4 p.m. daily from April through November) and Mount Wilson Observatory, or you can get serious and set off on one of the steep trails down its flank.

Chantry Flat, above Arcadia, is the hikers' hub on the lowland side. Chantry Flat is also the jumping-off spot for cabin owners who must walk down to their homes away from home in Big Santa Anita Canyon. At Chantry Flat, you'll find spacious (although often inadequate) parking space, a ranger station, a picnic ground, and a mom-and-pop refreshment stand. There's also a freight business—the last pack station operating year round in California. Almost daily, horses, mules, and burros carry building materials and other supplies to canyon residents.

A sturdy gate on Santa Anita Avenue just above Arcadia clangs shut every night at 10 p.m. and doesn't open till 6 a.m. the next morning. On the weekends, it's wise to arrive early at Chantry Flat; otherwise parking is hard to come by. It's also worth noting that—if the recent past is any guide—the road to Chantry Flat could be closed to cars due to any combination of fire, flood, or mudslide.

Several of the trips below (those originating on Angeles National Forest lands) require a National Forest Adventure Pass for trailhead parking. The pass costs $5 per day or $30 per year.

In August and September of 2009, Mount Wilson was the scene of dramatic battles between firefighters and the ever-shifting flames of the Station Fire. Mount Wilson Observatory and a large telecommunications facility nearby were saved during this effort. Santa Anita Canyon and Chantry Flat were untouched by the fire, though most of the area north of the Mount Wilson summit was thoroughly incinerated. Several trails described in this chapter have experienced serious damage. They are noted where appropriate in the individual trip descriptions in this chapter.

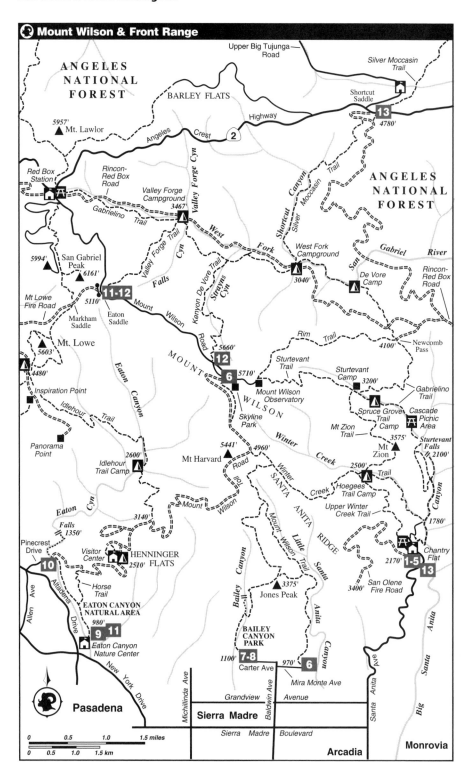

**Mount Wilson & Front Range**

# trip 1  Santa Anita Ridge

| | |
|---|---|
| **Distance** | 7.5 miles round trip, Out-and-back |
| **Hiking Time** | 3½ hours (round trip) |
| **Elevation Gain/Loss** | 1350'/1350' |
| **Difficulty** | Moderately strenuous |
| **Trail Use** | Suitable for mountain biking, dogs allowed |
| **Best Times** | November through May |
| **Agency** | ANF/LARD |
| **Optional Map** | USGS 7.5-min *Mt. Wilson* |
| **Notes** | Marked trails/obvious routes, easy terrain |

see map on p. 242

**DIRECTIONS** Exit Interstate 210 at Santa Anita Avenue in Arcadia. Drive north through Arcadia and Sierra Madre, and beyond the last subdivision at the foot of the mountains. You pass a vehicle gate (open 6 a.m. to 10 p.m.) and continue north on Santa Anita Canyon Road about 3 miles to reach the parking lots at Chantry Flat.

Winding its way lazily upward from the crowded parking lots at Chantry Flat, San Olene Fire Road leads to a shoulder of Santa Anita Ridge—the viewful divide between Big and Little Santa Anita canyons. From the top of the road, the sweeping view takes in the Santa Anita Park race track (only 3 miles to the south), a good chunk of the San Gabriel Valley, and parts of the San Gabriel Mountains' High Country to the north and northeast.

The road climbs 3.5 miles at an almost steady 6 percent grade—a bit tedious at walking pace; probably better for running or mountain biking. On clear days, the scenery is uniformly pleasant, especially after winter storms have dusted the surrounding summits. Edging along north-facing slopes much of the way, the road twists and turns through stands of mature chaparral and mini-groves of bay and maple. Best of all, you're likely to meet no one at all beyond the first half mile. The route is ideally suited for a late afternoon or early evening stroll. From the top you could catch the sunset, watch the city lights turn on, then return by the light of a three-quarter or full moon (but remember, the gate below Chantry Flat closes at 10 p.m. daily).

Route finding could scarcely be more simple. Follow the paved service road upward from the picnic area. At 0.7 mile you pass the Chantry Flat Air-Attack Station (heliport), where the pavement ends and a dirt road continues. (Those who would prefer a much shorter, but gut-busting, approach can follow an old fire break straight up the ridge west of the heliport. It leads to the uppermost hairpin turn on San Olene Fire Road.) At 3.5 miles the road levels. There's a microwave reflector structure on the left and a water tank signed SANTA ANITA RIDGE on the right. Proceed another quarter mile down the ridge to the south for the best view of the valley below.

**ANGELES FOREST**

# trip 2  Hoegees Loop

|  |  |
|---|---|
| **Distance** | 5.4 miles, Loop |
| **Hiking Time** | 2½ hours |
| **Elevation Gain/Loss** | 1300'/1300' |
| **Difficulty** | Moderate |
| **Trail Use** | Suitable for backpacking, dogs allowed |
| **Best Times** | All year |
| **Agency** | ANF/LARD |
| **Optional Map** | USGS 7.5-min *Mt. Wilson* |
| **Notes** | Marked trails/obvious routes, easy terrain |

see
map on
p. 242

**DIRECTIONS**  Exit Interstate 210 at Santa Anita Avenue in Arcadia. Drive north through Arcadia and Sierra Madre, and beyond the last subdivision at the foot of the mountains. You pass a vehicle gate (open 6 a.m. to 10 p.m.) and continue north on Santa Anita Canyon Road about 3 miles to reach the parking lots at Chantry Flat.

The canyons of Big Santa Anita and Winter Creek exist in a time warp. On foot is the only way in for the owners of the 82 cabins on Forest Service land here, dating from the early 1900s. Typical cabin amenities include kerosene lamps, drinking water carried in by the jugful, and one-hole privies. This ramble on rustic trails takes you through both of these secluded canyons, where trickling streams and rustling leaves make you forget you're anywhere near a big city.

On this looping hike to and from Hoegees Trail Camp on Winter Creek, you'll get a good feel for the riparian splendor that attracted early residents and day-trippers, and that still attracts legions of hikers today. (Since there are about a dozen stream crossings on the route without benefit of bridges, you'll want to avoid this trip after heavy rain.) Native alders, oaks, bays, and willows cluster along the bubbling, cascading streams. Ivy and vinca, planted by the early settlers, have run rampant in some areas, climbing high into the trees in a fashion reminiscent of the kudzu-vine invasion of the American Southeast. Both canyons have been plugged in many places with crib dams—check dams constructed of precast concrete logs—but many decades years of steady regrowth have softened their visual impact.

Start at the south edge of the lower parking lot at Chantry Flat, where a gated,

paved road (the Gabrielino Trail) starts descending into Big Santa Anita Canyon. After rounding the first sharp bend at 0.2 mile, veer right onto the narrow and precipitous First Water Trail. This was once

Winter Creek

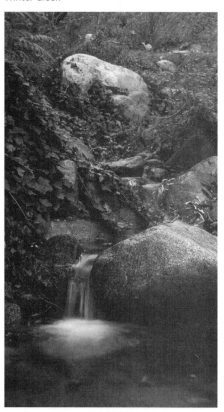

a lateral branch of the original Sturtevant Trail between the San Gabriel Valley and Sturtevant Camp (see Trip 4). Descend on precipitous switchbacks (watch your step!) to the stream below, where an appropriately named First Water Camp welcomed hot and footsore hikers in the 1920s and '30s. Turn left (upstream) and follow the rudiments of a trail amid streamside cabins and boulders to the confluence of Big Santa Anita Canyon and Winter Creek, where the paved trail comes down from Chantry Flat. A small restroom building occupies a flat area nearby (1780′) where the largest resort of the area, Roberts' Camp, sprawled in the early 1900s. During the peak of its popularity, a branch of the L.A. County Library and a post office were established here to serve guests and passing hikers.

From the confluence, head west into the steep-walled confines of Winter Creek. The well-traveled trail snakes upward, sometimes along the stream, otherwise up on the canyon walls in order to bypass crib dams or to swing by cabins. After 1.5 miles

(from the confluence) you come to Hoegees Trail Camp (tables, stoves), tucked into a shady nook on Winter Creek's south bank. Nearby are the scattered foundation ruins of Hoegees Trail Camp (later called Camp Ivy), a hiker's resort established in 1908, and destroyed by wildfire in 1953. Today, Hoegees is one of the more popular trail camps in the San Gabriels—charming, rustic, and easy to reach by either leg of our looping hike.

Your return is by way of the Upper Winter Creek Trail. From Hoegees, continue upstream on the north bank, passing the Mount Zion Trail on the right. Presently, the trail swings left to cross the stream and climb obliquely up Winter Creek's south canyon wall. In a short while you reach a signed junction—right toward Mount Wilson, left back to your starting point a crooked 2.6 miles away. About 0.3 mile from the end, the trail joins a paved section of San Olene Fire Road; it will take you down past the picnic area to the upper parking lot at Chantry Flat.

---

**trip 3** ## Sturtevant Falls

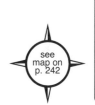

see map on p. 242

| | |
|---|---|
| **Distance** | 3.4 miles round trip, Out-and-back |
| **Hiking Time** | 1½ hours (round trip) |
| **Elevation Gain/Loss** | 700′/700′ |
| **Difficulty** | Moderate |
| **Trail Use** | Dogs allowed, good for kids |
| **Best Times** | All year |
| **Agency** | ANF/LARD |
| **Optional Map** | USGS 7.5-min *Mt. Wilson* |
| **Notes** | Marked trails/obvious routes, easy terrain |

**DIRECTIONS**  Exit Interstate 210 at Santa Anita Avenue in Arcadia. Drive north through Arcadia and Sierra Madre, and beyond the last subdivision at the foot of the mountains. You pass a vehicle gate (open 6 a.m. to 10 p.m.) and continue north on Santa Anita Canyon Road about 3 miles to reach the parking lots at Chantry Flat.

**A**t Sturtevant Falls, the waters of Big Santa Anita Canyon leap (or dribble, depending on the season) over a 50-foot precipice into a shallow pool. Sturtevant Falls ranks, along with falls of a similar stat-

ure in Millard and San Antonio canyons, as one of the more impressive and yet easily reached waterfalls in Southern California. A local attraction since the days of the early resorts, it still draws hundreds of visitors on

**ANGELES FOREST**

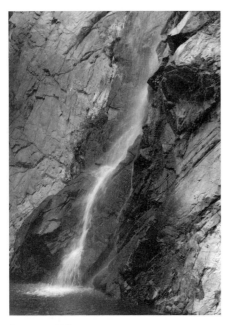

Sturtevant Falls

day, when flat lighting enhances the subdued colors of the rocks, the trees, and the frothing water.

From the south edge of the lower parking lot at Chantry Flat, hike the first, paved segment of the Gabrielino Trail down to the confluence of Winter Creek and Big Santa Anita Canyon (0.6 mile). Pavement ends at a metal bridge spanning Winter Creek. Pass the restrooms and continue up alder-lined Big Santa Anita Canyon on a wide road bed following the left bank. Edging alongside a number of small cabins, the deteriorating road soon assumes the proportions of a foot trail.

At 1.4 miles, amidst a beautiful oak woodland, you come to a four-way junction of trails. Take the right fork and continue upstream, boulder-hopping over the clear-flowing stream part of the way (and perhaps getting your feet wet for the first time), to the foot of the falls. Don't be tempted to climb the sidewalls; the two trails going left back at the four-way junction can take you safely past the falls if you want to press on farther up the canyon.

some fair-weather weekends. To avoid the crowds and gain some feeling of majesty in this special spot, it's best to pay a visit on a weekday. Better yet, come on an overcast

## trip 4  Mount Zion Loop

see map on p. 242

| | |
|---|---|
| **Distance** | 9.4 miles, Loop |
| **Hiking Time** | 5½ hours |
| **Elevation Gain/Loss** | 2100'/2100' |
| **Difficulty** | Moderately strenuous |
| **Trail Use** | Suitable for backpacking, dogs allowed |
| **Best Times** | October through June |
| **Agency** | ANF/LARD |
| **Optional Map** | USGS 7.5-min *Mt. Wilson* |
| **Notes** | Marked trails/obvious routes, easy terrain |

**DIRECTIONS** Exit Interstate 210 at Santa Anita Avenue in Arcadia. Drive north through Arcadia and Sierra Madre, and beyond the last subdivision at the foot of the mountains. You pass a vehicle gate (open 6 a.m. to 10 p.m.) and continue north on Santa Anita Canyon Road about 3 miles to reach the parking lots at Chantry Flat.

Sturtevant Camp is both the oldest (1893) and the only remaining resort of the Big Santa Anita drainage. Run by the Methodist Church as a retreat (but available to other groups by reservation), the camp remains accessible only by foot trail. Supplies are packed in from Chantry Flat on the backs of pack animals, not unlike a century ago. Today's pack trains ply the Gabrielino Trail up Big Santa Anita Canyon past Sturtevant Falls. Around the turn of the century, however, travelers and supplies came by way of a trail hacked out by Wilbur M. ("Sturde") Sturtevant and some associates. Beginning in Sierra Madre, this original Sturtevant Trail worked its way along the high, west wall of lower Big Santa Anita Canyon; crossed a shady spot later known as Chantry Flat; traversed Winter Creek at a point near today's Hoegees Trail Camp; ascended a hot, dry slope to a notch just below Mount Zion; and finally slanted downward to Sturtevant's camp in Big Santa Anita's headwaters.

In this scenic loop trip from Chantry Flat, you'll climb by way of the newer Gabrielino Trail to Sturtevant Camp, and return by way of the Mount Zion and Upper Winter Creek trails—the original Sturtevant route. Do it in a day, or take your time on an overnight backpacking trip, with a stay at Spruce Grove Trail Camp. The trail camp is a popular one, so plan to get there early to secure a spot on the weekend—or go on a weekday.

From the south edge of the lower parking lot at Chantry Flat, hike the first, paved segment of the Gabrielino Trail down to the confluence of Winter Creek and Big Santa Anita Canyon (0.6 mile). Pavement ends at a metal bridge spanning Winter Creek. Pass the restrooms and continue up alder-lined Big Santa Anita Canyon on a wide road bed following the left bank. Edging alongside a number of small cabins, the deteriorating road soon assumes the proportions of a foot trail.

At 1.4 miles, amidst a beautiful oak woodland, you come to a four-way junction of trails. The right branch goes up-canyon to Sturtevant Falls; the middle and left branches bypass the falls and join again about a mile upstream. The left, upper trail is recommended for horses. Take the middle, or lower, trail—the more scenic and exciting alternative—unless you fear heights. The lower trail slices across a sheer wall above the falls and continues through a veritable fairyland of miniature cascades and crystalline pools bedecked with giant chain ferns.

A half mile past the reconvergence of the upper and lower trails, you come upon Cascade Picnic Area (2.8 miles—tables and restrooms here), named for a smooth chute in the stream bottom just below. Press on

Gabrielino Trail above Winter Creek

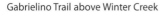

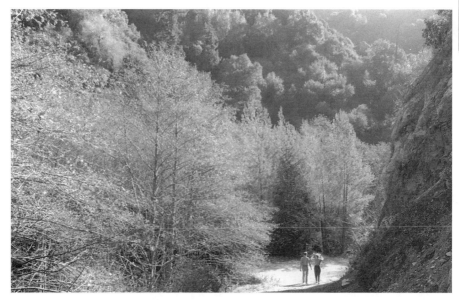

past a hulking crib dam to Spruce Grove Trail Camp (3.5 miles), named for the bigcone Douglas-fir trees that attain truly inspiring proportions hereabouts.

A little higher, the Gabrielino Trail forks right to climb toward Newcomb Pass (see Trip 13). You go left on the signed Sturtevant Trail. Go left again, 0.1 mile on, at the entrance to Sturtevant Camp. Cross above a crib dam to the opposite side of the creek from the camp, continue another 0.1 mile, and look for stone steps rising on the left—the beginning of the Mount Zion Trail (3.9 miles). This restored version of Sturtevant's original trail (reconstructed in the late 1970s and early '80s) winds delightfully upward across a ravine and then along timber-shaded, north-facing slopes.

When you reach the trail crest in a notch just northwest of Mount Zion, take the side path up through manzanita and ceanothus to the summit, where a broad if somewhat unremarkable view can be had of surrounding ridges and a small slice of the San Gabriel Valley.

Return to the main trail and begin a long, switchback descent (1000 feet of elevation loss in about 1.5 miles) down the dry, north canyon wall of Winter Creek—a sweaty affair if the day is sunny and warm. At the foot of this stretch you reach the cool canyon bottom and a T-intersection with the Winter Creek Trail (6.7 miles), lying just above Hoegees Trail Camp. Turn right, going upstream momentarily, follow the trail across the creek, and climb to the next trail junction. Bear left on the Upper Winter Creek Trail and complete the remaining 2.6 miles, cool and semi-shaded most of the way.

## trip 5  Mount Wilson Loop

see map on p. 242

| | |
|---|---|
| **Distance** | 13.8 miles, Loop |
| **Hiking Time** | 8 hours |
| **Elevation Gain/Loss** | 3300'/3300' |
| **Difficulty** | Strenuous |
| **Trail Use** | Suitable for backpacking, dogs allowed |
| **Best Times** | October through June |
| **Agency** | ANF/LARD |
| **Optional Map** | USGS 7.5-min *Mt. Wilson* |
| **Notes** | Marked trails/obvious routes, easy terrain |

**DIRECTIONS**  Exit Interstate 210 at Santa Anita Avenue in Arcadia. Drive north through Arcadia and Sierra Madre, and beyond the last subdivision at the foot of the mountains. You pass a vehicle gate (open 6 a.m. to 10 p.m.) and continue north on Santa Anita Canyon Road about 3 miles to reach the parking lots at Chantry Flat.

Basically an extension of Trip 4 above, this loop hike from Chantry Flat will take you all the way to Mount Wilson, where a host of roads and trails converge. Completion of the entire loop is a respectable achievement, even for those in excellent physical condition. Of course, those with a penchant for downhill walking only, and the wherewithal to arrange the necessary transportation, can utilize either the uphill or the downhill segments described here as a strictly one-way downhill route.

From the south edge of the lower parking lot at Chantry Flat, hike the first, paved segment of the Gabrielino Trail down to the confluence of Winter Creek and Big Santa Anita Canyon (0.6 mile). Pavement ends at a metal bridge spanning Winter Creek. Pass the restrooms and continue up alder-lined Big Santa Anita Canyon on a wide road bed following the left bank. Edging alongside a number of small cabins, the deteriorating road soon assumes the proportions of a foot trail.

At 1.4 miles, amidst a beautiful oak woodland, you come to a four-way junction of trails. The right branch goes up-canyon to Sturtevant Falls; the middle and left branches bypass the falls and join again about a mile upstream. The left, upper trail is recommended for horses. Take the middle, or lower, trail—the more scenic and exciting alternative—unless you fear heights. The lower trail slices across a sheer wall above the falls and continues through a veritable fairy-land of miniature cascades and crystalline pools bedecked with giant chain ferns.

A half mile past the reconvergence of the upper and lower trails, you come upon Cascade Picnic Area (2.8 miles—tables and restrooms here), named for a smooth chute in the stream bottom just below. Press on past a hulking crib dam to Spruce Grove Trail Camp (3.5 miles), named for the bigcone Douglas-fir trees that attain truly inspiring proportions hereabouts.

A little higher, the Gabrielino Trail forks right to climb toward Newcomb Pass (see Trip 13). You go left on the signed Sturtevant Trail. Just 0.1 mile ahead, at Sturtevant Camp, the Mount Zion Trail branches left; you keep straight on the Sturtevant Trail, continuing up though upper Big Santa Anita Canyon, in deep shade most of the while.

A series of switchbacks begins at about 4.6 miles as the trail tackles a steep slope consisting of crumbling outcrops and decomposed granite soil. Usually there's some kind of trail maintenance going on—or at least badly needed—here. (Take care not to hasten erosion yourself by breaking off the edge of the trail.)

"Halfway Rest" at 5.2 miles features a log bench in a restful, sylvan setting overlooking the uppermost reaches of Big Santa Anita Canyon. You're now exactly halfway between Sturtevant Camp, 1.4 miles below, and the top of the trail at Echo Rock on Mount Wilson's east shoulder. Switchbacks continue on the upper 1.4-mile segment, now mostly through sunny chaparral.

Echo Rock (6.6 miles) features a grandstand view of ridges marching east toward Mount San Antonio and south into the usual haze or smog blanket over the San Gabriel Valley. Continue west about 100 yards to a paved service road, and follow it west past the domes of the historic 60-inch and 100-inch reflector telescopes (each having held the distinction of being the world's largest telescope for a long period), the 150-foot-high solar telescope, and assorted smaller instruments. It was here that astronomer Edwin Hubble, using the great 100-inch Hooker Reflector in the 1920s and '30s, gathered evidence that supported the notion of an expanding universe populated by billions of galaxies—the accepted modern view. Today, operations at the observatory have diminished—light pollution has hampered its effectiveness—but the observatory still maintains a small museum (on your right, open 10 a.m. to 4 p.m.) for the convenience of visitors and travelers like yourself.

At 7.0 miles you'll come to the "Pavilion," centerpiece of Skyline Park, a small picnic-and-sightseeing facility, generally open to public access by road from April through November. A seasonal snack-bar concession may be found here. To the west lies a string of towering radio and TV antennas. Virtually every major broadcasting station in the L.A. area transmits its signal from here.

Exit through a gate to the west (one-way, westbound only for pedestrians from 4 p.m. to 10 a.m.) into a large, circular parking area. Two paths depart from the south side of this lot—a gated fire road (the old Mount Wilson Toll Road from Altadena) and a foot trail (signed MOUNT WILSON TRAIL) that switchbacks downward to join the old toll road on the saddle between Mount Wilson and Mount Harvard. Take the trail—it's shorter and more interesting.

ANGELES FOREST

On the saddle (7.8 miles), you'll find a cluster of Monterey pines and stone foundations, all that remains of Camp Wilson (aka Martin's Camp) a popular resort for hikers and sportsmen in the late 1800s and early 1900s. Continue downward on the old toll road 0.5 mile to the intersection of the Mount Wilson Trail on the left, just as the toll road begins curving west. You follow a fire break down about 100 yards, then pick up a narrow trail to the right offering a gentler descent. It follows the sunny ridgeline between Winter Creek and Little Santa Anita Canyon, known variously as Manzanita Ridge and Santa Anita Ridge. At 8.8 miles, stay left atop the ridge as the Mount Wilson Trail forks right and descends into Little Santa Anita Canyon. You're now on the Winter Creek Trail. At 9.6 miles, this trail veers left off the ridge and starts a long, crooked descent down Winter Creek's canyon wall. Hearty growths of live oak and bigcone Douglas-fir make this a cool and agreeable stretch, even though there's no relief from the jarring descent. Bigleaf maples near the bottom of the canyon herald your arrival at the junction (11.2 miles) with the trail to Hoegees on the left. Keep straight at this intersection and finish up the easy way—on the Upper Winter Creek Trail.

## trip 6   Mount Wilson to Sierra Madre

see map on p. 242

| | |
|---|---|
| **Distance** | 7.4 miles, Point-to-point |
| **Hiking Time** | 3½ hours |
| **Elevation Gain/Loss** | 100'/4800' |
| **Difficulty** | Moderately strenuous |
| **Trail Use** | Dogs allowed |
| **Best Times** | November through May |
| **Agency** | ANF/LARD |
| **Optional Map** | USGS 7.5-min *Mt. Wilson* |
| **Notes** | Marked trails/obvious routes, easy terrain |

**DIRECTIONS** *North End:* Exit Interstate 210 at Angeles Crest Highway in La Cañada-Flintridge. Drive 13.5 miles north and east to Red Box Station and the intersection of Mount Wilson Road. Turn right on Mount Wilson Road and proceed 4 miles to the parking lot at the end of the road. *South End:* From Interstate 210 in Arcadia, drive 1.5 miles north on Baldwin Avenue, and turn right on Mira Monte Avenue. Go two blocks east on Mira Monte to reach the Mount Wilson Trailhead on the left.

The lower part of the Mount Wilson Trail, which lies in the city of Sierra Madre, may close during periods of high fire danger, so check first with the forest service, or with Sierra Madre, whose website www.cityofsierramadre.com includes current information about the city's recreational areas.

On the Mount Wilson Trail you can almost feel the weight of history. This is the oldest and most direct route connecting Mount Wilson's summit and the San Gabriel Valley floor, and the first of many trails that were built to something resembling modern standards in the San Gabriel Mountains. In 1864, Benjamin Wilson widened and improved this former Indian path in order to exploit timber resources near the summit. Very little timber was actually cut, but the precipitous trail soon became popular among hikers and horsemen. By 1889, the first instrument placed on the mountaintop that would someday host the world's foremost observatory was hauled up in pieces on the same trail—a process that took a month to accomplish.

By 1891, a "new" Mount Wilson trail from the mouth of Eaton Canyon (Mount Wilson Toll Road) was constructed, largely preempting the shorter but steeper older trail. Still in use today, the old trail remains a viable route only by virtue of volunteers who maintain it.

From the south edge of the parking lot at the end of Mount Wilson Road, take the signed Mount Wilson Trail, which immediately starts zigzagging down a steep slope. After 0.7 mile you join Mount Wilson Toll Road. Continue on the old toll road 0.5 mile to the intersection of the Mount Wilson Trail on the left, just as the toll road begins curving west. Follow a fire break down about 100 yards, then pick up a narrow trail to the right offering a gentler descent. At 1.7 miles, the Mount Wilson Trail forks right and starts descending through chaparral into the headwaters of Little Santa Anita Canyon. Live oaks, sycamores, bigleaf maples, alders, and bigcone Douglas-firs cluster about the canyon bottom below. You cross the canyon bottom and descend along a shady, west-side slope for a while. Next, a set of tight switchbacks takes you down to a wooded glen along the canyon stream at 3.5 miles. There you'll find the founda-tion ruins of Orchard Camp (a resort), earlier known as Halfway House because it was located almost exactly halfway between Mount Wilson and the foot of the trail in Sierra Madre.

After a more-or-less level stretch under oaks, look for a side path to the left (4.3 miles) leading to an open spot—a some-time heliport—on the shoulder of a ridge overlooking the canyon. Thereafter, you begin an almost constant, steep descent across dry, chaparral slopes. In spring, sweet alyssum (a non-native escapee from foothill gardens) blooms along the path. The trail splits at 5.1 miles. An older, obscure branch goes down the canyon bottom to a spot called "First Water" and then up to the main trail again, while the newer branch stays high on the west slope. Below the reconvergence, retaining screens anchored to the canyon side have so far managed to keep the trail from slipping completely away.

The trail becomes a dirt road at 7.0 miles. Just beyond this point, take the path to the right, because the road ahead is private. You end up on a paved drive, and after 0.1 mile more reach the trailhead on Mira Monte Avenue in Sierra Madre.

## trip 7  Bailey Canyon

see map on p. 242

| | |
|---|---|
| **Distance** | 1.2 miles round trip, Out-and-back |
| **Hiking Time** | 1 hour (round trip) |
| **Elevation Gain/Loss** | 350'/350' |
| **Difficulty** | Easy |
| **Trail Use** | Dogs allowed, good for kids |
| **Best Times** | All year |
| **Agency** | COSM |
| **Optional Map** | USGS 7.5-min *Mt. Wilson* |
| **Notes** | Marked trails/obvious routes, easy terrain |

**DIRECTIONS** From Interstate 210 in Arcadia, drive 1.6 miles north on Baldwin Avenue, and turn left on Carter Avenue. Proceed 0.5 mile west to reach the small day-use parking lot at Bailey Canyon Park.

Sierra Madre's impeccably maintained Bailey Canyon Park includes a small, shady picnic area, and the lower part of a trail that now goes all the way to the Mount Wilson Trail above Orchard Camp. This little excursion within the park visits the narrow bottom of Bailey Canyon, which hosts an easy-to-reach small, seasonal waterfall.

From the west side of the parking lot, walk west under shade-giving trees to a gap in a chain link fence. Pick up a paved service road just beyond, and follow it uphill and around a debris basin lying at the mouth of Bailey Canyon. Follow the narrow Bailey Canyon Trail onward into the canyon.

A short distance ahead, stay left—as the trail to Jones Peak splits right—and continue following the sandy stream bottom. In a few minutes you'll come to the end of the line for easy hiking. A dike of dark, intrusive igneous rock, squeezed between lighter granite walls, lies ahead. This natural barrier forces any water flowing in the canyon to plunge about 15 feet over a precipice. The waterfall trills like a bird only after significant rain has fallen.

## trip 8  Jones Peak

see map on p. 242

| | |
|---|---|
| **Distance** | 7.0 miles round trip, Out-and-back |
| **Hiking Time** | 4 hours (round trip) |
| **Elevation Gain/Loss** | 2300'/2300' |
| **Difficulty** | Moderately strenuous |
| **Trail Use** | Dogs allowed |
| **Best Times** | October through May |
| **Agency** | COSM |
| **Optional Map** | USGS 7.5-min *Mt. Wilson* |
| **Notes** | Marked trails/obvious routes, easy terrain |

**DIRECTIONS** From Interstate 210 in Arcadia, drive 1.6 miles north on Baldwin Avenue, and turn left on Carter Avenue. Proceed 0.5 mile west to reach the small day-use parking lot at Bailey Canyon Park.

Jones Peak is nowhere near the loftiest of the many named summits you can climb in the sharply rising Front Range of the San Gabriel Mountains. But its elevated position—barely 1 mile by crow's flight from the fringe of the vast Los Angeles Basin metropolitan sprawl—affords you a 180-degree-plus view of a big chunk of Southern California. That view is nothing less than commanding during the best clear-air episodes characteristic of the late fall and winter seasons. The view is not, of course, anywhere near as impressive if the basin is choked in smog.

From the west side of the Bailey Canyon Park lot, walk west under shade-giving trees to a gap in a chain link fence. Pick up a paved service road just beyond, and follow it uphill and around a debris basin lying at the mouth of Bailey Canyon. Follow the narrow Bailey Canyon Trail onward into the canyon.

A short distance ahead, a spur trail to a small, seasonal waterfall in Bailey Canyon splits left. Stay right and commence a crooked, unforgivingly steep ascent up the east wall of the canyon. As you climb, note the distant downtown Los Angeles skyline positioned over the mission-style buildings of a Passionist Fathers monastery right down below.

At 2.2 miles, the trail reaches a level about even with the seasonal stream flowing in the upper reaches of Bailey Canyon. A cabin foundation lies just below the trail on a small flat just above the stream. That's a good place to take a breather, since the remaining 1.3 miles of the hike are again steep. Proceed generally east up a series of tight switchbacks, and arrive at a saddle.

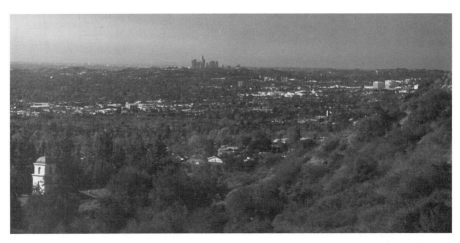

L.A. Basin vista en route to Jones Peak

Swing right and scamper up a sketchy path to the Jones Peak summit, where you can take in the comprehensive view.

On the clearest days, the tree-dotted urban plain rolls out like a shaggy carpet toward the Pacific Ocean, which takes on a silvery sheen in late fall and winter. Look for as many as three of the Channel Islands punctuating the horizon: Santa Catalina Island (often obvious); San Clemente Island (sometimes glimpsed to the left of the left-most tip of Santa Catalina); and tiny Santa Barbara Island (well to the right of Santa Catalina).

## **trip 9** Eaton Canyon Falls

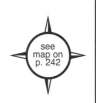

see map on p. 242

ANGELES FOREST

| | |
|---|---|
| **Distance** | 3.4 miles round trip, Out-and-back |
| **Hiking Time** | 1½ hours (round trip) |
| **Elevation Gain/Loss** | 400'/400' |
| **Difficulty** | Moderate |
| **Trail Use** | Dogs allowed |
| **Best Times** | All year |
| **Agency** | ECNA |
| **Optional Map** | USGS 7.5-min *Mt. Wilson* |
| **Notes** | Marked trails/obvious routes, moderate terrain |

**DIRECTIONS** From Interstate 210 on the east side of Pasadena, take the Madre Street/Sierra Madre Villa Avenue exit. Go north on Sierra Madre Villa and its extension, New York Drive, for a total of 2.3 miles. Turn right on Altadena Drive, and immediately right again into Eaton Canyon Natural Area. Park next to the Nature Center.

On October 27, 1993, the floor of lower Eaton Canyon (along with 118 homes in surrounding neighborhoods) was reduced to white ash and black cinders by the fast-moving Altadena Fire. By the following spring, which came on the heels of a wetter-than-average rainy season, visitors to the 184-acre Eaton Canyon Natural Park could only gasp in wonder as they beheld millions of wildflowers, swaying in the breeze, on the canyon floor. It is a California truism that from what seems the worst

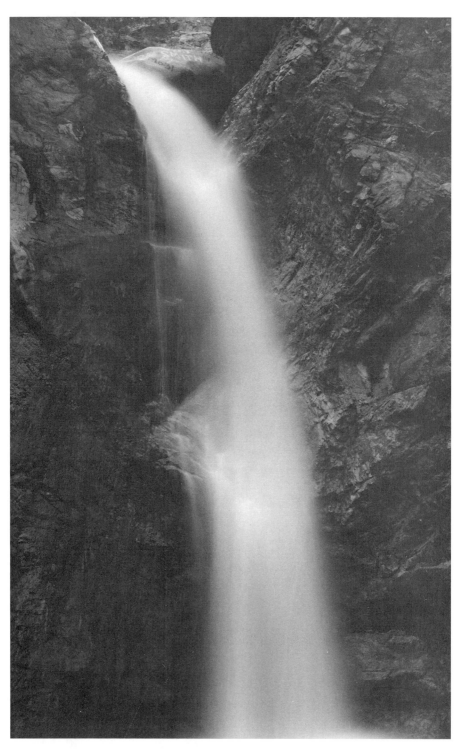

Eaton Canyon Falls

possible disaster, new life—and hope—can emerge triumphantly.

The brash, fire-following wildflowers have diminished with every passing season, and the oaks and chaparral shrubbery on the canyon rim have fully regenerated by now. A new Nature Center building, replacing the earlier one that burned, was dedicated in 1998. Either sooner or later, history will likely repeat itself when another Santa-Ana-wind-driven fire blows into town.

Upstream from the park, where the waters of Eaton Canyon have carved a raw groove in the San Gabriel Mountains, you'll discover Eaton Canyon Falls. Impressive only during the wetter half of the year, the falls possesses, as John Muir once put it, "a low sweet voice, singing like a bird." The falls are well worth visiting, especially in the aftermath of a larger winter storm, if only to witness the power of large (by meager Southern California standards anyway) volumes of falling water.

From the parking lot at Eaton Canyon Nature Center, follow the Eaton Canyon Trail upstream along the canyon's cobbled flood plain or stream. Beyond, the trail sticks to an elevated stream terrace, passing some beautiful live-oak woods. At 1.1 miles you rise to meet the Mount Wilson Toll Road bridge over Eaton Canyon. Cross to the west end of the bridge, descend on the upstream side, and make your way up the canyon bottom (don't do this if the stream is too lively and dangerous to ford). You'll skip across rocks in the stream several times, or perhaps resort to wading. Except for a line of alders along part of the stream and some live oaks on terraces just above the reach of floods, the canyon bottom and the precipitous walls are desolate and desertlike. After a half mile of canyon-bottom travel, you come to the falls, where the water slides and then free-falls a total of about 35 vertical feet down a narrow chute in the bedrock.

## trip 10  Henninger Flats

|  |  |
|---|---|
| **Distance** | 5.4 miles round trip, Out-and-back |
| **Hiking Time** | 3 hours (round trip) |
| **Elevation Gain/Loss** | 1400'/1400' |
| **Difficulty** | Moderately strenuous |
| **Trail Use** | Suitable for backpacking, suitable for mountain biking, dogs allowed, good for kids |
| **Best Times** | October through June |
| **Agency** | HFFS |
| **Optional Map** | USGS 7.5-min *Mt. Wilson* |
| **Notes** | Marked trails/obvious routes, easy terrain |

see map on p. 242

**ANGELES FOREST**

**DIRECTIONS** From Interstate 210 in Pasadena, go north on Allen Avenue 2.6 miles to the intersection of Altadena Avenue. Go straight across at this intersection onto Pinecrest Drive. Continue 0.5 mile to the Mount Wilson Toll Road Trailhead on the left (at 2260 Pinecrest Drive).

Park-like Henninger Flats is a pleasant surprise to come upon after the sunny, often sweaty climb up the lower end of Mount Wilson Toll Road. The flats and slopes hereabouts have been the site of an experimental forest for more than 80 years now, with seedlings of pine, cypress, cedar, and other trees raised for reforestation projects. Run by the Los Angeles County Fire Department, the area encompasses four delightful camp and picnic areas, a visitor center, a pioneer museum, a short nature trail, and a seedling nursery. The visitor center features a large relief model of the Mount Wilson/Front Range area, and outside there's a diminutive lookout structure that stood on C–astro Peak in the Santa Monica Mountains during 1925–71. Henninger Flats' half-mile-high elevation perched directly over the edge of the city gives it a commanding view—by day and especially by night. Backpackers register with the ranger on duty. Campfire permits and wood are usually available.

The old toll road is now a fire road used by fire-department or forestry trucks, and plenty of self-propelled travelers of all sorts. Walk through the gate on Pinecrest Drive (typically open between sunrise and one hour after sunset) and proceed down across a bridge over Eaton Canyon. Dogged determination, and hopefully the inspiration of fabulous views over the big city below, will get you up the moderately steep and steady grade ahead. This well-engineered road/former trail was built and improved

(among other reasons) to haul telescope parts to the summit of Mount Wilson, including those of the 100-inch Hooker Reflector—the world's largest telescope for 31 years.

You can easily use up a couple of extra hours at Henninger Flats poking around the museum and the visitor center and taking short side trips to check out the groves of trees. For the best view of the surroundings, try climbing a little higher to Henninger Ridge: Continue upward on Mount Wilson Toll Road another 0.6 mile, and turn left on the dirt road that loops around to a heliport. This puts you on the shoulder of a ridge perched 400 feet above the groves of Henninger Flats, where the view of the city below stretches 180 degrees. From the north side of the ridge, Mount Wilson rears up starkly, 2.5 miles away. After a winter storm, the spike-shaped antennas on its crest look exactly like upside-down icicles.

Mt. Wilson from Henninger Ridge

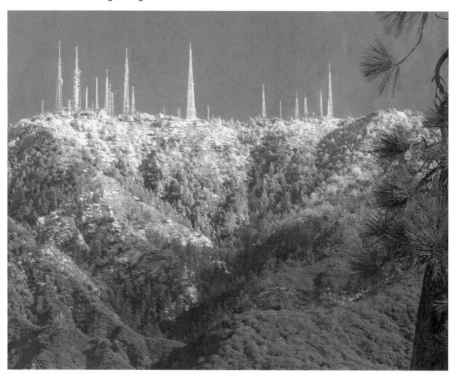

## trip 11  Idlehour Descent

| | |
|---|---|
| **Distance** | 10.8 miles, Point-to-point |
| **Hiking Time** | 5½ hours |
| **Elevation Gain/Loss** | 1200'/5300' |
| **Difficulty** | Strenuous |
| **Trail Use** | Suitable for backpacking, dogs allowed |
| **Best Times** | October through June |
| **Agency** | ANF/LARD |
| **Optional Map** | USGS 7.5-min *Mt. Wilson* |
| **Notes** | Marked trails/obvious routes, easy terrain |

see map on p. 242

**DIRECTIONS** *North End:* Exit Interstate 210 at Angeles Crest Highway in La Cañada-Flintridge. Drive 13.5 miles north and east to Red Box Station and the intersection of Mount Wilson Road. Turn right on Mount Wilson Road and proceed 2.4 miles to a roadside parking area at Eaton Saddle. *South End:* From Interstate 210 on the east side of Pasadena, take the Madre Street/Sierra Madre Villa Avenue exit. Go north on Sierra Madre Villa and its extension, New York Drive, for a total of 2.3 miles. Turn right on Altadena Drive, and immediately right again into Eaton Canyon Natural Area.

Not an idle descent at all, this one-way hike passes through some of the most varied and interesting terrain in the Front Range. From shady canyon to mountainside view, the landscape is ever changing along the way. Over a distance of almost 11 miles on roads and trails, you journey 4 air-line miles from the crest of the Front Range at Eaton Saddle all the way down to the edge of the L.A. Basin at Eaton Canyon County Park. The name "Idlehour" comes from Idlehour Trail Camp, formerly a trail resort, passed at the midway point of the hike.

From Eaton Saddle, follow Mount Lowe Fire Road 0.5 mile west to Markham Saddle, where trails intersect left and right. Bear left on the Mount Lowe Trail. At a trail junction ahead (1.3 miles) the Mount Lowe west trail comes in acutely from the right. Keep straight to remain on the shorter, better-maintained east-side route down along the flank of the mountain. At 2.1 miles you can either drop to the fire road on your right or stay on the trail another 0.2 mile to meet the same fire road farther south. Continue walking south on the fire road, curving left toward Inspiration Point as the road on the right descends to Mount Lowe Trail Camp. About 100 feet farther, turn left on the Idlehour Trail (2.4 miles).

Descend through scattered north-slope groves of live oak and bigcone Douglas-firs to a crossing of a west fork of Eaton Canyon, 3.7 miles. You then climb a bit to cross a chaparral-covered divide to the east, and begin a switchback descent into Eaton Canyon. Look for the fault-like discontinuity in

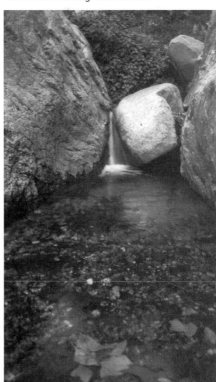

Mini-waterfall along Idlehour Trail

the igneous rock exposed on Eaton Canyon's sheer east wall.

At the bottom (4.8 miles) the trail goes down-canyon and becomes intermittently lost in a refreshingly chilly wonderland of crystal-clear cascades, overarching oaks and maples, and crispy carpets of orange and brown leaf-litter. Cabin foundation ruins can be found under the trees, a reminder that even in this inviting hideaway, no construction is spared for long the ravages of fire and flood—or in this case removal by the Pasadena Water Department. After some easy boulder-hopping, you come to Idlehour Trail Camp (5.4 miles), nestled on an oak-shaded flat lying next to a rock fin, with vertical striations, dividing Eaton Canyon from its aforementioned west fork. Naturally, this is the best place for a picnic if you're day-hiking, or home for the night if you're backpacking the route.

The narrow, wild section of Eaton Canyon below the camp was eschewed by trail builders in favor of a route up the east canyon wall to Mount Wilson Toll Road. (Some people have followed the dangerous lower canyon route, including John Muir, who later described the front face of the San Gabriels as "rigidly inaccessible.") The safe and easy Idlehour Trail goes east up a tributary (Harvard Branch) momentarily, then climbs up and over a ridge to meet Mount Wilson Toll Road (6.9 miles).

Descend on the old toll road past Henninger Flats (8.1 miles) to a hairpin turn (9.8 miles), where an equestrian trail (sign says EATON CANYON TRAIL) takes off down the slope to the left. Switchbacks, steep at times, take you down 0.5 mile to the wide Eaton Canyon Trail following Eaton Canyon wash. Turn left and complete the remaining 0.5 mile to the nature center at Eaton Canyon Natural Area.

The first (upper) one-third of the Idlehour Descent lies within the burn zone of the 2009 Station Fire. Access to the fire roads and trails originating at Eaton Saddle may be affected for some time to come.

## trip 12  Valley Forge & DeVore Trail

see map on p. 242

| | |
|---|---|
| **Distance** | 7.6 miles, Point-to-point |
| **Hiking Time** | 4 hours |
| **Elevation Gain/Loss** | 1750'/2300' |
| **Difficulty** | Moderately strenuous |
| **Trail Use** | Suitable for backpacking, dogs allowed |
| **Best Times** | October through June |
| **Agency** | ANF/LARD |
| **Optional Maps** | USGS 7.5-min *Mt. Wilson, Chilao Flat* |
| **Notes** | Marked trails/obvious routes, easy terrain |

**DIRECTIONS** *East End:* Exit Interstate 210 at Angeles Crest Highway in La Cañada-Flintridge. Drive 13.5 miles north and east to Red Box Station and the intersection of Mount Wilson Road. Turn right on Mount Wilson Road and proceed 4 miles to where the road splits and becomes a one-way loop around the antenna-spiked Mount Wilson ridgeline. Parking space is available in a roadside turnout to the west. *West End:* The hike ends at Eaton Saddle, 2.4 miles up Mount Wilson Road from Red Box.

The Falls Canyon Research Natural Area on the north slope of Mount Wilson helps protect a steeply sloping, 1000-acre block of land covered by magnificent stands of bigcone Douglas-fir and canyon live oak. The point-to-point route described here circumnavigates that area by way of the Kenyon DeVore (formerly Rattlesnake), Gabrielino, and Valley Forge trails, completing about four-fifths of a circle. (You

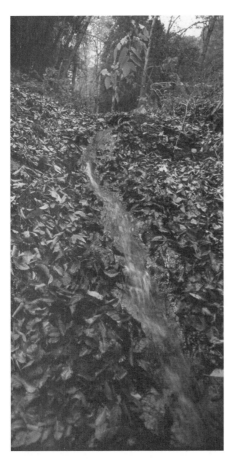

Strayns Canyon flow over autumn leaves, before the Station Fire

the main canyon or tributaries at least four times. (The canyon's name is apparently a corruption of the name of A.G. Strain, who operated a tourist camp on Mount Wilson's north slope in the 1890s.) Deeply shaded by alders and bigleaf maples down along the stream, this is a thoroughly enjoyable stretch.

At 3.0 miles there's an easy-to-miss junction. The combined DeVore/Gabrielino Trail continues down-canyon, on the right-hand side of the stream, to Rincon-Red Box Road. You go left, across the stream, westbound on the Gabrielino Trail. On it you contour, more or less, through shady glens or through sunny thickets of chaparral highlighted by big, gorgeous manzanitas.

At 4.9 miles you come to an intersection with the Valley Forge Trail, which is your route back up to Mount Wilson Road. On the Gabrielino Trail, just beyond this junction, there's a side path to Valley Forge Campground down along the bank of West Fork San Gabriel River. This makes a good overnight campsite for trail travelers, as the road from Red Box is now gated year round and there's always peace and quiet here.

On the Valley Forge Trail you go up through the semi-shade of oaks, bay laurels, and tall chaparral—first on switchbacks, then on a straighter course high on the west wall of Falls Canyon. At 7.6 miles you reach the Eaton Saddle parking lot on Mount Wilson Road, only 2 miles west of your starting point.

The area described in this trip was thoroughly burned during the 2009 Station Fire. Check with the Forest Service to determine if trails in the area are open.

can make this a full-circle hike by walking some 2 miles along the narrow shoulder of possibly busy Mount Wilson Road.)

From the turnout on Mount Wilson Road, the Kenyon DeVore Trail descends on long and sometimes poorly maintained switchbacks. You're following the drainage of Strayns Canyon, crossing the stream of

**ANGELES FOREST**

# trip 13 Angeles Crest to Chantry Flat

see map on p. 242

| | |
|---|---|
| **Distance** | 11.0 miles, Point-to-point |
| **Hiking Time** | 7 hours |
| **Elevation Gain/Loss** | 1800'/4400' |
| **Difficulty** | Strenuous |
| **Trail Use** | Suitable for backpacking, dogs allowed |
| **Best Times** | October through June |
| **Agency** | ANF/LARD |
| **Recommended Maps** | USGS 7.5-min *Chilao Flat, Mt. Wilson* |
| **Notes** | Navigation required, easy terrain |

**DIRECTIONS** *North End:* Exit Interstate 210 at Angeles Crest Highway in La Cañada-Flintridge. Drive 18.5 miles north and east to Shortcut Saddle. Look for the spot where the Silver Moccasin Trail crosses Angeles Crest Highway, mile 43.3 according to the mile-markers. *South End:* Exit Interstate 210 at Santa Anita Avenue in Arcadia. Drive north through Arcadia and Sierra Madre, and beyond the last subdivision at the foot of the mountains. You pass a vehicle gate (open 6 a.m. to 10 p.m.) and continue north on Santa Anita Canyon Road about 3 miles to reach the parking lots at Chantry Flat.

This wide-ranging traverse takes you from Shortcut Saddle to Chantry Flat, through wooded and fern-draped canyons, and over a major divide. The closure of the Rincon-Red Box Road to motor vehicles has made this area effectively more remote from civilization (and any form of help in an emergency) than it has been for decades.

The drive between start and end points takes well over an hour at best, so a good arrangement would be to line up someone to drop you off on Angeles Crest Highway and later pick you up at Chantry Flat.

Shortcut Saddle is considered to be on the nebulous dividing line between the "Front Range" of the San Gabriels, south and west, and the "High Country," of which Charlton-Chilao Recreation Area (see Chapter 22), just north, is a part.

You start off on the Silver Moccasin Trail, which dates from 1942, when Boy Scouts mapped out what is now a 52-mile route from Chantry Flat to Vincent Gap near Mount Baden-Powell. Today it combines with parts of the Pacific Crest and Gabrielino trails. The part of the Silver Moccasin Trail you'll be traveling on was originally Newcomb's Trail, a turn-of-the-century shortcut route for hikers and sportsmen between Big Santa Anita Canyon and the High Country.

From Shortcut Saddle, follow the southbound Silver Moccasin Trail as it zigzags down 120 vertical feet to a dirt road. Turn right, go 0.1 mile along the road, and then turn left on the continuation of the trail. You now descend hot, south-facing, chaparral-covered slopes, finally settling into the aptly named Shortcut Canyon (1.5 miles). There's only a trickle here winter through spring, but more and more water ahead. At one point, the trail passes directly beneath the exposed root system of a bigleaf maple that will surely tumble in the next great flood. Manmade improvements in the form of gabions (rock-filled, wire-mesh structures used to stabilize the banks) are seen not long before you reach Shortcut Canyon's confluence with the West Fork San Gabriel River.

Cross West Fork to reach West Fork Campground (3.2 miles) and the site of a historic ranger station built in 1900, now removed to Chilao. Either this camp or De-Vore Camp ahead is good for an overnight layover if you are backpacking the route.

From West Fork Campground, go east (downstream), fording the river again almost immediately. Your sometimes-obscure trail meanders down one of the most beautiful riparian stretches in the county. The stream slides over and around smooth boulders, while sunlight filtering though the tall alders and maples glances off lens-like convexities and concavities on the water surface.

At DeVore Camp (4.2 miles), you turn away from the river and head south—very steeply at first—up along a shady draw to the south. Soon the upgrade eases. Endless switchbacks take you 1300 vertical feet up past a crossing of Rincon-Red Box Road to Newcomb Pass (5.7 miles), where a couple of picnic tables have been thoughtfully placed. Ignoring both the Rim Trail to Mount Wilson to the right, and the spur of a fire road to the left, continue south into the watershed of Big Santa Anita Canyon.

The gradual descent across a sun-baked chaparral slope (great views from here on a clear day), then through oak and bay woods, leads to a trail junction (7.6 miles), deep in the shaded bowels of Big Santa Anita. Turning downstream on a now-well-traveled stretch of the Gabrielino Trail, you pass Spruce Grove Trail Camp, Cascade Picnic Area, and Sturtevant Falls. From the Winter Creek confluence, follow the crowds up the paved road to Chantry Flat.

Note: The upper (north) half of the Angeles Crest to Chantry Flat traverse was burned in the 2009 Station Fire. Check with the Forest Service to determine if access to the entire route is available.

Big Santa Anita Canyon below Spruce Grove

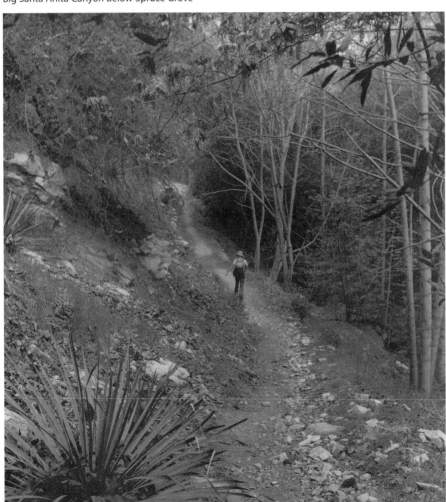

ANGELES FOREST

# chapter 22

# Angeles Forest:
# Charlton-Chilao Recreation Area

Gateway to the High Country of the San Gabriel Mountains, the Charlton-Chilao Recreation Area draws a good fraction of the travelers headed east on Angeles Crest Highway from Los Angeles. On the way up there are scattered trees aplenty along the highway, but at Charlton Flats the traveler first comes upon what looks like true forest—stately pines, firs, and cedars. It's plain to see the Forest Service has gone all-out to accommodate large numbers of visitors.

Three miles beyond Charlton Flats is a turnoff for the Chilao Visitor Center, open Wednesday through Sunday, generally from spring through fall, and closed during the winter season. Here you'll find exhibits, lots of free printed information, books for sale, scheduled summer activities, and knowledgeable rangers on duty. Three short interpretive trails start from here and loop outward into the forest.

The blacktop road to the visitor center continues past spacious camp and picnic grounds, and returns to the highway. Newcomb's Ranch Cafe, the first commercial establishment on Angeles Crest Highway up from La Cañada, is around the corner from the visitor center. (Important note: your car should be gassed up before driving to the High Country; there are no service stations on the 60-mile stretch between La Cañada and Wrightwood.)

Winter snows may block access (by car) from the highway to Charlton Flats and part of the Chilao complex, but that's no reason not to come. Both areas, with their meandering, gently graded access roads, are perfect for cross-country skiing after the bigger winter storms. Unplowed Santa Clara Divide Road from Three Points is another good bet. (Hint: go on weekdays or arrive early in the morning on weekends and holidays.)

All trips below require a National Forest Adventure Pass ($5 per day, $30 per year) for trailhead parking.

Note: The Charlton Flats Picnic Area and portions of the camp and picnic grounds near Chilao Visitor Center were burned in the 2009 Station Fire. Not all trails in the area may be open.

Vetter Mountain lookout, before the Station Fire

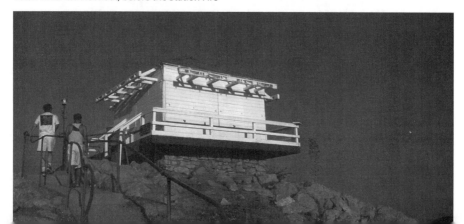

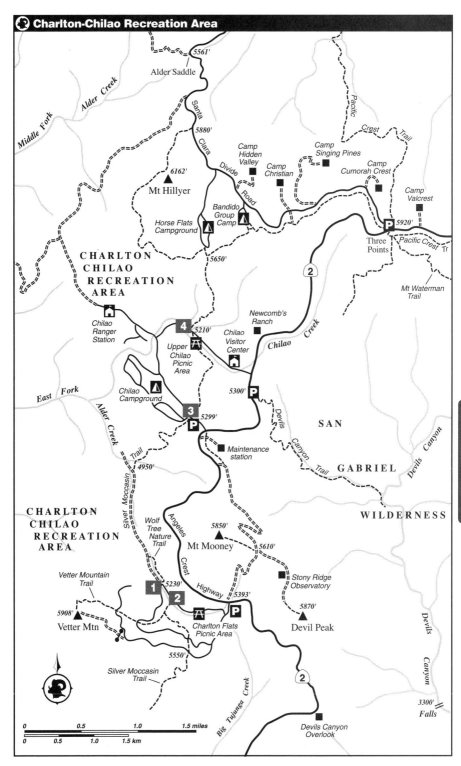

**Charlton-Chilao Recreation Area**

5561'
Alder Saddle

Alder Creek

Middle Fork

Santa Clara Divide Road

5880'

6162'
Mt Hillyer

Camp Hidden Valley
Camp Christian
Camp Singing Pines
Camp Cumorah Crest
Camp Valcrest

Pacific Crest Trail

Bandido Group Camp

Horse Flats Campground

P 5920'
Three Points
Pacific Crest Tr

5650'

2

Mt Waterman Trail

CHARLTON CHILAO RECREATION AREA

Chilao Ranger Station

Newcomb's Ranch

4 5210'
Upper Chilao Picnic Area
Chilao Visitor Center

Chilao Creek

East Fork

Chilao Campground

Alder Creek

5300'  P

Trail
4950'

3 5299'
P

Maintenance station

Devils Canyon Trail

SAN

GABRIEL

Devils Canyon

WILDERNESS

CHARLTON CHILAO RECREATION AREA

Silver Moccasin Trail

Wolf Tree Nature Trail

Angeles Crest Highway

5850'
Mt Mooney

5610'

Stony Ridge Observatory

Vetter Mountain Trail

1 5230'
2

5393'

5870'
Devil Peak

5908'
Vetter Mtn

A
Charlton Flats Picnic Area
P

5550'

Silver Moccasin Trail

Big Tujunga Creek

2

Devils Canyon

3300'
Falls

Devils Canyon Overlook

0    0.5    1.0    1.5 miles
0    0.5    1.0    1.5 km

**ANGELES FOREST**

# trip 1  Wolf Tree Nature Trail

see map on p. 263

| | |
|---|---|
| **Distance** | 0.5 mile, Loop |
| **Hiking Time** | ½ hour |
| **Elevation Gain/Loss** | 50'/50' |
| **Difficulty** | Easy |
| **Trail Use** | Dogs allowed, good for kids |
| **Best Times** | All year |
| **Agency** | ANF/LARD |
| **Optional Map** | USGS 7.5-min *Chilao Flat* |
| **Notes** | Marked trails/obvious routes, easy terrain |

**DIRECTIONS**  Exit Interstate 210 at Angeles Crest Highway in La Cañada-Flintridge. Drive 22.6 miles north and east to the turnoff for Charlton Flats Picnic Area on the left. After turning into the picnic area, swing right at the first intersection and continue on pavement 0.6 mile to a gate.

Tucked away in a far corner of the sprawling Charlton Flats Picnic Area is the Wolf Tree Nature Trail, one of the more interesting self-guiding trails in the National Forest. The trail starts beyond the gate, 0.6 mile in from the highway. (During the winter season, when the picnic area is typically closed to auto traffic, you could walk the additional distance to the trailhead from the highway.)

The trail runs along a conifer-shaded draw, wet only during times of snowmelt. Among other features, the interpretive plaques point out clear evidence of a fire in 1878. While other woods have long since rotted away, fallen logs and standing snags of durable incense cedar are still in evidence.

The "wolf tree"—the dominant tree of the forest—is in this case an outsized (roughly 100 feet tall) Coulter pine. Since Coulter pine cones are the largest and heaviest of the native conifers (up to 14 inches in length and 5 pounds), you would not want to spend much time beneath that wolf tree.

The 2009 Station Fire burned the area encompassed by the Charlton Flat Picnic Area, including the Wolf Tree Nature Trail. It will be interesting to see if the Coulter pines and other trees in this area will stage a comeback in the years ahead, and if so how long that will take.

Coulter pine cone

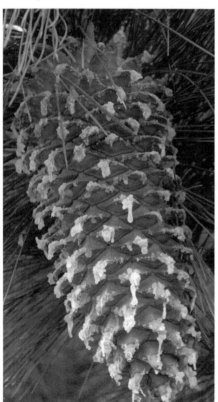

## trip 2 Vetter Mountain

| | |
|---|---|
| **Distance** | 3.3 miles, Loop |
| **Hiking Time** | 1½ hours |
| **Elevation Gain/Loss** | 700'/700' |
| **Difficulty** | Moderate |
| **Trail Use** | Dogs allowed, good for kids |
| **Best Times** | All year |
| **Agency** | ANF/LARD |
| **Optional Map** | USGS 7.5-min *Chilao Flat* |
| **Notes** | Marked trails/obvious routes, easy terrain |

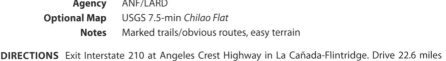

see map on p. 263

**DIRECTIONS** Exit Interstate 210 at Angeles Crest Highway in La Cañada-Flintridge. Drive 22.6 miles north and east to the turnoff for Charlton Flats Picnic Area on the left. After turning into the picnic area, swing right at the first intersection and continue on pavement 0.6 mile to a gate.

Vetter Mountain's pint-sized fire-lookout building—before it was destroyed in the 2009 Station Fire—perched atop Vetter's rounded summit and offered a 360-degree view over the midsection of the San Gabriels. The historic lookout building, which was reopened for service in 1998 after an 18-year hiatus, was a popular weekend destination for hikers of all ages. Today, the same panoramic summit view can be enjoyed, though much of the surrounding landscape will look pretty desolate for a while. There is considerable interest in historic fire lookouts in most of the nation's national forests, and hopefully this one (the only active lookout in the San Gabriels when it was destroyed) will be rebuilt.

Aside from visiting Vetter's summit, this loop hike also swings around through Charlton Flats' formerly lush, heterogeneous forest of live oak, Coulter pine, Jeffrey pine, sugar pine, incense cedar, and bigcone Douglas-fir. In the years to come it will be interesting to observe the pattern of plant succession, and to learn just how much of the forest has survived, and which kinds of trees will be favored in the post-fire environment.

Drive, or walk, to the start of the Wolf Tree Nature Trail (see Trip 1 above). Across the road to the west, starting up the south side of a ravine, is a signed path to Vetter Mountain, uphill all the way. About 200 yards up the path, the Silver Moccasin Trail swings left—don't take it; this is your return route. Keeping straight, you ascend through mixed forest and then scattered pines, crossing paved service roads twice. A final switchbacking stretch through chaparral leads to the lookout site, 1.3 miles from the start.

Looking north and east from the lookout perch, you'll spot Pacifico Mountain, Mount Williamson, Waterman Mountain, Twin Peaks, Old Baldy, and other High Country summits. The Front Range sprawls west and south, blocking from view most of the city.

When it's time to descend, follow the dirt road downhill instead of the trail. After 0.7 mile you'll meet a paved service road. Continue straight (east) on the pavement for another 0.6 mile and look carefully for the crossing of the Silver Moccasin Trail. Turn left on the trail, cross pavement again in a short while, and complete the final, mostly level stretch across a forested slope.

ANGELES FOREST

# trip 3  Chilao & Charlton Loop

see map on p. 263

| | |
|---|---|
| **Distance** | 5.4 miles, Loop |
| **Hiking Time** | 3 hours |
| **Elevation Gain/Loss** | 800'/800' |
| **Difficulty** | Moderately strenuous |
| **Trail Use** | Suitable for mountain biking, dogs allowed, good for kids |
| **Best Times** | October through June |
| **Agency** | ANF/LARD |
| **Optional Maps** | USGS 7.5-min *Chilao Flat, Waterman Mtn.* |
| **Notes** | Marked trails/obvious routes, easy terrain |

**DIRECTIONS** Exit Interstate 210 at Angeles Crest Highway in La Cañada-Flintridge. Drive 24.8 miles north and east to the turnoff for Chilao Campground (mile 49.7 on Angeles Crest Highway) on the left. Drive 0.2 mile to a small parking area where the signed Silver Moccasin Trail crosses the road.

This trip makes use of a variety of dirt roads, paved roads, and trails to accomplish a circumnavigation of Mount Mooney, one of several small summits rising above the flats of Charlton-Chilao. If the air is crystal-clear, an optional side trip to either Mount Mooney or Devil Peak (involving extra mileage) is highly recommended as well.

On the Silver Moccasin Trail, go south up along a brushy hill overlooking some campsites (the trail is easy to lose at first) and then crookedly down along a brushy ravine. At 0.9 mile, you reach an attractive pine-fringed valley—East Fork Alder Creek. Here you pick up a dirt road and continue south up along the East Fork to join a hairpin curve on a paved service road (1.9 miles) just below the edge of Charlton Flats Picnic Area. Bear left and continue uphill on pavement to the restroom building at the entrance to the picnic area (2.8 miles). From there, walk across Angeles Crest Highway and pick up a dirt road (not directly across the highway, but a little to the left) going north. This road takes you up to a saddle (3.5 miles) on the ridge between Mount Mooney and Devil Peak.

Both peaks are dotted with Jeffrey and Coulter pines, making them good sites for a picnic, but the view from Devil is far superior as it includes more of the rugged San Gabriel Wilderness and also (when the smog is lying low) Santa Catalina Island. Both peaks have climbers' registers, although few people sign in at Devil Peak. The side trip to Devil is 0.8 mile each way, first on a dirt road and then on a steep fire break. Mooney's ascent from the saddle is just 0.4 mile by way of a steep trail.

From the saddle, your circle route continues north on the fire road down a sparsely wooded slope. After two hairpin turns and a stretch through chaparral, the road swings back to Angeles Crest Highway (4.8 miles). Just short of where the road reaches the highway, turn right onto the old trail that contours through chaparral alongside the highway. This is really a piece of the original highway (dirt road) that preceded the present paved highway. Follow this to an access road leading to a Caltrans maintenance station. Jog left on the access road, right on Angeles Crest Highway, and left on the entrance road to Chilao Campground.

Note: The majority of the Chilao & Charlton loop hike was swept by the flames of the 2009 Station Fire.

# trip 4  Mount Hillyer

| | |
|---|---|
| **Distance** | 5.8 miles, Loop |
| **Hiking Time** | 3 hours |
| **Elevation Gain/Loss** | 1100'/1100' |
| **Difficulty** | Moderately strenuous |
| **Trail Use** | Dogs allowed, good for kids |
| **Best Times** | All year |
| **Agency** | ANF/LARD |
| **Optional Map** | USGS 7.5-min *Chilao Flat* |
| **Notes** | Marked trails/obvious routes, easy terrain |

see map on p. 263

**DIRECTIONS**  Exit Interstate 210 at Angeles Crest Highway in La Cañada-Flintridge. Drive 25.7 miles north and east to the turnoff for the Chilao Visitor Center on the left. Drive 0.6 mile (passing the visitor center) to a small parking area for the Silver Moccasin Trail on the right.

Lovers of the high Sierra Nevada may get some sense of deja vu atop the rounded ridge known as Mount Hillyer. The breeze sings in the branches of sugar pines, Jeffrey pines, Coulter pines, and bigcone Douglas-firs. Angular outcrops and large boulder piles lie on the slopes. The granite here is not so fractured and pulverized as it is in other parts of the San Gabriels. The view is only fair; the main attractions are the peace and quiet, and the pine-scented air.

Granite boulders on Mount Hillyer

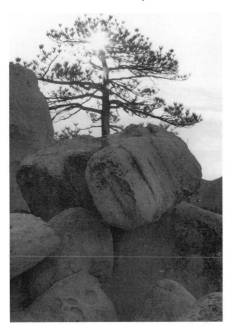

For small kids the complete loop route described here is long, steep in parts, and challenging, but you can customize the hike to suit your needs. Horse Flats Campground can be reached by car in the warmer part of the year from Three Points. You could start the Hillyer climb from the campground, or end a trip there by making use of a car shuttle.

Start hiking north on the Silver Moccasin Trail, using switchbacks to gain a slope covered by scattered pines and dense, sweet-smelling chaparral. From just south of Horse Flats Campground (1.1 mile), the Silver Moccasin Trail continues over a low ridge to the east, but you veer left (west) toward Mount Hillyer's south ridge. Well-beaten, sometimes steep switchbacks take you to a rounded summit area, where two high points (6200+ feet) lie. Continue down the ridge to the northeast, passing a 6162-foot knoll labeled Mount Hillyer on the topo map.

Due north of the 6162-foot knoll, an old road bed goes sharply downhill. Follow it to paved Santa Clara Divide Road (3.5 miles), which carries no traffic during the off-season, and light traffic otherwise. Turn right, walk south on the road 0.5 mile to the Horse Flats Campground turnoff, then go 0.7 mile to the south end of the campground. There you can pick up the Silver Moccasin Trail and retrace your steps back to Chilao.

ANGELES FOREST

# chapter 23

# Angeles Forest:
# Crystal Lake Recreation Area

**H**istorian/author John Robinson compares the form of the San Gabriel River's mountain watershed to a "colossal live oak, standing squat on a stout trunk, with an erect center limb and long horizontal branches extending outward in both directions." The West and East forks form the horizontal branches, while the center branch, the North Fork, drains the top of the tree—Crystal Lake Recreation Area. Highway 39 goes north from Interstate 210 at Azusa and travels up the "trunk" and the center limb—the main San Gabriel Canyon—and then dead-ends just beyond the Crystal Lake turnoff.

The spacious, oak- and conifer-dotted flats that make up Crystal Lake Recreation Area are quite a rarity in the tectonically active San Gabriels. Here, too, is found bantam-sized Crystal Lake, the only permanent natural lake on the south slopes of the San Gabriels. The area was first opened to visitors as a county park in 1932; after World War II it reverted to Forest Service administration. Now, as then, it caters mostly to day trippers and campers seeking a quick escape from the big city.

As you drive up San Gabriel Canyon toward the Crystal Lake basin, it may be interesting to recall some of the canyon's tortured history. John Robinson's book *The San Gabriels II* covers in fascinating detail the efforts to exploit and tame the canyon for mineral riches, water resources, flood control, electrical power, transportation, and recreation. Many of these attempts ended in monumental failures that could easily be blamed entirely on "acts of God"—fire, flood, and landslide—were it not for human arrogance and stupidity.

Perhaps the biggest fiasco was the abortive and costly attempt in the late 1920s to erect below the West and East forks what would have been (for a time) the world's largest dam. A massive landslide during construction put that project to rest. (Later, the much smaller San Gabriel and Morris dams were successfully completed downstream.)

The history of California Highway 39, the only road link between Crystal Lake and the outside world, is a story of dashed hopes as well. It took 1½ years to rebuild this highway after torrential flooding in 1938. About 40 years ago, an ambitious effort to realign a narrow, cliff-hanging section of the highway south of Crystal Lake was aborted when road crews bored through 200 feet of canyon wall without finding solid bedrock suitable for anchoring a bridge. You can see the ugly scars of this experiment below the recreation area near Coldbrook Campground.

A dubious scheme to extend Highway 39 northward to Angeles Crest Highway by way of the sheer, unstable upper slopes of Bear Canyon actually came to fruition in 1961. The road remained in service intermittently until 1978, when a landslide swept away a 500-foot-long section. Since then, hundreds of other slides have occurred in the area. As of 2009 there's a study going on to ascertain the possibility and the cost (probably $30 million) to return the upper section of Highway 39 to use by the motoring public.

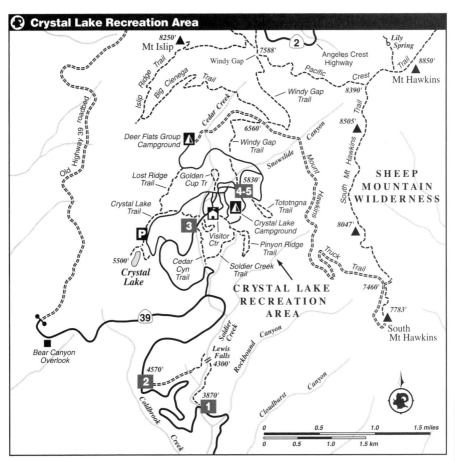

Meanwhile, the Crystal Lake area—and Highway 39—have suffered from the effects of the 2002 Curve Fire and subsequent flooding and earth movements. Up until 2009, Crystal Lake Recreation Area was closed to public use, and so was Highway 39 above Coldbrook Ranger Station. Caltrans and the Forest Service hope to have the highway and recreation area back open by sometime after 2009. All of the following hike descriptions assume that the recreation area has reopened.

At the trailheads below, you will need to post a National Forest Adventure Pass on your parked car ($5 per day, $30 per year). These permits can be obtained at the San Gabriel Information Station on Highway 39 near the mouth of the canyon just north of Azusa, and at most 24-hour businesses in the Azusa area.

# trip 1 Lewis Falls

see map on p. 269

| | |
|---|---|
| **Distance** | 0.8 mile round trip, Out-and-back |
| **Hiking Time** | ½ hour (round trip) |
| **Elevation Gain/Loss** | 300'/300' |
| **Difficulty** | Easy |
| **Trail Use** | Dogs allowed, good for kids |
| **Best Times** | All year |
| **Agency** | ANF/SGRD |
| **Optional Map** | USGS 7.5-min *Crystal Lake* |
| **Notes** | Marked trails/obvious routes, moderate terrain |

**DIRECTIONS** Exit Interstate 210 at Azusa Avenue (Highway 39) in Azusa. Go north on Azusa Avenue, which becomes San Gabriel Canyon Road. Continue a total of about 20 miles. Use the roadside mileage markers to identify the starting point—a small, shaded turnout on the right at mile 34.8, where Soldier Creek tumbles through a culvert under the highway.

On the precipice called Lewis Falls, Soldier Creek shoots (or cascades, or merely dribbles) some 50 feet down a two-tiered rock face. The volume of water splattering on rocks and sand below is seldom dramatic; but the cool spray and the sounds of falling water are refreshing. The hike to the base of the falls is short—only about 15 minutes, a manageable adventure (with some assistance) for small children.

From the turnout, make your way up a well-beaten trail on the east side of the creek, under shade-giving oaks, bays, and bigcone Douglas-firs. Near the last cabin upstream, the trail virtually disappears in the flood-scoured bed of Soldier Creek. A final, 200-yard scramble along the stream takes you to the base of the falls.

Most of the year Soldier Creek is a tame brook, easily jumped by the average adult. But a major storm, or a rapid thaw in the snowpack above, could produce runoff deep and swift enough to be hazardous—at least for kids.

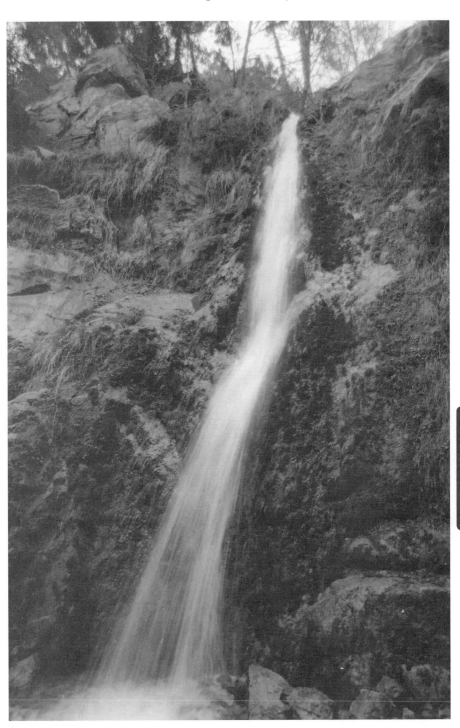

Lewis Falls

# trip 2  Upper Soldier Creek

| | |
|---|---|
| **Distance** | 1.4 miles round trip, Out-and-back |
| **Hiking Time** | 1 hour (round trip) |
| **Elevation Gain/Loss** | 250'/250' |
| **Difficulty** | Moderate |
| **Trail Use** | Dogs allowed |
| **Best Times** | All year |
| **Agency** | ANF/SGRD |
| **Optional Map** | USGS 7.5-min *Crystal Lake* |
| **Notes** | Marked trails/obvious routes, moderate terrain |

see map on p. 269

**DIRECTIONS**  Exit Interstate 210 at Azusa Avenue (Highway 39) in Azusa. Go north on Azusa Avenue, which becomes San Gabriel Canyon Road. Continue a total of about 22 miles. Use the roadside mileage markers to identify the starting point—a wide, gated fire road that goes east at mile 36.8. Park on the shoulder of Highway 39 so as not to block any traffic or block the gate itself.

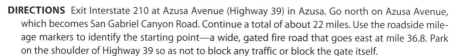

Just above Lewis Falls—but not accessible by way of Trip 1 above—is a beautiful stretch of Soldier Creek featuring a half dozen small cascades. Deeply shaded by oaks and conifers, and adorned with ferns, this rugged little hideaway is, again, just a short walk away from Highway 39.

On foot, follow the wide dirt road 0.5 mile east to its end. This stub of a road was part of a projected realignment of Highway 39 that would have been in place sometime in the 1970s if it hadn't been for insurmountable construction difficulties.

From the road end, find the narrow trail, on the left, that contours through manzanita brush. It leads about 300 yards to the cascades that lie upstream from Lewis Falls. Parts of the narrow trail edge precariously along steep, erodible slopes, so watch your step.

Soldier Creek above Lewis Falls

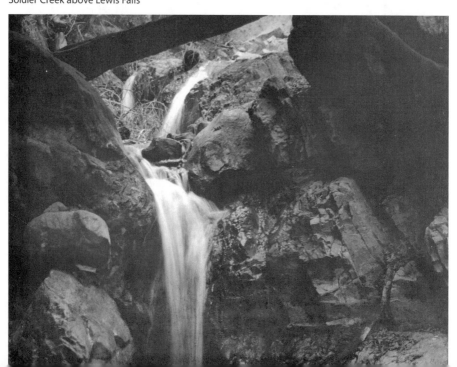

# **trip 3** Crystal Lake Nature Trails

| | |
|---|---|
| **Distance** | ½ to 1 mile (per trail) |
| **Hiking Time** | Varies |
| **Difficulty** | Easy to moderate |
| **Trail Use** | Dogs allowed, good for kids |
| **Best Times** | All year (whenever accessible) |
| **Agency** | ANF/SGRD |
| **Optional Map** | USGS 7.5-min *Crystal Lake* |
| **Notes** | Marked trails/obvious routes, easy to moderate terrain |

see map on p. 269

**DIRECTIONS** Exit Interstate 210 at Azusa Avenue (Highway 39) in Azusa. Go north on Azusa Avenue, which becomes San Gabriel Canyon Road. Continue a total of about 25 miles to the Crystal Lake Recreation Area on the right. Drive in 1 mile and park near the visitor center.

Briefly stated, the several short nature trails of Crystal Lake Recreation Area offer one of the best introductions to the high, forested country of the San Gabriel Mountains. You won't ever get very far away from the sounds of auto traffic or happy campers on these trails, but you can certainly learn quite a bit about the area's natural features.

Stop by the visitor center to obtained detailed maps of the trails and campground access roads of the Crystal Lake area, and self-guiding leaflets for some of the trails listed below. Note that as of 2009 the entire Crystal Lake Recreation Area was closed due to storm damage, but that a reopening is anticipated.

The **Tototngna Trail**, a self-guiding, 0.7-mile walk, starts from the main trailhead parking area 0.5 mile beyond (northeast of) the visitor center. *Tototngna*, "place of the stones" in the Gabrielino tongue, refers to the boulder-filled gullies sweeping down toward the Crystal Lake basin from the steep mountain walls surrounding it. On this oak-shaded walk, you'll discover such minutiae as lichens, oak galls, and a small geologic fault. Note: As of 2009 the Tototngna Trail was severely damaged.

The **Golden Cup Trail**, starting halfway between the visitor center and the main trailhead parking lot, loops for 0.3 mile through a grove of golden cup oaks, better known as canyon live oaks. The more colorful of the two names comes from the golden color of the shallow pod cup that holds the acorn. Other names for this tree are iron oak and maul oak, allusions to the great density and durability of its wood.

The **Pinyon Ridge Trail**, starting just southeast of the visitor center, travels 1 mile through habitats ranging from the lush oak-and-conifer forest to barren, sun-baked slopes. This 20-stop, self-guiding loop trail climbs to a high and dry ridge dominated by an isolated colony of pinyon pines. These stunted pines seem quite at home in their local microhabitat, but actually they're quite far from their normal range on the desert-facing slopes of the San Gabriel Mountains.

The **Soldier Creek Trail** diverges from the Pinyon Ridge Trail at a small footbridge just below the starting point. You can make a 1.5-mile loop by descending the Soldier Creek Trail to its junction with the **Cedar Canyon Trail**, climbing the Cedar Canyon Trail to meet the main entrance road into the recreation area, and following the entrance road east past the visitor center over to where you started. Both trails are deeply shaded by live oaks, incense cedars, and other trees. "Soldier Creek Trail" is a bit of a misnomer because the trail actually follows a tributary of Soldier Creek. Both this creek and Cedar Creek turn into delightful, tumbling brooks during times of snowmelt—typically winter through early spring.

ANGELES FOREST

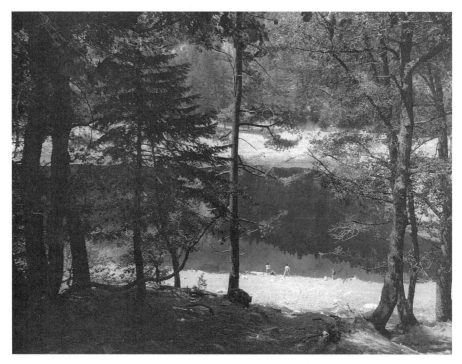

Crystal Lake

Just east of the starting point for the Pinyon Ridge Trail, on the lower entrance road to campground loop C, is a 100-yard-long side trail to the Goliath Oak. Set amid a thicket of lesser oaks, this giant canyon live oak measures 20 feet in trunk circumference and 82 feet in height.

The **Half Knob Trail** starts on the south side of the entrance road, just west of the visitor center. It loops halfway around and then back (0.6 mile total) along the side of a wooded knoll—or "knob" if you prefer.

The **Lake Trail** allows you to hike from the visitor center to Crystal Lake, 1.0 mile one-way. On the way you'll pass the Lost Ridge Trail, which climbs along a sharply defined ridgeline and joins the paved access road to Deer Flats Group Campground. If you follow the Lost Ridge Trail, you could loop back to the visitor center by way of the access road and the Windy Gap Trail (see Trips 4 and 5 for more on the Windy Gap Trail).

# trip 4 | Mount Islip—South Approach

|  |  |
|---|---|
| **Distance** | 7.0 miles round trip, Out-and-back |
| **Hiking Time** | 4 hours (round trip) |
| **Elevation Gain/Loss** | 2200'/2200' |
| **Difficulty** | Moderately strenuous |
| **Trail Use** | Suitable for backpacking, dogs allowed |
| **Best Times** | May through November |
| **Agency** | ANF/SGRD |
| **Optional Map** | USGS 7.5-min *Crystal Lake* |
| **Notes** | Marked trails/obvious routes, easy terrain |

see map on p. 269

**DIRECTIONS**  Exit Interstate 210 at Azusa Avenue (Highway 39) in Azusa. Go north on Azusa Avenue, which becomes San Gabriel Canyon Road. Continue a total of about 25 miles to the Crystal Lake Recreation Area on the right. Drive in 1.5 miles to the main hikers' parking lot, 0.5 mile beyond the Crystal Lake Recreation Area visitor center.

The south approach of Mount Islip feels a bit like real mountain climbing, despite the rather straightforward ascent by way of marked trails. You begin amid spreading oaks and tall conifers in Crystal Lake basin, rise through progressively smaller and sparser timber, and finally reach the nearly bald and often windblown summit. There, a comprehensive view both north over the Mojave Desert and south over the metropolis is offered on clear days. For the slight effort of nearly a mile on the way up or down, you can spend the night at Little Jimmy Campground, one of the nicest trail camps in the San Gabriels.

From the trailhead, follow the Windy Gap Trail north. You cross Mount Hawkins Truck Trail twice, and then tackle the steep, upper slopes of the cirque-like rim overlooking the Crystal Lake basin. At 2.5 miles you reach Windy Gap, which is the lowest spot on the north side of that rim.

At Windy Gap you meet the Pacific Crest Trail, which joins from the right (east). Continue briefly north on the PCT to the next junction. Going left takes you more directly to the summit of Mount Islip, while going right would lead you to Little Jimmy Campground and a more roundabout ascent of the mountain. In either case, you'll end up on the trail that follows the sunny east ridge of Mount Islip to its summit. (Note: Hard snow or ice can linger on the steep, north-facing slopes north of Windy Gap until sometime in May. You might avoid that stretch if need be by going straight up the east shoulder of Mount Islip from Windy Gap; that route becomes snow-free earlier in the season.)

Old stone cabin on Mount Islip

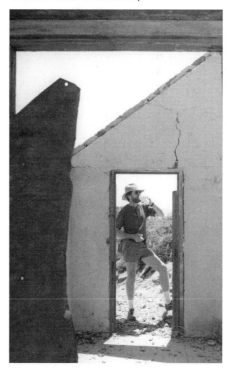

ANGELES FOREST

On the summit (3.5 miles) you'll discover the shell of an old stone cabin, and footings of a fire lookout tower that stood on Islip from 1927 until 1937, when the lookout was moved to a better site to the southeast—South Mount Hawkins. That structure was completely destroyed in the 2002 Curve Fire, but plans are afoot to rebuild it, again on South Mount Hawkins.

On your return, for the sake of variety, you can follow the Islip Ridge and Big Cienega trails. Two switchbacks below the summit of Mount Islip, turn right on the Islip Ridge Trail, which goes down Islip's south ridge. A future extension of that trail may go south and east all the way to Crystal Lake. You, however, travel just 1.0 mile down Islip Ridge Trail and then veer east on Big Cienega Trail. After another 2.0 miles of gradual descent along wooded south-facing slopes, you join the Windy Gap Trail just north of the upper crossing of Mount Hawkins Truck Trail. Turn right and return to the hikers' parking lot.

## trip 5  Mount Hawkins Loop

see map on p. 269

| | |
|---|---|
| **Distance** | 11.5 miles, Loop |
| **Hiking Time** | 7 hours |
| **Elevation Gain/Loss** | 3400'/3400' |
| **Difficulty** | Strenuous |
| **Trail Use** | Suitable for backpacking, dogs allowed |
| **Best Times** | May through November |
| **Agency** | ANF/SGRD |
| **Recommended Map** | USGS 7.5-min *Crystal Lake* |
| **Notes** | Navigation required, moderate terrain |

**DIRECTIONS** Exit Interstate 210 at Azusa Avenue (Highway 39) in Azusa. Go north on Azusa Avenue, which becomes San Gabriel Canyon Road. Continue a total of about 25 miles to the Crystal Lake Recreation Area on the right. Drive in 1.5 miles to the main hikers' parking lot, 0.5 mile beyond the Crystal Lake Recreation Area visitor center.

The completion of the South Mount Hawkins Trail along the high, east rim of Crystal Lake basin in the late 1980s made the popular traverse between Mount Hawkins and South Mount Hawkins considerably easier than before. On this trip you'll start at the main Windy Gap Trailhead down in the basin, climb to South Mount Hawkins, climb north to the higher Mount Hawkins, and return by looping back on the Pacific Crest and Windy Gap trails.

Most years, the route becomes snow-free sometime in May. Don't be fooled if the slopes visible from Crystal Lake basin appear to be clear of snow in April or early May; icy passages with seemingly bottomless runouts could still await you on the high, north end of the Hawkins ridge. Check first at the visitor center, or with a ranger.

Start by taking the Windy Gap Trail north to the second crossing of the Mount Hawkins Truck Trail, 1.0 mile. Turn right and follow the dirt road as it climbs steadily and moderately across the steep slopes east of Crystal Lake Basin. If it's summer, it's best if you can cover these 3 miles of somewhat tedious road-walking before the morning sun breaks over the high crest to the east.

On a sparsely wooded saddle at 3.9 miles, you'll get your first glimpse east into some of the rugged canyons of Sheep Mountain Wilderness. From the saddle, you can take the foot trail going south along the ridge to the South Hawkins summit, rather than staying

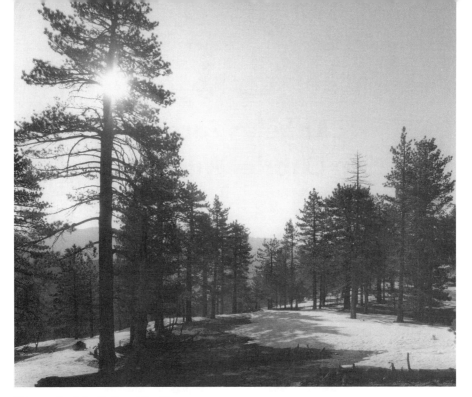

Ridge north of South Mount Hawkins

on the road. Prior to the 2002 Curve Fire, a whitewashed lookout tower perched here. There are plans to rebuild the structure.

The South Hawkins summit presides over a wrinkled landscape of dry, sinuous ridges and steeply plunging canyons. One way or another, nearly all the mountainous terrain in your field of view sheds water into the San Gabriel River.

After your visit to South Hawkins, retrace your steps back to the saddle (4.7 miles). Take the spur road curving north to the site of an old heliport, and continue north on the South Mount Hawkins Trail, which is cut high along the east-facing slope of the Hawkins ridge. The singed remains of Jeffrey pines, sugar pines, and white firs cling to the slopes, serving as picturesque frames for the wraith-like profiles of lower ridges engulfed in fog or smog.

At 6.9 miles, you reach a junction with the Pacific Crest Trail. A second side trip is necessary if you want to reach Mount Hawkins, one of several rounded summits defining the crest of what's known as the middle High Country—Mount Islip to Mount Baden-Powell. Turn east and head for the obvious promontory a half mile away. You'll scramble up the last 300 yards or so through scattered pines. To the east, the rounded summits of Troop Peak, Mount Burnham, and Mount Baden-Powell can be seen curving to the right. In the north, beyond lesser summits, spreads the flat Mojave Desert floor.

You return to Crystal Lake by way of the shortest route—west on the Pacific Crest Trail to the trail junction at Windy Gap, then left down the Windy Gap Trail.

# chapter 24

# Angeles Forest:
# San Gabriel Wilderness

San Gabriel Wilderness was first set aside as a protected area in 1932—well before the advent of the National Wilderness Preservation System in 1964. Its 36,137 acres encompass some extremely rugged terrain, with elevations ranging from under 2000 feet to over 8000 feet. Many areas in this wilderness are characterized by slopes steeper than 100 percent, that is, steeper than a 45-degree incline.

Green ribbons of riparian vegetation cling to the narrow bottoms of the two principal drainages—Bear Creek and Devils Canyon—while dense chaparral forms an almost impenetrable cover on the lower canyon walls. Scattered bigcone Douglas-firs at lower elevations gradually give way to statuesque ponderosa, Jeffrey, Coulter, lodgepole, and sugar pines; incense cedars; and white firs on the higher slopes of Waterman Mountain and Twin Peaks.

This varied, rough, and remote habitat harbors mule deer, Nelson bighorn sheep, black bear, and mountain lions. You're most likely to see the former two, less likely to encounter bears (they love to hang around camp- and picnic areas), and least likely to encounter a mountain lion. Grizzly bears, once a common hazard, were hunted to extinction here by about the turn of the 20th Century.

Although a trans-mountain Indian trail once followed the length of Bear Creek, no such trails cross San Gabriel Wilderness today. The currently maintained hiking trails only graze the edges of the wilderness, leaving the interior (especially south of Twin Peaks) virtually unexplored in modern times.

You can easily enter San Gabriel Wilderness at least six ways, as described in the trips listed below. Once inside the boundary the trails tend to fade, but the possibilities

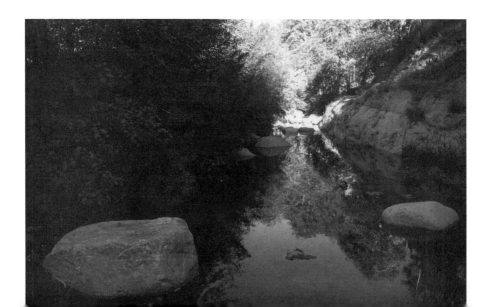

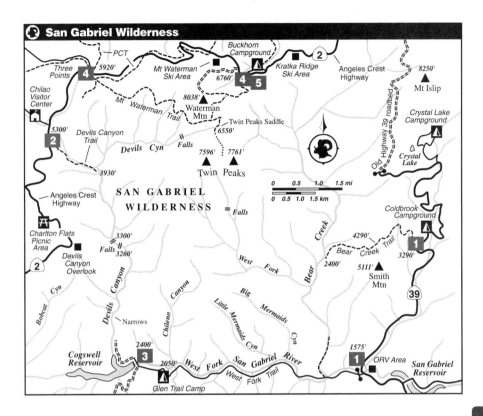

for further exploration (mostly of a very rugged kind) are almost endless. At present, you may enter San Gabriel Wilderness without having the usual wilderness permit that is required for most other wilderness areas around the state. This does not absolve you from obtaining a fire permit, if applicable. If you do plan to venture well off the beaten track, then for your own safety it would be wise to consult with a ranger first.

All trips below require a National Forest Adventure Pass ($5 per day, $30 per year) for trailhead parking.

The 2009 Station Fire in its closing stages burned into the west half of the San Gabriel Wilderness, affecting Trips 2, 3 and 4 in this chapter. Before you hike here, be sure to get the latest update from Angeles National Forest personnel.

ANGELES FOREST

Quiet pool in Bear Creek canyon

**trip 1** # Bear Creek Trail

see map on p. 279

| | |
|---|---|
| **Distance** | 9.7 miles, Point-to-point |
| **Hiking Time** | 7 hours |
| **Elevation Gain/Loss** | 1100'/2800' |
| **Difficulty** | Moderately strenuous |
| **Trail Use** | Suitable for backpacking, dogs allowed |
| **Best Times** | October through June |
| **Agency** | ANF/SGRD |
| **Recommended Map** | USGS 7.5-min *Crystal Lake* |
| **Notes** | Navigation required, moderate terrain, bushwhacking |

**DIRECTIONS** *North End:* Exit Interstate 210 at Azusa Avenue (Highway 39) in Azusa. Go north on Azusa Avenue, which becomes San Gabriel Canyon Road. After about 12 miles you cross the West Fork San Gabriel River bridge; the spacious West Fork trailhead/staging area lies to the left. Continue north on Highway 39 another 5.5 miles to the start of the Bear Canyon Trail at the edge of a large roadside turnout, mile 32.2 according to the roadside mile markers. *South End:* The hike ends at the West Fork trailhead/staging area.

**B**ear Creek and its myriad tributaries drain about half of San Gabriel Wilderness—roughly 25 square miles of steeply plunging ravines and canyons. Virtually none of this convoluted landscape ever experiences the tread of hiking boots except for the lower stretch of Bear Creek, reached by way of the Bear Creek Trail from Highway 39. The one-way route described here takes you into the heart of this wild area and includes almost 4 miles of boulder-hopping along perennially flowing Bear Creek. A short car-shuttle along Highway 39 can be used to connect the two ends of the hike.

Wide and easy at first, the Bear Canyon Trail twists and turns up through sun-struck chaparral, gaining 1000 feet in a

Old cabin foundation, lower Bear Creek canyon

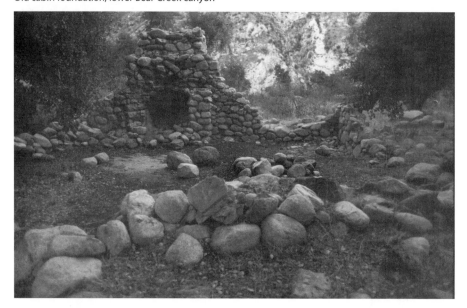

moderately easy 2.5 miles. Traffic noise from the highway below gradually fades as you climb higher.

The 4290-foot saddle at the top of that grade marks the high point on the hike as well as the wilderness boundary. Down the other side you descend quickly on a narrower and rougher trail, and all vestiges of civilization (save an occasional passing aircraft) instantly disappear from view. Tall, nearly impenetrable chaparral on the steep north slopes keeps most of the sunlight away during the fall and winter months. To the northwest, the Twin Peaks ridge soars impressively over the far wall of Bear Creek canyon. Caution is in order in a couple of spots where the trail crosses perpetually eroding ravines.

The descent concludes with a zigzag passage down along a ridge between two steep ravines. You arrive at Bear Creek's east bank, where blackened boulders indicate a small trail camp, 4.7 miles. (A spectacular narrow section of Bear Creek canyon, with vertical granite walls, begins 0.3 mile upstream from this point—worth a look if you have time for the side trip.)

Little hint of any trail can be found in the next 4 miles as you follow the stream to its confluence with West Fork San Gabriel River. Narrow and vegetation-choked at first, the canyon becomes wider, flatter, and talus-filled as you press on ahead. Once the stream has room to meander across the canyon floor, it curves from wall to wall, forcing you to plunge into the streamside alders and boulder-hop or wade across the water. You'll repeat that process about 25 times.

Atop low, oak-shaded terraces at 5.7 miles (at the West Fork Bear Creek confluence) and at 7.5 miles (next to the remains of a stone cabin), you'll find plenty of room to

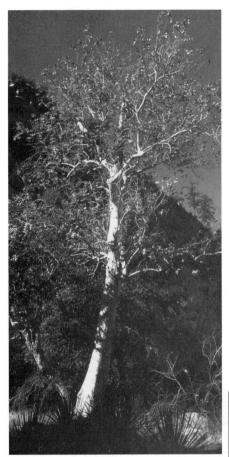

Sycamore in Bear Creek canyon

set up a tent in a picturesque, shady setting. Below the lower campsite, a well-beaten but intermittent path helps improve your speed for the last mile or so. At 8.7 miles, you cross West Fork San Gabriel River and join the paved West Fork National Recreation Trail, which is the main access road to Cogswell Reservoir, doubling as a bike and hike trail. Turn left and walk a mile out to Highway 39 and your waiting car.

ANGELES FOREST

# trip 2  Upper Devils Canyon

| | |
|---|---|
| **Distance** | 9.8 miles round trip, Out-and-back |
| **Hiking Time** | 7 hours (round trip) |
| **Elevation Gain/Loss** | 2100'/2100' |
| **Difficulty** | Moderately strenuous |
| **Trail Use** | Suitable for backpacking, dogs allowed |
| **Best Times** | October through June |
| **Agency** | ANF/SGRD |
| **Optional Maps** | USGS 7.5-min *Chilao Flat, Waterman Mtn.* |
| **Notes** | Marked trails/obvious routes, moderate terrain |

see
map on
p. 279

see map on p. 279

**DIRECTIONS** Exit Interstate 210 at Angeles Crest Highway in La Cañada-Flintridge. Drive 25 miles north and east to the Devils Canyon Trailhead on the right, mile 50.4, just south of the Chilao Visitor Center turnoff.

If you stand at Devils Canyon Overlook (just below Charlton Flat on Angeles Crest Highway) on a warm spring day, a withering updraft fans your face like the hot breath of a furnace. There's no hint of the clear, cascading stream and the cool, shady microenvironment hidden in the deep crease of the canyon 2000 feet below.

Getting down there isn't bad at all; most of the effort comes in getting back up. I'd recommend spending a full day (or parts of two days) exploring the canyon. You can splash around in some of the shallow pools (in May or June, when the water warms), watch ducks and water ouzels at work or play, fish for trout (you'll need a state license) and/or trek down to the upper of two waterfalls in the canyon. If the weather's warm, you should plan to wait until the sun sinks to the west before making the long climb back up the afternoon-shaded west canyon wall.

The trail starts at the Devils Canyon Trailhead, not the roadside Devils Canyon Overlook mentioned above. Your zigzagging descent on the trail takes you across slopes clothed alternately in chaparral and mixed conifer forest. By 1.5 miles you reach a branch of what will soon become a trickling stream—one of the several tributaries that contribute to Devils Canyon's ample springtime flow. The deeply shaded trail leads to the main canyon (be sure to mark this spot or take note of surrounding landmarks so you can recognize this place when it's time to head back up the trail), 2.6 miles, and then downstream a bit farther to the site of a former trail camp on a flat bench west of the Devils Canyon stream. In accordance with the philosophy of returning designated wilderness areas to as natural a condition as possible, this former trail camp, as well as all others within the wilderness borders, have had their stoves and tables removed.

Downstream, you follow a fairly distinct path in places; otherwise you boulder-hop and wade. Mini-cascades feed pools 3-4 feet deep harboring elusive brook trout. Water-loving alders and sycamores cluster along the stream, while patriarchal live oaks and bigcone Douglas-firs stand on higher and dryer benches and slopes, waiting in the wings, as it were, for the next big flood to sweep the upstarts away. Watch for poison oak as the canyon walls narrow; and keep an eye out for a silvery, two-tier waterfall at the mouth of a side canyon coming in from the east, mile 4.5.

Beyond the two-tier fall, 0.4 mile of rock scrambling and wading takes you to a constriction in the canyon where water slides down a sheer incline some 20 vertical feet. Avoiding the slippery lip of these falls,

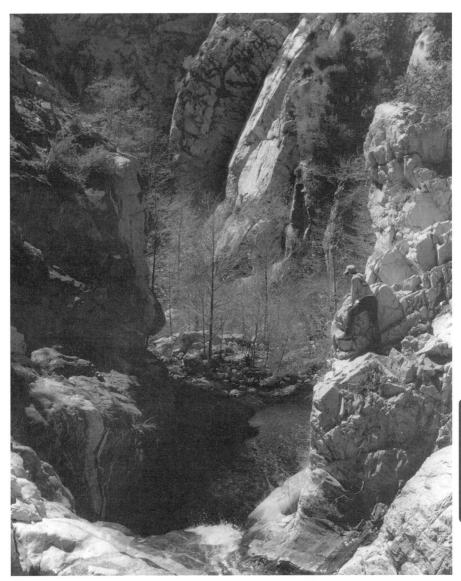

Top of upper fall in Devils Canyon

you can climb the rock wall to the right for an airy view of the cascade and shallow pool below. Without rappelling gear, this is basically the end of the line (a second waterfall just below this one can be reached from Cogswell Reservoir below—see Trip 3). You'll have to return by the same route.

Note: The 2009 Station Fire burned over most of the area detailed in this trip. It may take some time before the Devils Canyon Trail reopens, and some years will be required for the riparian vegetation in the bottom of the canyon to recover.

### trip 3  Lower Devils Canyon

see map on p. 279

| | |
|---|---|
| **Distance** | 9.4 miles round trip, Out-and-back (from Cogswell Reservoir) |
| **Hiking Time** | 7 hours (round trip) |
| **Elevation Gain/Loss** | 1200'/1200' |
| **Difficulty** | Strenuous |
| **Trail Use** | Suitable for backpacking, dogs allowed |
| **Best Times** | November through May |
| **Agency** | ANF/SGRD |
| **Optional Maps** | USGS 7.5-min *Azusa, Waterman Mtn.* |
| **Notes** | Marked trails/obvious routes, difficult terrain, bushwhacking |

**DIRECTIONS**  Exit Interstate 210 at Azusa Avenue (Highway 39) in Azusa. Go north on Azusa Avenue, which becomes San Gabriel Canyon Road. After about 12 miles you cross the West Fork San Gabriel River bridge and arrive at the spacious West Fork trailhead/staging area on the left.

In the lower reaches of Devils Canyon, a vociferous little stream darts over an obstacle course of rounded boulders perpetually shaded by thickets of alder and sycamore. Now and again the water slackens in transparent pools of Zen-like simplicity, cupped in naked granite. Skittish trout lurk in the watery depths, while a great blue heron stalk the shallows. Hawks wheel through the sky overhead, ever-watchful of the movements of small, furry creatures below. This is quintessential wilderness—remote, pristine, and in this case devilishly difficult to reach.

The journey into lower Devils Canyon almost necessarily begins with . . . a bike ride! If you don't have bike wheels, then you necessarily face 15 miles of round-trip walking on pavement in addition to the 9.4 miles of hiking described here. You should allow more than an extra hour for the pedaling part.

From the south end of the bridge, wheel your bike around the vehicle gate onto the West Fork National Recreation Trail. This paved service road/bike path meanders up the beautiful West Fork canyon bottom to the top of Cogswell Dam 7.5 miles away. Once you get past the first graffiti-scarred half mile, the remainder of the ride is a refreshing prelude to the Devils Canyon hike. (The epilogue for the hike is even nicer—you hardly have to pedal at all when coasting back to your car.)

After 6.3 miles of riding—nearly 500 feet of elevation gain—you reach Glen Campground (hike-in or bike-in; first-come, first

Biking along the West Fork National Recreation Trail

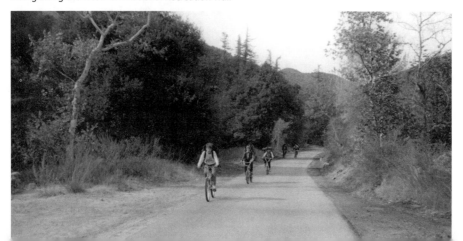

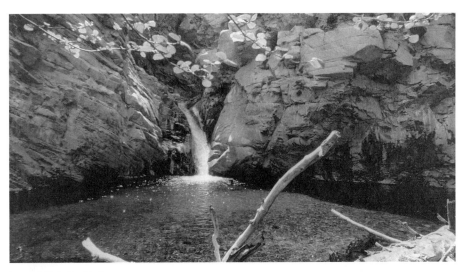

Lower falls in Devils Canyon

ANGELES FOREST

served). You then continue another 1.2 miles (350 feet gain) to Cogswell Dam. (The dam and reservoir were off-limits to public visitation for some years following 9/11, and it is possible this closure could be imposed again.)

You're allowed to walk or ride your bike across the dam to gain access to the dirt road along the far (north) side. If you have a road bike, secure it at the dam (or somehow conceal it) and continue on foot—Cogswell Dam is our assumed starting point for the hike. If you have a mountain bike, you can continue riding on dirt for another 1.5 miles.

Either way, the rapidly deteriorating road at 1.5 miles will force you to scramble, one way or another, down about 80 feet to the wide, sand- and boulder-filled floor of Devils Canyon. This barren, often-bone-dry stretch bears no resemblance to what you'll find only a mile up-canyon. The first small pools, where water sinks below the surface and percolates into the porous substratum, will probably be found a short distance ahead.

At 2.3 miles, the canyon floor suddenly narrows and you must somehow get past a moat-like pool, about 10 feet deep, squeezed between nearly vertical rock walls. Beyond lies a veritable Shangri-La of crystalline pools and miniature cascades. A half-rotten log helped me get across the moat and into the narrows ahead. You, however, should count on the possibility of having to swim; take along a water-proof plastic bag you can use to package your clothes and other gear you can't afford to get wet.

The barest hint of an animal trail threads through the canyon ahead. Mostly you'll scramble, boulder-hop, and wade. This part of the canyon is much like upper Devils Canyon (Trip 2), except the pools are more grand. The best one (at 2.8 miles), about 10 feet deep and bounded by water-polished granite and banded metamorphic rock, is a sensational swimming hole. There are lots of alder trees and some sycamores down along the stream; oaks, incense cedars, and scattered poison oak a little higher above the stream; and hardy bigcone Douglas-firs clinging to the slopes.

At about 3.5 miles the canyon floor widens considerably. High and dry campsites can be found in the next mile. At 4.5 miles the canyon narrows again, and just ahead of that, progress comes to a halt because of an unclimbable waterfall. This is the lower of two closely spaced falls that rock climbers have been able to descend by means of rappelling. Here, the waters of Devils Canyon funnel though a sheer-walled constriction in the canyon floor and drop about 20 vertical feet into a pool about 40 feet wide and 4 feet deep.

Note: Much of the San Gabriel Wilderness east of Cogswell Dam was swept by the flames of the 2009 Station Fire. Access to lower Devils Canyon may therefore be restricted for a time. Sediment deposited in the Devils Canyon streambed in future rainy seasons could make reaching the lower falls easier than as described above, at least for while.

## trip 4  Mount Waterman Trail

| | |
|---|---|
| **Distance** | 7.8 miles, Point-to-point |
| **Hiking Time** | 4½ hours |
| **Elevation Gain/Loss** | 1400'/2250' |
| **Difficulty** | Moderately strenuous |
| **Trail Use** | Suitable for backpacking, dogs allowed |
| **Best Times** | May through November |
| **Agency** | ANF/SGRD |
| **Optional Map** | USGS 7.5-min *Waterman Mtn.* |
| **Notes** | Marked trails/obvious routes, easy terrain |

see map on p. 279

**DIRECTIONS** *East End:* Exit Interstate 210 at Angeles Crest Highway in La Cañada-Flintridge. Drive 33 miles north and east to the Buckhorn Trailhead on the left, at mile 58.0 on Angeles Crest Highway. *West End:* The hike ends at Three Points Trailhead, located at the intersection of Santa Clara Divide Road, mile 52.8 on Angeles Crest Highway.

The Mount Waterman Trail traverse across the north rim of San Gabriel Wilderness provides almost constant views of statuesque pines, yawning chasms, and distant, hazy ridges. You start near the entrance to Buckhorn Campground and you end up half-circling broad-shouldered Waterman Mountain by the time you arrive at Three Points, 5 miles away by car. Snow can linger on the easternmost mile of the trail until May, but it tends to disappear much earlier on the remaining (mostly south-facing) parts of the trail. This is one of the most popular High Country summer hikes—heartily recommended for all but the warmest days.

Pick up the Mount Waterman Trail on the south side of Angeles Crest Highway, opposite the Buckhorn Trailhead. Follow the well-graded foot trail—not the old road bed that parallels the trail at first—along a shady slope. After 1.0 mile of easy ascent through gorgeous mixed-conifer forest, you come to a saddle overlooking Bear Creek. The trail turns west, follows a viewful ridge, and then ascends on six long switchbacks to a trail junction, 2.1 miles. A trail to Waterman Mountain's rounded summit goes right; you stay left and contour west about a half mile, then zigzag south down to a second junction, 3.5 miles. Twin Peaks saddle, a spacious camping spot, lies below to the left. If you're simply day-hiking this stretch, then stay right (west).

The remaining 4+ miles take you gradually downhill (steeper at the very end) along Waterman Mountain's south flank. You wind in and out of broad ravines, either shaded by huge incense cedars and vanilla-scented Jeffrey pines, or exposed to the warm sunshine on chaparral-covered slopes. The older cedar trees are gnarled veterans of past fires.

Near the end, you hook up briefly with the Pacific Crest Trail. On it you swing down to cross Angeles Crest Highway, and climb up to Three Points Trailhead.

Note: The majority of the Mount Waterman Trail was burned during the 2009 Station Fire.

# trip 5 Waterman Mountain & Twin Peaks

| | |
|---|---|
| **Distance** | 11.8 miles round trip, Out-and-back |
| **Hiking Time** | 7½ hours (round trip) |
| **Elevation Gain/Loss** | 4000'/4000' |
| **Difficulty** | Strenuous |
| **Trail Use** | Suitable for backpacking, dogs allowed |
| **Best Times** | May through November |
| **Agency** | ANF/SGRD |
| **Recommended Map** | USGS 7.5-min *Waterman Mtn.* |
| **Notes** | Navigation required, moderate terrain |

see map on p. 279

**DIRECTIONS** Exit Interstate 210 at Angeles Crest Highway in La Cañada-Flintridge. Drive 33 miles north and east to the Buckhorn Trailhead on the left, at mile 58.0 on Angeles Crest Highway.

The "top of the world" views from Waterman Mountain and especially Twin Peaks ridge are among the best in the San Gabriel Mountains. This peak-bagging extravaganza visits both Waterman Mountain's summit and the east summit of Twin Peaks (11.8 miles out-and-back for the whole trip). You can, however, easily customize this hike to include more or include less, to suit your ability and desire.

From the trailhead start by crossing over to the south side of Angeles Crest Highway. Follow the well-graded Mount Waterman Trail—not the old road bed that parallels the trail at first—along a shady slope. After 1.0 mile of easy ascent through gorgeous mixed-conifer forest, you come to a saddle overlooking Bear Creek. The trail turns west, follows a viewful ridge, and then ascends on six long switchbacks to a trail junction, 2.1 miles. A right turn here starts you on the way to the summit of Waterman Mountain, 0.7 mile west. The trail itself swings around the north side of a lesser summit, crosses a saddle, and then bypasses, on the north, the true 8038-foot summit. You leave the trail and walk about 200 yards up a sparsely treed slope to the summit plateau. A summit register has been in place here since 1924.

When you arrive back at the first trail junction, turn west and continue following the Mount Waterman Trail. You contour west for about a half mile, then start zigzag-ging down a forested south slope to a second trail junction. Make a hard left here and continue descending a more primitive trail to Twin Peak Saddle (6550'), the lowest point on the divide separating upper Devil Canyon from upper Bear Creek. You could pitch a tent here, but there's much more room—and a better view—atop a 6816-foot knob 0.3 mile southeast.

Setting up at Buckhorn Campground

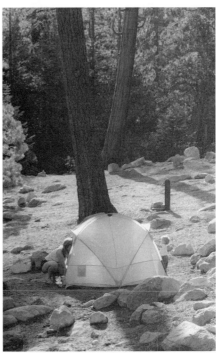

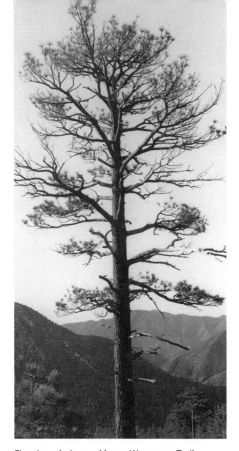

Fire-singed pine on Mount Waterman Trail

distance east to bag the 7761-foot eastern peak. If you drop a short way down to rock outcrops south and east, just below the summit, you'll have a dizzying view of the secret, upper reaches of Bear Creek's West Fork. Serrated ridges of shattered diorite, a rock-climber's nightmare, seem to tumble into the pit below. Quite often you can look out over a low-lying blanket of smog in the L.A. Basin and see Santa Catalina Island floating out at sea beyond the hazy dome of Palos Verdes. The Santa Anas, Palomar Mountain, the Santa Rosas, San Jacinto Peak and Old Baldy arc around the horizon from south to east. Also clearly in view, unfortunately, is the east wall of upper Bear Creek canyon, ripped apart during the grading for the now-closed upper segment of Highway 39.

Before returning to Buckhorn, consider visiting the 7596-foot west summit of Twin Peaks. From there, the view south is even more vertiginous, and the ugly scars of Highway 39 are hidden by the slightly higher eastern peak. Just west of the west summit is a superbly situated small campsite—a flat, sandy hollow amid boulders and scattered pines. According to the summit registers on both peaks, more than 100 people climb the east peak every year, while only about a dozen make the west peak. Hikers signing in frequently report sightings of bighorn sheep.

From Twin Peaks Saddle, the now-sketchy trail contours south to reach a second saddle (6580′) at the north base of Twin Peaks ridge. From there, you simply go straight up the slope, dodging boulders and trees, until you arrive on the ridgeline between the two peaks. Climb a short

# chapter 25

# Angeles Forest:
# High Country & North Slope

North of Angeles Crest Highway and down the slopes toward Devil's Punch-bowl country, the San Gabriel Mountains meld into desert in a most pleasant way. Timbered slopes dominate the cool crest, while on the warmer desert flats below, Joshua trees and high-desert scrub vegetation clearly hold sway. In between these two extremes there thrives an enigmatic mixture of oak and conifer forest, pinyon-juniper woodland, chaparral, and (in the bigger watercourses) riparian vegetation.

The trail system through these parts is somewhat underutilized as compared to trails farther west that are closer to the metropolis. The Pacific Crest Trail skims the crest of the range here, never straying too far from Angeles Crest Highway, while the High Desert National Recreation Trail probes the wild ridges and canyons of the slopes to the north. Not really a single trail, the High Desert Trail consists of several connected trails: Burkhart Trail, Punch-bowl Trail, South Fork Trail, and Manzanita Trail. I've described trips along each of the segments, as a day hiker would walk them to the best advantage, except for the Manzanita Trail, which is the least interesting of the four. Serious backpackers could put together a marathon-length (26-mile) loop on the High Desert Trail by including the leg of the PCT that stretches from Islip Saddle to Little Rock Creek.

Roadside campgrounds in the area include Angeles Crest's seasonally open Buckhorn Campground, which was used as a high-country sportsman's camp long before Angeles Crest Highway permitted easy access to it. On the desert side, there are two campgrounds, Sycamore Flats and South Fork—both located in the Big Rock Creek drainage. These latter two are among the better sites for stargazing in the San Gabriels, as they're shielded by the mountains from much (but not all) of the L.A. Basin light pollution.

In winter, snow often closes the upper parts of Angeles Crest Highway (particularly east of Kratka Ridge Ski Area) and lesser roads in the area, so you'll want to check with the Forest Service before you

PCT below Mount Islip

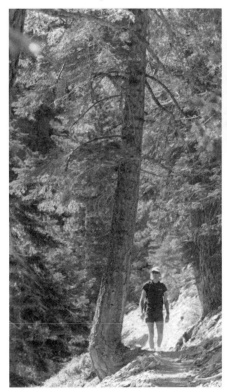

ANGELES FOREST

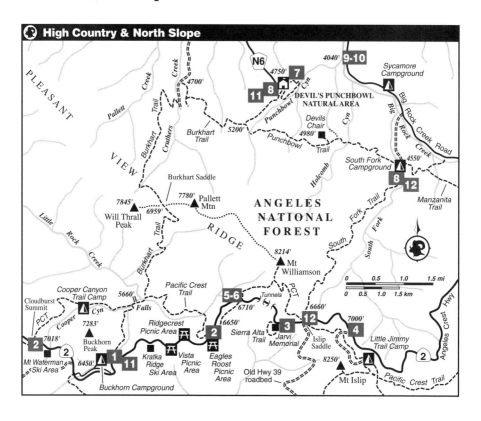

head up there early in the season. If you're a cross-country skier, you'll want to take advantage of any and all unplowed roads while the snow is fresh.

All trailheads below—except the parking lot inside Devil's Punchbowl Natural Area—require a National Forest Adventure Pass ($5 per day, $30 per year) for parking.

# trip 1  Cooper Canyon Falls

see map on p. 290

| | |
|---|---|
| **Distance** | 3.0 miles round trip, Out-and-back |
| **Hiking Time** | 1½ hours (round trip) |
| **Elevation Gain/Loss** | 800′/800′ |
| **Difficulty** | Moderate |
| **Trail Use** | Dogs allowed |
| **Best Times** | April through November |
| **Agency** | ANF/SCMRD |
| **Optional Map** | USGS 7.5-min *Waterman Mtn.* |
| **Notes** | Marked trails/obvious routes, easy terrain |

**DIRECTIONS** Exit Interstate 210 at Angeles Crest Highway in La Cañada-Flintridge. Drive 33 miles north and east to the turnoff for Buckhorn Campground on the left, at mile 58.3 on Angeles Crest Highway. Drive all the way through the campground to the far (northeast) end, where a short stub of dirt road leads to a trailhead parking area.

Cooper Canyon Falls roars with the melting snows of early spring, then settles down to a quiet whisper by June or July. You can cool off in the spray of the 25-foot cascade, or at least sit on a water-smoothed log and soak your feet in the chilly, alder-shaded pool just below the base of the falls. In the right season (April or May most years) these falls are one of the best unheralded attractions of the San Gabriel Mountains. The trail takes you quickly to the falls, downhill all the way, and then uphill all the way back. The forest hereabouts is dense enough to give plenty of cool shade for most of the unrelenting climb back up.

From the trailhead, the Burkhart Trail takes off down along the west wall of an unnamed, usually wet canyon garnished by two waterfalls. The first, at 6220 feet in the canyon bottom, is easy to reach by descending from the trail—this little gem of a cascade drops 10 feet into a rock grotto. The second, 30 feet-high falls, at 6050 feet, is very hazardous to approach from above, but is reachable from below by scrambling up the canyon bottom from Cooper Canyon.

At 1.2 miles, the trail bends east to follow Cooper Canyon's south bank. Continue another 0.3 mile, down past the junction of the trail (Pacific Crest Trail) that doubles back to follow the north bank upstream. Look or listen for water plunging over the rocky declivity to the left. A rough pathway leads down off the trail to the alder-fringed pool below.

ANGELES FOREST

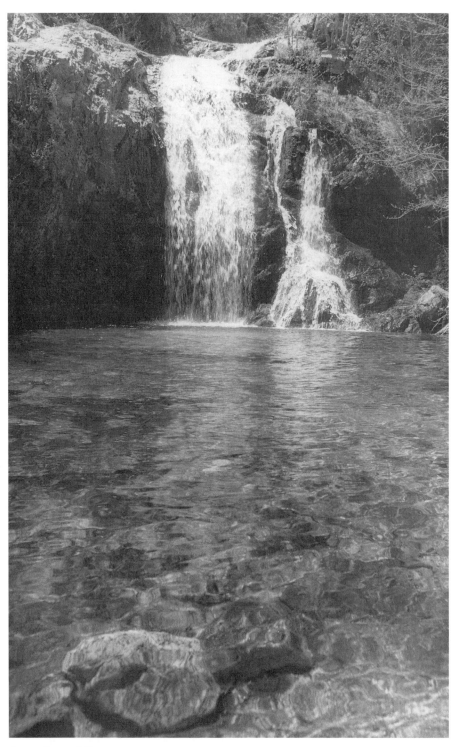

Cooper Canyon Falls

# trip 2 Cooper Canyon & Rattlesnake Trail

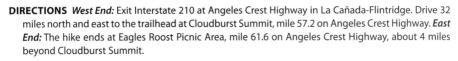

see map on p. 290

| | |
|---|---|
| **Distance** | 6.3 miles, Point-to-point |
| **Hiking Time** | 3 hours |
| **Elevation Gain/Loss** | 1200'/1550' |
| **Difficulty** | Moderate |
| **Trail Use** | Suitable for backpacking, dogs allowed |
| **Best Times** | April through November |
| **Agency** | ANF/SCMRD |
| **Optional Map** | USGS 7.5-min *Waterman Mtn.* |
| **Notes** | Marked trails/obvious routes, easy terrain |

**DIRECTIONS** *West End:* Exit Interstate 210 at Angeles Crest Highway in La Cañada-Flintridge. Drive 32 miles north and east to the trailhead at Cloudburst Summit, mile 57.2 on Angeles Crest Highway. *East End:* The hike ends at Eagles Roost Picnic Area, mile 61.6 on Angeles Crest Highway, about 4 miles beyond Cloudburst Summit.

This delightful stretch of the PCT, one of the best in Southern California, is best hiked one-way. If you set this up as a car shuttle, leave one car at or outside Eagles Roost Picnic Area, and take the other to Cloudburst Summit, where the PCT begins as a disused fire road that contours north.

Snowmelt and spring waters flow into Little Rock Creek from hundreds of small rivulets and creases in the High Country, giving rise to the happy stream that tumbles, forthwith, toward the thirsty floor of the Mojave Desert. Here, amidst magnificent groves of pine, fir, cedar, and oak, the Pacific Crest Trail deigns to descend from the high and dry ridgelines and, for a brief while, tracks Little Rock Creek and its main upper tributary—Cooper Canyon.

Once on the trail, you soon start descending along sparsely wooded slopes. After a sharp hairpin turn at 1.2 miles, the trail settles alongside a moist ravine blanketed by bracken fern. Presently you arrive at Cooper Canyon Trail Camp (1.6 miles), which features a huge fire ring, and quiet campsites—if the Scouts aren't whooping it up around the campfire.

Your descent continues along the north bank of year-round Cooper Canyon. Colorful patches of lupine dot the sunny clearings, and columbines nod in the air set in motion by the flowing water. At 2.7 miles,

you swing across the creek to meet the Burkhart Trail.

Bearing left, you continue down-canyon past Cooper Canyon Falls (see Trip 1) and reach the shady confluence of Little Rock Creek at 3.1 miles. This is the nadir of your trip—you mostly climb from now on. The Burkhart Trail splits to the north here; you go east on the PCT, a section formerly known as the Rattlesnake Trail. Setting a course well above trickling Little Rock Creek, the trail winds along the slope to the north, circuitously contouring around every ravine. You pass just below a seasonal spring in a ravine at 3.6 miles, and below even-less-dependable Rattlesnake Spring at 4.5 miles.

After a slight descent, you meet Little Rock Creek again (5.1 miles), and swing sharply right to commence the final uphill grind to Eagles Roost Picnic Area. To the north (mostly behind you as you climb) looms the white- and pink-tinted rock outcrop known as Eagles Roost.

Note: The Rattlesnake section of the PCT was closed from 2006 through 2009 in order to protect critical habitat for a rare species of frog. Check with the Forest Service to see if this section has reopened. During the closure period, through-hikers on the PCT have been allowed to follow an alternate route.

ANGELES FOREST

## trip 3  Sierra Alta Nature Trail

see map on p. 290

| | |
|---|---|
| **Distance** | 0.3 mile, Loop |
| **Hiking Time** | ¼ hour |
| **Elevation Gain/Loss** | 100'/100' |
| **Difficulty** | Easy |
| **Trail Use** | Dogs allowed, good for kids |
| **Best Times** | April through November |
| **Agency** | ANF/SGRD |
| **Optional Map** | USGS 7.5-min *Crystal Lake* |
| **Notes** | Marked trails/obvious routes, easy terrain |

**DIRECTIONS** Exit Interstate 210 at Angeles Crest Highway in La Cañada-Flintridge. Drive 38 miles north and east to the Jarvi Memorial on the right, at mile 63.6 on Angeles Crest Highway.

Jarvi Memorial Vista offers motorists a great view of both the yawning gorges of Bear Creek to the south and a sheer, fractured slope to the north punctured by two closely spaced tunnels on the highway. The memorial honors Sim Jarvi, former Angeles National Forest supervisor, and also serves as a trailhead for the Sierra Alta Nature Trail.

The trail, strictly good for education, not exercise, features plaques highlighting some examples of ponderosa pine, Jeffrey pine, and canyon live oaks, as well as views in various directions. Clear-day vistas can include the ocean, as well as Santa Catalina and San Clemente islands.

## trip 4  Mount Islip—North Approach

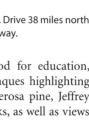

see map on p. 290

| | |
|---|---|
| **Distance** | 5.6 miles round trip, Out-and-back |
| **Hiking Time** | 3 hours (round trip) |
| **Elevation Gain/Loss** | 1250'/1250' |
| **Difficulty** | Moderate |
| **Trail Use** | Suitable for backpacking, dogs allowed, good for kids |
| **Best Times** | May through November |
| **Agency** | ANF/SGRD |
| **Optional Map** | USGS 7.5-min *Crystal Lake* |
| **Notes** | Marked trails/obvious routes, easy terrain |

**DIRECTIONS** Exit Interstate 210 at Angeles Crest Highway in La Cañada-Flintridge. Drive 40 miles north and east to start of a gated fire road on the right, at mile 65.5 on Angeles Crest Highway.

The ascent of Mount Islip from Crystal Lake to the south was described in Chapter 23. The north approach described here—via an easier and shortest-possible route—takes you through aromatic pine- and fir-forest most of the way. The gradual climb is well suited for children or anyone else who can handle moderate altitudes and hiking distances. If need be, you can shorten

the hike by turning back at Little Jimmy Campground, 1.5 miles up the slope.

You begin on the shoulder of Angeles Crest Highway, opposite the site of the now-removed Pine Hollow Picnic Area shown on older maps. Walk up the pine-cone-strewn gated road to where the Pacific Crest Trail crosses it, 0.5 mile up and 350 feet higher. Both the road and the PCT

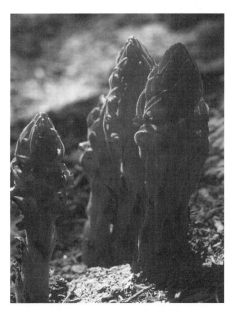

Snow plant

Jimmy Swinnerton (creator of the "Little Jimmy" comic strip), who summered here in 1909, nestles comfortably in a little flat shaded by statuesque pines. Tables and stoves make this a convenient spot for a picnic or an overnight layover. Down the trail contouring south toward Windy Gap (below the trail a quarter mile away) is year-round Little Jimmy Spring.

From the campground, the summit trail goes uphill (west at first), and continues looping upward to gain Mount Islip's east shoulder (stay right where a trail slants left and descends to meet the PCT). You ascend along this shoulder, swing around two switchbacks just below the summit, and arrive at the old hut and lookout site on top.

Note: The section of Angeles Crest Highway between Islip Saddle and Vincent Gap may close for years at a time due to storm damage and landslides. If this is the case, you can begin your hike at Islip Saddle, following the PCT all the way to Little Jimmy Campground.

go south and east to Little Jimmy Campground, but the trail is nicer.

Little Jimmy Campground, which honors early-century newspaper cartoonist

see map on p. 290

ANGELES FOREST

---

## trip 5  Mount Williamson

| | |
|---|---|
| **Distance** | 3.4 miles round trip, Out-and-back |
| **Hiking Time** | 2 hours (round trip) |
| **Elevation Gain/Loss** | 1500'/1500' |
| **Difficulty** | Moderately strenuous |
| **Trail Use** | Suitable for backpacking, dogs allowed |
| **Best Times** | April through November |
| **Agency** | ANF/SCMRD |
| **Optional Map** | USGS 7.5-min *Crystal Lake* |
| **Notes** | Marked trails/obvious routes, easy terrain |

**DIRECTIONS** Exit Interstate 210 at Angeles Crest Highway in La Cañada-Flintridge. Drive 37 miles north and east to the large, north-side turnout on Angeles Crest Highway at mile 62.5—this is 0.3 mile west of the western tunnel entrance on the highway.

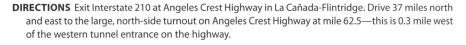

**M**ount Williamson isn't the highest peak on the San Gabriels' crest, but it hovers more closely over the desert than Mounts Islip, Hawkins, Baden-Powell, and others south of Angeles Crest Highway. From the bare patch at the

summit, you look down upon the obviously linear traces of the San Andreas and Punchbowl faults, and often over thousands of square miles of Mojave Desert. During the very best visibility, the southernmost Sierra Nevada can be seen, as well as Telescope Peak high on the west rim of Death Valley.

The hike to the top is short and sweet, but involves steady elevation gain from a starting point at an elevation of nearly 7000 feet. You start by walking northwest on an old road bed, but soon veer right on the narrow Pacific Crest Trail. That trail wastes no time in switchbacking up the steep, sparsely forested southwest flank of Mount Williamson. Behind you, from time to time, you can catch a great view of Bear Creek's V-shaped chasm and Twin Peaks to the south.

After only 1.3 miles (but 1200 feet higher) you arrive at a trail junction on the south ridge of Mount Williamson. The PCT continues straight ahead, descending to Islip Saddle in 1.6 miles—that PCT segment can be used as an alternative route to or from Williamson. You then go left on the unmaintained but well-beaten path up the rocky ridge toward the summit.

In a cairn at the top you'll find a register, where you can dutifully add your name (and any comments) to the hundreds of other signatures recorded here annually. If you want to spend the night, there's plenty of room on the open summit to pitch a tent or lay out to watch the stars. If you do so, don't miss the spectacle of the sun rising as a fiery orange ball over the desert floor, May through August.

Mount Williamson summit, looking east

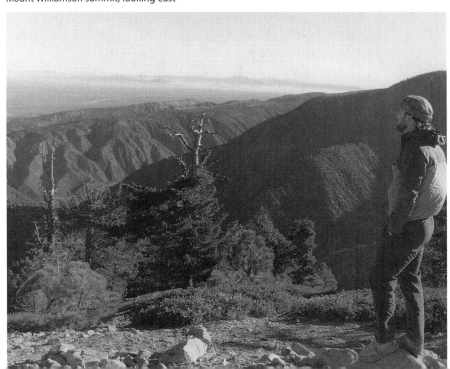

## trip 6  Pleasant View Ridge

| | |
|---|---|
| **Distance** | 10.2 miles, Out-and-back |
| **Hiking Time** | 8 hours |
| **Elevation Gain/Loss** | 4200'/4200' |
| **Difficulty** | Strenuous |
| **Trail Use** | Suitable for backpacking, dogs allowed |
| **Best Times** | May through November |
| **Agency** | ANF/SCMRD |
| **Recommended Maps** | USGS 7.5-min *Crystal Lake, Valyermo, Juniper Hills* |
| **Notes** | Navigation required, moderate terrain, bushwhacking |

see map on p. 290

**DIRECTIONS** Exit Interstate 210 at Angeles Crest Highway in La Cañada-Flintridge. Drive 37 miles north and east to the large, north-side turnout on Angeles Crest Highway at mile 62.5—this is 0.3 mile west of the western tunnel entrance on the highway.

From the conifer-clad heights of Pallett Mountain and Will Thrall Peak, Pleasant View Ridge delivers what its name promises. When north or northeast winds sweep smog and humid air away from Southern California, the ever-changing panoramas on this hike take in everything from sail-flecked Santa Monica Bay and the Channel Islands to the mind-stretching sweep of the Mojave Desert floor.

Earlier editions of this book described a one-way hike down from the high peaks of Williamson, Pallet and Will Thrall to the Little Rock Recreation Area down near the desert floor. Due to a long-time closure of that latter area for the purpose of protecting critical habitat, this hike has been revised here to include only the high part of the ridge. Due to the excessive up and downs accumulated on the round-trip, the elevation gains and losses area considerable on this essentially all-day hike.

The hike begins as it does in Trip 5 above. Start by walking northwest on an old road bed, but soon veer right on the narrow Pacific Crest Trail. That trail wastes no time in switchbacking up the steep, sparsely forested southwest flank of Mount Williamson. After only 1.3 miles (but 1200 feet higher) you arrive at a trail junction on the south ridge of Mount Williamson. The PCT continues straight ahead, and you go left on the unmaintained but well-beaten path up

the rocky ridge toward the 8214-foot Williamson summit, 1.7 miles. There's a hikers' register on top.

Now you make your way northwest along the undulating spine of Pleasant View Ridge, following only hints of trail, heading northwest from Mount Williamson. You pass over two slightly higher but unnamed points—8244 feet and 8248 feet—at 2.0 and 2.3 miles respectively, then begin the first of the many very sharp, rocky descents that characterize much of this trip. Over sparse pines and firs to the north, you'll look down upon some upthrust sandstone slabs known as Sandrocks—a part of the same Punchbowl Formation that is abundantly exposed at Devil's Punchbowl Natural Area.

At around 2.7 miles, look for the glittering wreckage of an aircraft caught near the top of a ridge 0.5 mile north. At 3.0 miles the Pleasant View ridgeline turns abruptly left (west) at a high point. (The wreckage lies about 0.2 mile northeast of here.) You descend, then climb again, to Pallett Mountain (4.0 miles), where you'll find another summit register.

You then descend a well-worn climber's path to Burkhart Saddle, cross the Burkhart Trail, and continue straight up the ridge west toward Will Thrall Peak. The peak (5.1 miles), which offers the most pleasant view everything, also features a plaque honoring

ANGELES FOREST

Will H. Thrall, editor of the Depression-era *Trails Magazine*. Will was an inveterate hiker of the San Gabriels from the 1920s through the 1950s.

There's a long, almost-never-visited segment of Pleasant View Ridge stretching northwest from Will Thrall Peak—a great area for some truly remote trail camping. The views, however, will not improve ahead—so Will Thrall Peak is the point for most hikers to turn around and return by way of the same route.

## trip 7  Devil's Punchbowl Loop Trail

see map on p. 290

| | |
|---|---|
| **Distance** | 1.0 mile, Loop |
| **Hiking Time** | ½ hour |
| **Elevation Gain/Loss** | 300'/300' |
| **Difficulty** | Easy |
| **Trail Use** | Dogs allowed, good for kids |
| **Best Times** | All year |
| **Agency** | DPNA |
| **Optional Map** | USGS 7.5-min *Valyermo* |
| **Notes** | Marked trails/obvious routes, easy terrain |

**DIRECTIONS** From the Antelope Valley Freeway (Highway 14) south of Palmdale, exit at Pearblossom Highway. Follow Pearblossom Highway for 14 miles to the small community of Pearblossom. At Pearblossom, turn right on Longview Road (County N6) and follow signs for the Devil's Punchbowl, which lies 7 miles ahead.

Tens of millions of years in the making, Devil's Punchbowl is without a doubt L.A. County's most spectacular geological showplace. An observer looking down into this 300-foot-deep chasm immediately senses the enormity of the forces that pro-duced the tilted and tangled collection of beige sandstone slabs.

The Punchbowl is caught between two active faults—the main San Andreas Fault and an offshoot, the Punchbowl Fault—along which old sedimentary formations

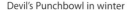

Devil's Punchbowl in winter

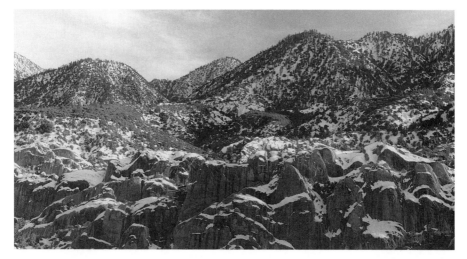

have been pushed upward and crumpled downward, as well as transported horizontally. Erosion has put the final touches on the scene, roughing out the bowl-shaped gorge of Punchbowl Canyon and carving, in a host of unique ways, the rocks exposed at the surface.

Operated by the county as a special-use area under permit from Angeles National Forest, the 1310-acre park includes a superb nature center, a couple of short nature walks (including the loop trail described here), and the Punchbowl Trail—a part of the High Desert National Recreation Trail. Devil's Punchbowl is open 7 days a week from sunrise to sunset, no admission charge.

The Devil's Punchbowl Loop Trail is a perfect introduction to this fascinating area.

It begins just behind the nature center, zigzags down off the rim to touch the seasonal creek in Punchbowl Canyon, and then climbs back out of the canyon opposite some of the tallest upright formations in the park. Near the start of the trail is a side path—the 0.3-mile Pinon Pathway—a self-guiding nature trail that loops through the pinyon-juniper forest along the Punchbowl rim.

During winter, occasional snowfalls dust the 4000-foot elevation of the Punchbowl itself and leave a lingering mantle of white on the pine-dotted slopes of the San Gabriel Mountains right above. During these episodes the trail can become muddy and slippery, and therefore probably not suitable for small children.

## trip 8  Devil's Chair

see map on p. 290

| | |
|---|---|
| **Distance** | 5.5 miles, Point-to-point |
| **Hiking Time** | 3 hours |
| **Elevation Gain/Loss** | 1200'/1400' |
| **Difficulty** | Moderate |
| **Trail Use** | Suitable for backpacking, dogs allowed |
| **Best Times** | September through June |
| **Agency** | DPNA |
| **Optional Map** | USGS 7.5-min *Valyermo* |
| **Notes** | Marked trails/obvious routes, easy terrain |

**ANGELES FOREST**

**DIRECTIONS** *West End:* From the Antelope Valley Freeway (Highway 14) south of Palmdale, exit at Pearblossom Highway. Follow Pearblossom Highway for 14 miles to the small community of Pearblossom. At Pearblossom, turn right on Longview Road (County N6) and follow signs for the Devil's Punchbowl, which lies 7 miles ahead. *East End:* From Longview Road, 2.5 miles south of Pearblossom, turn east on Fort Tejon Road. Drive 2.1 miles to Valyermo Road and turn right (south). Continue 2.9 miles and turn right on Big Rock Creek Road. Drive 3.5 miles more and look for the dirt-road turnoff for South Fork Campground, on the right. Continue 1 mile into the campground itself.

The fenced viewpoint at Devil's Chair presides over what looks like frozen chaos—a vast assemblage of sandstone chunks and slabs tipped at odd angles, bent, seemingly pulled apart here, compressed there. This is really not so surprising when you realize that the Devil's Chair sits practically astride the "crush zone" of the Punchbowl Fault.

Devil's Chair can be reached with equal ease by starting either from Devil's Punch-

bowl Natural Area on the west or from South Fork Campground on east. With a little help from a friend, perhaps, you can do the whole traverse in a one-way direction, as we suggest here. The west-to-east direction has a slight downhill advantage. You'll need a permit, free from the ranger at Devil's Punchbowl Natural Area's nature center, if you'll be camping along the trail.

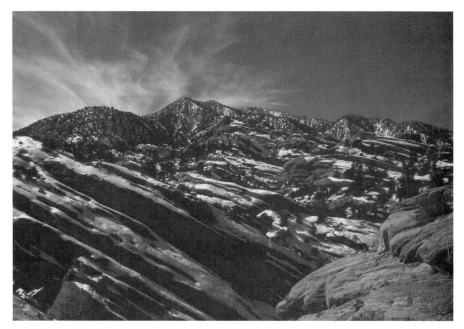

Inside the Punchbowl

If snow is present, check at the nature center to see if the route is safe. You should be aware that snow closes South Fork Campground, and that South Fork Big Rock Creek (next to the campground) could be difficult to ford after a big storm.

From the south side of the Devil's Punchbowl parking lot, find and follow the signed Burkhart Trail as it climbs northwest along the rim of the punchbowl. You're actually following the upper (south) edge of a downward sloping terrace—part of an alluvial fan left high and dry when the Punchbowl creek began carving a new course northeast. You join an old road at 0.5 mile, pass a small reservoir at 0.7 mile, and arrive at a trail junction at 0.8 mile. Here, in a Coulter-pine grove, bear left on the Punchbowl Trail leading east. The delightful, contouring path takes you around several shady ravines, all draining into the Punchbowl. After some sharply descending switchbacks, you reach a trail junction (3.0 miles) from where a 0.1-mile spur goes west and then north over a narrow, rock-ribbed ridge to the high perch known as Devil's Chair. Protective fencing furnishes some psychological comfort for the nervous-making traverse.

East of the junction the trail keeps dropping, touches a saddle, descends crookedly past large manzanita shrubs, and crosses a small stream in the bottom of pine- and oak-shaded Holcomb Canyon (3.7 miles). Flat areas suitable for camping can be found hereabouts.

Continue east up chaparral-smothered slopes to a saddle, then down the other side for a crooked mile to South Fork Campground.

## trip 9   Lower Punchbowl Canyon

| | | |
|---|---|---|
| **Distance** | 2.0 miles round trip, Out-and-back | |
| **Hiking Time** | 1½ hours (round trip) | |
| **Elevation Gain/Loss** | 400'/400' | |
| **Difficulty** | Moderate | |
| **Trail Use** | Suitable for backpacking, dogs allowed | |
| **Best Times** | October through June | |
| **Agency** | ANF/SCMRD | |
| **Optional Map** | USGS 7.5-min *Valyermo* | |
| **Notes** | Marked trails/obvious routes, moderate terrain | |

see map on p. 290

**DIRECTIONS** From the Antelope Valley Freeway (Highway 14) south of Palmdale, exit at Pearblossom Highway. Follow Pearblossom Highway for 14 miles to the small community of Pearblossom. At Pearblossom, turn right on Longview Road (County N6). After 2.5 miles turn left (east) on Fort Tejon Road. Drive 2.1 miles to Valyermo Road and turn right. Continue 2.9 miles and turn right on Big Rock Creek Road. After another 0.5 mile you pass the Angeles National Forest boundary (large sign). Go 0.2 mile farther to a parking turnout.

On this trip you enter Devil's Punchbowl by a little-known back way—the mouth of Punchbowl Canyon. Once above the lower canyon portals, you'll find yourself in a maze-like wonderland reminiscent of the "slickrock" country of southern Utah, save for the reddish hues. The hike is best done in winter or early spring, when snowmelt or runoff courses down the canyon and its tributaries.

At the parking turnout you'll see a gated, private footbridge spanning Big Rock Creek. Don't use it. Instead ford the creek where you can, and start boulder-hopping up the narrow gorge to the west—Punchbowl Canyon. The canyon divides at 0.3 mile; stay right, in the main fork. Soon the familiar Punchbowl Formation rocks are all around you. The slabs of pebbly sandstone rise dramatically to the south—if you're game for it, scramble up for a great view of the brooding San Gabriels. Caution is in order when the rock is wet; it tends to disintegrate grain by grain much as Utah's slickrock does.

A small waterfall about 1 mile up the meandering canyon blocks any further easy walking. You can head back at this point, or you can find a way to scramble around it and reach the Devil's Punchbowl Loop Trail a short distance above.

ANGELES FOREST

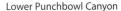
Lower Punchbowl Canyon

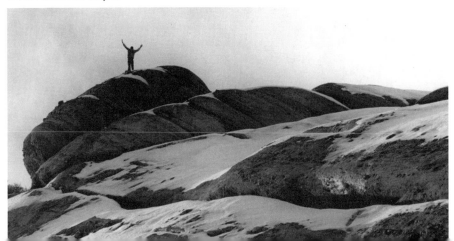

## trip 10 Holcomb Canyon

| | |
|---|---|
| **Distance** | 3.7 miles, Loop |
| **Hiking Time** | 3½ hours |
| **Elevation Gain/Loss** | 700'/700' |
| **Difficulty** | Moderately strenuous |
| **Trail Use** | Suitable for backpacking, dogs allowed |
| **Best Times** | October through June |
| **Agency** | DPNA |
| **Recommended Map** | USGS 7.5-min *Valyermo* |
| **Notes** | Navigation required, moderate terrain, bushwhacking |

see map on p. 290

**DIRECTIONS** From the Antelope Valley Freeway (Highway 14) south of Palmdale, exit at Pearblossom Highway. Follow Pearblossom Highway for 14 miles to the small community of Pearblossom. At Pearblossom, turn right on Longview Road (County N6). After 2.5 miles turn left (east) on Fort Tejon Road. Drive 2.1 miles to Valyermo Road and turn right. Continue 2.9 miles and turn right on Big Rock Creek Road. After another 0.5 mile you pass the Angeles National Forest boundary (large sign). Go 0.2 mile farther to a parking turnout.

Much of the fascination of the Devil's Punchbowl area lies in its trailless canyons, where the erosive forces of water have carved deep furrows in the soft sandstone. This beautiful loop trip, off-trail and requiring navigational skills almost the whole way, includes alder-shaded Holcomb Canyon as well as the large tributary

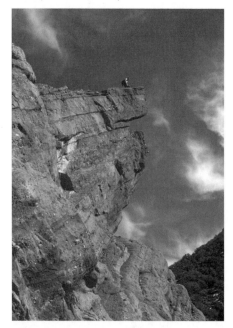

Outcrop in Holcomb Canyon

of Punchbowl Canyon overlooked by the Devil's Chair.

Walk down the shoulder of the road 0.3 mile to another turnout, cross Big Rock Creek wherever most expedient, and start following the rocky banks of a tributary creek heading due south into Holcomb Canyon. A nice mountain-desert mix of vegetation pervades the area: alder, willow and sycamore along the creek banks; live-oak, incense cedar and mountain mahogany higher on the banks; pinyon pine dotting the dry slopes. The bedrock here is mostly the San Francisquito Formation—a marine sandstone formed about 60 million years ago. The Punchbowl Formation, which is a nonmarine sandstone only about 8 million years old, is seen briefly on the right (west) in the form of a blocky outcrop soaring over a pinched section of the canyon, 1.1 miles from the start. Soon you'll return to the Punchbowl Formation and stay in it for most the remainder of the trip.

At 1.6 miles, you'll notice a shallow draw on the left (east). Look for the crossing of the Punchbowl Trail a short distance ahead. Use it to climb 0.3 mile west via switchbacks to a saddle. You then leave the trail and descend cross-country, northwest through manzanita and scrub oak, into the head of a ravine. Proceed down the ravine to a three-way junction of ravines in a small flat just below the stony gaze of the Devil's Chair, 2.1 miles. From there on, you simply continue down-canyon (north) and

eventually hook up with the lower end of Punchbowl Canyon, 0.3 mile short of your car. Meanwhile, there are lots of interesting rock formations to explore along the way. Don't forget your camera!

## trip 11  Burkhart Trail

| | |
|---|---|
| **Distance** | 12.2 miles, Point-to-point |
| **Hiking Time** | 7 hours |
| **Elevation Gain/Loss** | 2000'/3700' |
| **Difficulty** | Moderately strenuous |
| **Trail Use** | Suitable for backpacking, dogs allowed |
| **Best Times** | April through November |
| **Agency** | ANF/SCMRD |
| **Optional Maps** | USGS 7.5-min *Waterman Mtn., Juniper Hills, Valyermo* |
| **Notes** | Marked trails/obvious routes, easy terrain |

see map on p. 290

**DIRECTIONS** *South End:* Exit Interstate 210 at Angeles Crest Highway in La Cañada-Flintridge. Drive 33 miles north and east to the turnoff for Buckhorn Campground on the left, at mile 58.3 on Angeles Crest Highway. Drive all the way through the campground to the far (northeast) end, where a short stub of dirt road leads to a trailhead parking area. *North End:* From the Antelope Valley Freeway (Highway 14) south of Palmdale, exit at Pearblossom Highway. Follow Pearblossom Highway for 14 miles to the small community of Pearblossom. At Pearblossom, turn right on Longview Road (County N6) and follow signs for the Devil's Punchbowl, which lies 7 miles ahead.

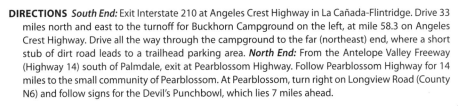

**F**ar from sight and sound of the city, the Burkhart Trail blazes a lonely path over Pleasant View Ridge and down into the upper margins of the Mojave Desert. Here the natural landscape is not marred by canyon-carving highways and fire roads, not blemished by powerlines, and mercifully free, for the most part, from the noxious clouds of air pollution that drift across the county. Here the clean, dry air bears the melded exudations of both pines and desert sage.

Although this is certainly one of the better hiking routes in the San Gabriels, relatively few hikers make the long climb, descent and traverse all the way to Devil's Punchbowl Natural Area. Of course, you'll need to solve some transportation problems first. At best, you can have someone drop you off at the start, Buckhorn Campground, and pick you up later at Devil's Punchbowl. The shortest way around is via Vincent Gap and Big Rock Creek Road

(partly dirt) to the east. The second shortest way is via Big Pines and Big Pines Road (paved all the way).

Start off from Buckhorn Campground by descending to Cooper Canyon Falls, and descending farther to Little Rock Creek, 1.7 miles. After crossing the creek, bear left and commence a long climb to Burkhart Saddle—a gap on the high crest of Pleasant View Ridge. You wind steadily upward on sparsely forested slopes lacking underbrush, but resplendent (in springtime) with blue and white lupines, red and blue penstemons, sunflowers, and other wildflowers. Little Rock Creek lies below, its stream coursing through a thirsty-looking gorge.

Around 2.8 miles the trail crosses a perpetually sliding slope of sheared metamorphic rock, then gains better footing as it angles over to and finally crosses a tributary of Little Rock Creek. A series of long switchbacks takes you up the slope to the west,

ANGELES FOREST

across the tributary once more, then up to Burkhart Saddle, 5.0 miles. There, a cool, dry breeze chills your sweat-soaked skin and clothing as you contemplate whether it's worth it to climb (as a side trip) either Pallett Mountain or Will Thrall Peak for a better view of what you can already see of the desert below.

Down the other side, conifer forest grades into chaparral as you drop north down along a canyon wall overlooking the upper gorge of Cruthers Creek. After a couple of zigzags near the bottom you join a ranch road (8.3 miles). Its crooked course takes you down along the creek, then east onto a gently sloping hillside. Look for the signed trail veering right toward Devil's Punch-

bowl Natural Area (the road itself continues north into the private Lewis Ranch).

You climb about 500 feet, then contour for almost 2 miles across the northern spurs of the San Gabriels, passing an odd but agreeable mix of beavertail cactus and sage, manzanita-rich chaparral, and scattered Coulter, pinyon, and Jeffrey pines. Views of the broad desert expanses below are frequent and inspiring. When you reach a dirt road at 11.5 miles where Punchbowl Trail keeps contouring ahead, bear left (northeast) on the road and walk down to a narrow trail continuing northeast along the rim of Punchbowl Canyon. The trail leads to the parking lot at Devil's Punchbowl Natural Area.

## trip 12  South Fork Trail

see map on p. 290

| | |
|---|---|
| **Distance** | 5.2 miles, Point-to-point |
| **Hiking Time** | 2½ hours |
| **Elevation Gain/Loss** | 100'/2200' |
| **Difficulty** | Moderate |
| **Trail Use** | Dogs allowed |
| **Best Times** | April through November |
| **Agency** | ANF/SCMRD |
| **Optional Maps** | USGS 7.5-min *Crystal Lake, Valyermo* |
| **Notes** | Marked trails/obvious routes, easy terrain |

**DIRECTIONS** *South End:* Exit Interstate 210 at Angeles Crest Highway in La Cañada-Flintridge. Drive 39 miles north and east to the Islip Saddle Trailhead, at mile 64.1 on Angeles Crest Highway. *North End:* From the Antelope Valley Freeway (Highway 14) south of Palmdale, exit at Pearblossom Highway. Follow Pearblossom Highway for 14 miles to the small community of Pearblossom. At Pearblossom, turn right on Longview Road. Go south 2.5 miles and turn left (east) on Fort Tejon Road. Drive 2.1 miles to Valyermo Road and turn right (south). Continue 2.9 miles and turn right on Big Rock Creek Road. Drive 3.5 miles more and look for the dirt-road turnoff for South Fork Campground, on the right. Continue 1 mile into the campground itself.

The easy-going descent of the South Fork Trail doesn't take much effort; you simply put one foot in front of the other and let gravity do the rest. The well-graded trail descends (or ascends if you'd rather get more exercise and reverse the directions given here) along the west wall of the V-shaped gorge cut by Big Rock

Creek's South Fork. Narrow, but seldom steep, the trail follows a natural, swaying contour as it curves around more than a dozen ravines indenting the canyon wall. South Fork creek murmurs far below (at least when swollen by melting snows), accompanied by the doleful trills of canyon wrens.

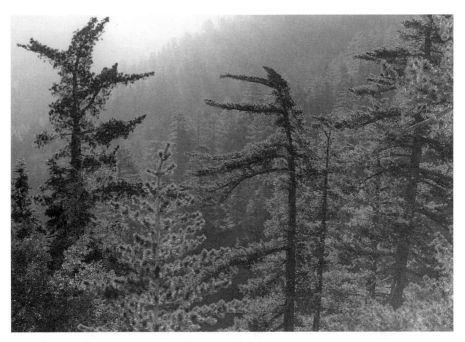

Bigcone Dougas-firs at the upper end of South Fork Trail

The hike is not difficult, but the transportation from one end to the other may be problematical. The shortest way around is via Vincent Gap and Big Rock Creek Road (partly dirt) to the east. The second shortest way is via Big Pines and Big Pines Road (paved all the way).

From Islip Saddle, take the trail contouring to the north, not the sharply ascending Pacific Crest Trail, which climbs northwest toward Mount Williamson's summit. Traffic noises fade quickly as you begin descending through a heterogeneous forest of Jeffrey pine, sugar pine, incense cedar, live oak, and bigcone Douglas-fir. As you descend, the high-country forest thins; pinyon pine, manzanita, mountain mahogany, and blue- and white-blossoming ceanothus clothe the dry and rocky slopes.

The trail loses elevation faster than the South Fork creek, so by 4.4 miles you'll be traversing a sheer slope only 200 feet above the stream. A couple of short switchbacks at 4.9 miles take you down to meet the alder- and sycamore-shaded creek. Cross over to the other side and continue walking through South Fork Campground until you reach the trailhead parking area just below (north of) the campsites.

South Fork Campground is one of Angeles National Forest's more pleasant and secluded drive-in campgrounds. During April and May, flannel bush, or fremontia, blooms on the broad, alluvial terraces along the creek, opposite and downstream from the campground. Considered one of the showiest of California native plants, the fremontias here stand up to 15 feet high and bear thousands of large, waxy, yellow flowers.

If you have time for further exploration, climb southeast from the campground on the Manzanita Trail about 0.5 mile to some sandstone (Punchbowl Formation) outcrops. You'll get a great view of both the South Fork canyon and the main Big Rock Creek wash.

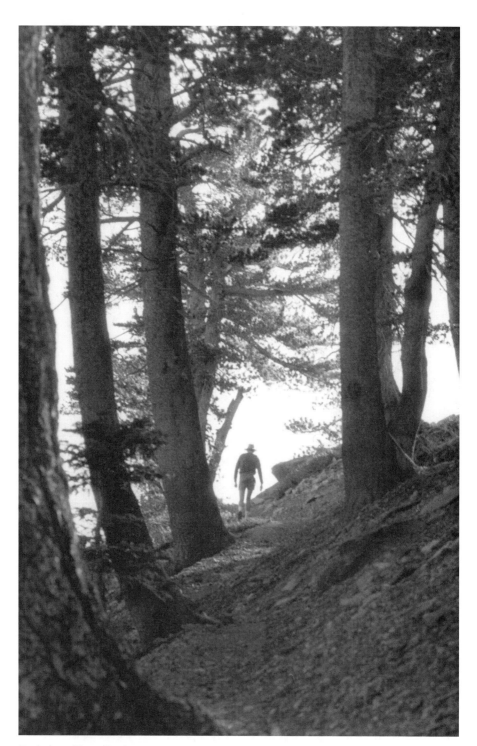

North slope, Mount Burnham

# chapter 26

# Angeles Forest: Big Pines & Sheep Mountain Wilderness

On the eastern extremity of the Angeles Crest, quite removed from L.A.'s often smoggy blanket of air, lies the Big Pines Recreation Area, an area set aside by the Forest Service specifically for year-round recreation. Blanketed by a heterogeneous mixture of pines, firs, and oaks, and perched high above the desert, Big Pines boasts the clean, dry, evergreen-scented air and crystal-line blue skies characteristic of the melding of mountain and desert environments.

During the winter months, Big Pines' snowplay venues (Mountain High and Ski Sunrise) draw crowds of snow-starved skiers and snowboarders from the cities below who would rather not drive an extra 250 miles or more to reach the major-league Sierra Nevada ski resorts. In summer, several campgrounds, picnic areas, and interpretive trails serve the needs of visitors escaping the lowland heat. Ironically, relatively few people come up during seasons when the area is really most beautiful—spring and fall. Daytime temperatures are most pleasant then, and the colors of the foliage are bold and vibrant.

From most of the Los Angeles Basin, the most expedient way to get to the Big Pines area is by way of an eastern route: Interstate 15 and Highway 138 to Angeles Crest Highway, and then through Wrightwood. The tedious west approach along Angeles Crest Highway from La Cañada-Flintridge may involve winter closures due to snow cover, and sometimes long-term closures as a result of storm damage.

Big Pines and Wrightwood share the distinction of lying smack dab on the San Andreas Fault. The crossroads of Big Pines itself (4 miles west of Wrightwood) marks the highest surface trace of the entire fault—6862 feet. Jackson Lake, a "sag pond" in geologic parlance, fills a small, natural depression along the fault 2 miles northwest of Big Pines. Wrightwood, one of the most attractive communities in Los Angeles County and the largest settlement in the San Gabriel Mountains, sprawls across another, much larger fault-caused depression called Swarthout Valley. Unfortunately for its roughly 5000 (summer) residents, Wrightwood is acutely susceptible to destruction not only by Southern California's incipient Great Quake, likely to occur on this stretch of the San Andreas within a century, but also by fire, flooding, and mudslides.

At Big Pines you'll find the Grassy Hollow Visitor Center, housed in a corner of the former Swarthout Lodge. The lodge once

Plaque at Big Pines

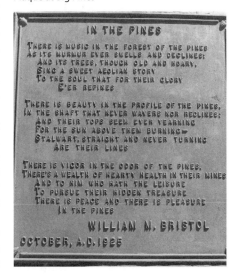

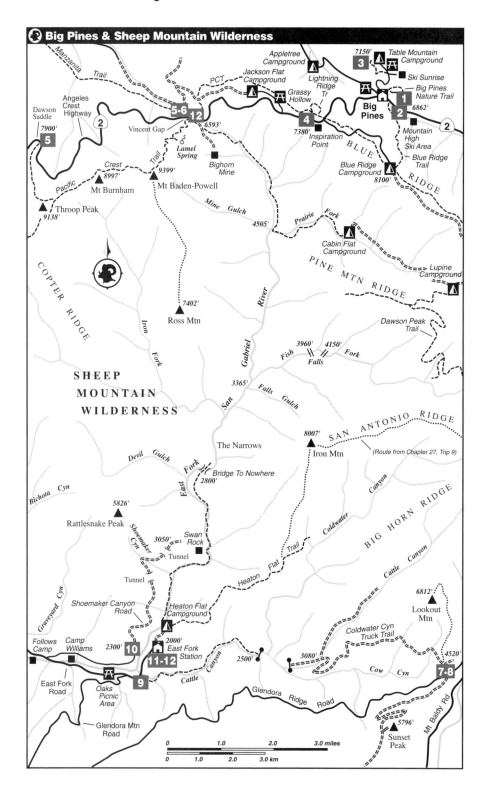

**Big Pines & Sheep Mountain Wilderness**

served as headquarters for Big Pines County Park, which was open from 1923 to 1940. Unable to afford the cost of administering the park, Los Angeles County deeded the property to the Forest Service in 1940. The County had spent about $4 million creating a first-class recreational complex consisting of campgrounds, cabins, picnic areas, organizational camps, a swimming pool, an ice-skating rink, tennis courts, toboggan and ski runs, and more. An arched pedestrian overpass, built of native stone, was built over the access road, its twin towers containing barred holding cells for drunks and troublemakers. Only the north tower stands today near the visitor center.

After falling into disuse during and after World War II, Big Pines experienced a resurgence of attention in the 1950s. New facilities for campers and day-users were constructed, and winter-sports areas were expanded and modernized. The use of snow-making machines today ensures that some of the ski slopes stay usable through much of the winter.

South of Big Pines, sprawling over some 44,000 acres, Sheep Mountain Wilderness is the largest and most recently (1984) designated federal wilderness in the San Gabriel Mountains. The name refers to the Nelson bighorn sheep, which are quite abundant throughout the area, and also to Iron Mountain—sometimes called Sheep Mountain—which lies near the geographic center of the wilderness.

The wilderness lies almost entirely in the grip of the many-branched, upper watershed of East Fork San Gabriel River. Rapid uplift and erosion have created topographical relief on a prodigious scale here. Boulder-strewn ridges dotted with sturdy conifers and clothed in tough blankets of chaparral fall thousands of feet to streams that tumble down V-shaped gorges. Elevations within the wilderness area range from 2400 feet on the East Fork near Swan Rock to 10,064 feet at Old Baldy's summit, which lies on the east boundary.

From the 1850s until the early 1900s, gold mining was king on the East Fork, with important ore-producing prospects located high on the slopes of Mount Baden-Powell and Old Baldy and on some of the steep slopes overlooking the East Fork. On the banks of the East Fork itself, mountains of gold-bearing alluvium were literally washed away during a spate of hydraulic mining activity in the 1870s. A fascinating history of East Fork's mining heyday can be read in John Robinson's slender book *Mines of the East Fork*. Mining for gold and tungsten continues today at a number of sites within the wilderness; this is because certain mining claims were legally "grandfathered" when the area was declared a wilderness.

Most trails of Sheep Mountain Wilderness don't penetrate very far into its interior; however, cross-country hiking through the canyons and along many of the high ridges is possible. Three of the routes detailed below (Trips 5, 9, and 10) lie outside Sheep Mountain Wilderness, but are included here because of their proximity to it.

It is not necessary to obtain a wilderness permit for entry into Sheep Mountain Wilderness, except when you start from the end of East Fork Road. Permits can be obtained from the East Fork Ranger Station, or you can fill out a self-issuing permit at the entrance to the station.

Even when a permit is not required, you should consult with an Angeles National Forest ranger to check on the latest snow conditions, stream levels, or other possible hazards if you're planning a long trip to the interior of the wilderness. You should also be aware that the trailheads on Angeles Crest Highway (Vincent Gap and Dawson Saddle) can be unreachable by car for several months out of the year—and sometimes for a stretch of years—because of adverse weather conditions or storm damage.

All trips below require a National Forest Adventure Pass ($5 per day, $30 per year) for trailhead parking.

ANGELES FOREST

## trip 1  Big Pines Nature Trail

see map on p. 308

| | |
|---|---|
| **Distance** | 0.5 mile, Loop |
| **Hiking Time** | ½ hour |
| **Elevation Gain/Loss** | 200'/200' |
| **Difficulty** | Easy |
| **Trail Use** | Dogs allowed, good for kids |
| **Best Times** | All year |
| **Agency** | ANF/SCMRD |
| **Optional Map** | USGS 7.5-min *Mescal Creek* |
| **Notes** | Marked trails/obvious routes, easy terrain |

**DIRECTIONS** From Interstate 15, north of San Bernardino, exit at Highway 138 and turn west. Drive 8.6 miles to Angeles Crest Highway, and turn left. Continue through Wrightwood; stay on Angeles Crest Highway for a total of 10 miles until you reach Big Pines and the Grassy Hollow Visitor Center.

The short and easy, self-guiding Big Pines Nature Trail highlights many of the native trees and shrubs of the Big Pines area. The trail originates behind the Grassy Hollow Visitor Center and starts by winding up through a sparse grove of centuries-old Jeffrey pines. If you aren't, as yet, very familiar with the local flora, this is a good trail to further your education.

Along the way, you'll be introduced to the canyon live oak and black oak, four kinds of pines, and shrubs such as ceanothus (mountain lilac), manzanita, yerba santa, flannel bush, service berry, and mountain mahogany. Interpretive plaques cover some of the uses of these native plants by the Gabrielino, Serrano, and Cahuilla Indians.

Manzanita blossoms

Yerba santa

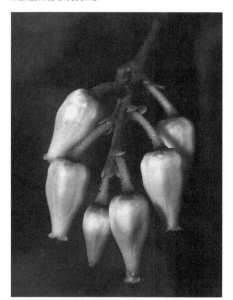

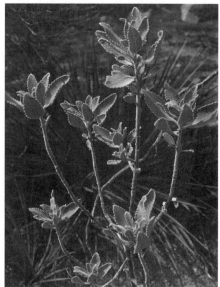

## trip 2  Blue Ridge Trail

| | |
|---|---|
| **Distance** | 4.6 miles round trip, Out-and-back |
| **Hiking Time** | 2½ hours (round trip) |
| **Elevation Gain/Loss** | 1300'/1300' |
| **Difficulty** | Moderate |
| **Trail Use** | Dogs allowed, good for kids |
| **Best Times** | May through November |
| **Agency** | ANF/SCMRD |
| **Optional Maps** | USGS 7.5-min *Mescal Creek, Mount San Antonio* |
| **Notes** | Marked trails/obvious routes, easy terrain |

see map on p. 308

**DIRECTIONS** From Interstate 15, north of San Bernardino, exit at Highway 138 and turn west. Drive 8.6 miles to Angeles Crest Highway, and turn left. Continue through Wrightwood; stay on Angeles Crest Highway for a total of 10 miles until you reach Big Pines and the Grassy Hollow Visitor Center.

Tall, aromatic pines and firs, and thin air (elevation averages 7500 feet) lend a High-Sierra-feel to the north slope of Blue Ridge. The nicely maintained Blue Ridge Trail climbs about 1000 feet up this slope to meet the Pacific Crest Trail just outside Blue Ridge Campground. From there you can climb a bit farther for a panoramic view of Mts. San Antonio, Baden-Powell, and other giants on the roofline of the Angeles Forest.

You have a lot of flexibility on this hike: From the campground you can return the way you came, walk down the PCT to Angeles Crest Highway, or arrange to get a ride down the Blue Ridge road (assuming the road is snow-free and open to traffic).

The Blue Ridge Trail starts near the restrooms opposite Grassy Hollow Visitor Center, and heads south. About halfway up the slope (1.0 mile), the trail crosses an old road bed and continues climbing. To the north, on Table Mountain, you'll spot the white domes of the Table Mountain and Smithsonian observatories. After several switchbacks, you meet the Blue Ridge road at Blue Ridge Campground. The PCT swings around the far side of the campground; you can join it by walking southeast about 0.1 mile on the road. Head southeast on the PCT, uphill along a ski run for another quarter mile. Then veer right to the top of a sage-covered rise dotted in spring and early summer with paintbrush and wallflower blossoms. There you'll have a panoramic view of Old Baldy's north slope—streaked with snow and often wreathed in cottony clouds in springtime.

That's a good spot to turn around, and to go back the way you came.

Mount Baldy seen from Blue Ridge Trail

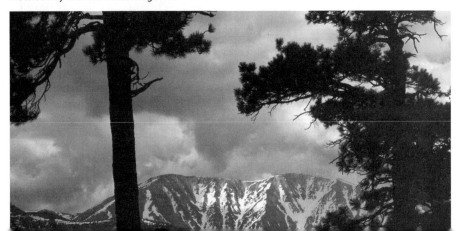

ANGELES FOREST

**trip 3** # Table Mountain Nature Trail

| | |
|---|---|
| **Distance** | 1.0 mile, Loop |
| **Hiking Time** | ½ hour |
| **Elevation Gain/Loss** | 200'/200' |
| **Difficulty** | Easy |
| **Trail Use** | Dogs allowed, good for kids |
| **Best Times** | April through November |
| **Agency** | ANF/SCMRD |
| **Optional Map** | USGS 7.5-min *Mescal Creek* |
| **Notes** | Marked trails/obvious routes, easy terrain |

see map on p. 308

**DIRECTIONS**  From Interstate 15, north of San Bernardino, exit at Highway 138 and turn west. Drive 8.6 miles to Angeles Crest Highway, and turn left. Continue through Wrightwood; stay on Angeles Crest Highway for a total of 10 miles until you reach the crossroads of Big Pines. As you pass the Grassy Hollow Visitor Center, turn right on Table Mountain Road and drive uphill to Table Mountain Campground.

The Table Mountain Nature Trail swings down a hillside below the entrance of Table Mountain Campground and later climbs back up to the campground's edge. You'll be introduced to Jeffrey pines, canyon live oaks, black oaks, and several other plants and trees that grow in the immediate area. Numbered posts correspond to the entries on the self-guiding leaflet available at the Grassy Hollow Visitor Center.

As you're traversing the south-facing slope traveled by the trail, you'll spot Mount Baden-Powell rising impressively in the west, and Blue Ridge, complete with the scars of ski runs, in the southeast. Blue Ridge was logged many decades ago, accounting for the even-aged appearance of the trees on its slopes.

Watch out for false paths that take off from some of the switchback corners of the trail; it's easy to lose the main trail. At trail's end, make a right on the paved campground road and walk back to the entrance.

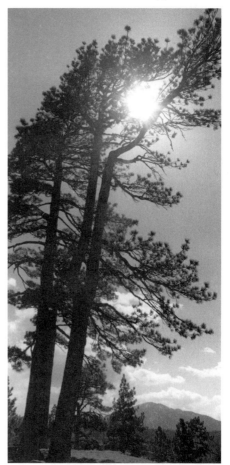
Pine forest at Table Mountain Campground

# trip 4  Lightning Ridge Nature Trail

|  |  |
|---|---|
| **Distance** | 0.8 mile, Loop |
| **Hiking Time** | ½ hour |
| **Elevation Gain/Loss** | 250'/250' |
| **Difficulty** | Easy |
| **Trail Use** | Dogs allowed, good for kids |
| **Best Times** | April through November |
| **Agency** | ANF/SCMRD |
| **Optional Map** | USGS 7.5-min *Mount San Antonio* |
| **Notes** | Marked trails/obvious routes, easy terrain |

see map on p. 308

**DIRECTIONS** From Interstate 15, north of San Bernardino, exit at Highway 138 and turn west. Drive 8.6 miles to Angeles Crest Highway, and turn left. Continue through Wrightwood and Big Pines; stay on Angeles Crest Highway for a total of 12 miles until you reach the trailhead for the Lightning Ridge Trail on the right (across from Inspiration Point, which is on the left).

The Lightning Ridge Nature Trail contours through the cool precincts of a wooded northeast-facing slope, then switchbacks upward to meet the Pacific Crest Trail on a windblown crest. You'll see Jeffrey pines, sugar pines, and white firs, and pass right through a beautiful glade of black oaks called Oak Dell—very nice in October when the leaves turn crispy gold and acorns fall. Near the crest are a number of stunted and distorted trees battered by winds and flattened by snow drifts that can pile up 10 feet high.

When you reach the PCT junction, try stepping off the trail and walking a short distance over to the top of the ridgecrest. The view from there is similar to that from Inspiration Point below, only a bit more panoramic. Old Baldy and Mount Baden-Powell rise like massive sentinels, bracketing the rugged slopes and canyons of Sheep Mountain Wilderness. To the south you look straight down the V-shaped, linear gorge of East Fork San Gabriel River.

Oak Dell on the Lightning Ridge Trail

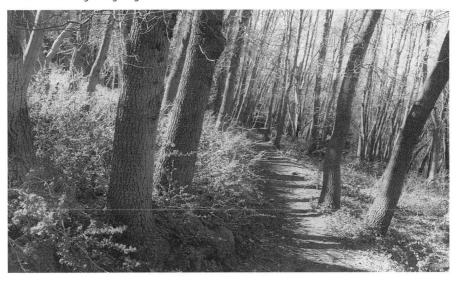

**ANGELES FOREST**

# trip 5 Mount Baden-Powell Traverse

see map on p. 308

| | |
|---|---|
| **Distance** | 9.2 miles, Point-to-point |
| **Hiking Time** | 5½ hours |
| **Elevation Gain/Loss** | 2400′/3700′ |
| **Difficulty** | Strenuous |
| **Trail Use** | Suitable for backpacking, dogs allowed |
| **Best Times** | May through November |
| **Agency** | ANF/SGRD |
| **Recommended Map** | USGS 7.5-min *Crystal Lake* |
| **Notes** | Navigation required, moderate terrain |

**DIRECTIONS** *East End:* From Interstate 15, north of San Bernardino, exit at Highway 138 and turn west. Drive 8.6 miles to Angeles Crest Highway, and turn left. Continue through Wrightwood and Big Pines; stay on Angeles Crest Highway for a total of 15 miles until you reach the large trailhead parking lot at Vincent Gap (mile 74.8 on Angeles Crest Highway). *West End:* The west-end starting point is mile 69.6 on Angeles Crest Highway, just east of Dawson Saddle, which is 5 miles west of Vincent Gap.

**N**amed in honor of Lord Baden-Powell, the British Army officer who started the Boy Scout movement in 1907, massive Mount Baden-Powell stands higher than any other mountain in the San Gabriels—except the Mount San Antonio complex to the east. Many thousands of hikers troop to Baden-

Looking down from Mount Baden-Powell Ridge

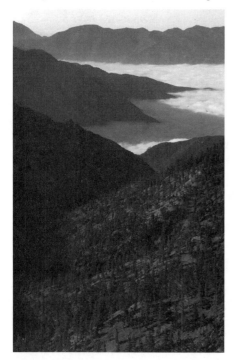

Powell's summit yearly, mostly by way of Vincent Gap on Angeles Crest Highway.

Baden-Powell's summit is the last major milestone on the 52-mile trek from Chantry Flat to Vincent Gap known as the Silver Moccasin Trail (in this part of the range it coincides with the Pacific Crest Trail). The five-day-long Silver Moccasin backpack is a rite-of-passage for L.A.-area Scouts.

If you want to climb Mount Baden-Powell in a most interesting way, try this one-way hike from Dawson Saddle to Vincent Gap. The effort involved is only little more than what's involved in the usual round trip from Vincent Gap, and you'll visit two other peaks as well. All three peaks offers their own unique and panoramic perspective of the rugged Sheep Mountain Wilderness below. The shuttle between ending and starting points (which can be done conveniently enough on a bicycle) is only 5 miles long. The following remarks assume that Angeles Crest Highway is open to vehicles west of Vincent Gap. Parts of this 5-mile stretch are notoriously susceptible to storm damage, and in the past landslides have closed the highway year round.

You begin right at mile 69.6, just east of Dawson Saddle, where there's parking space on the north side of the highway. Cross the highway to get to the trail, which goes south along the top of a long, ascending ridge. You

And, of course, limber pines have those characteristically flexible branches.

At 1.8 miles, near the bench mark 8789′, you join the Pacific Crest Trail. Head southwest on the PCT, then climb cross-country about 300 yards to reach the summit of Throop Peak. Hikers' registers are found here, as well as on the other two peaks you'll be visiting.

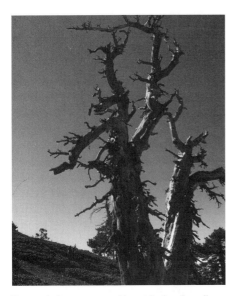

Battered pine snag atop Mount Baden-Powell

Return to the Dawson Saddle Trail junction and continue northeast on the PCT, which follows the main ridgeline. You descend to a saddle, then ascend to Mount Burnham's north flank, where switchbacks take you over to Burnham's east shoulder. You can make an easy side trip to Burnham's summit from the east shoulder.

After bagging Burnham, continue east, climbing a breathless 400 feet more, to reach the impressive Boy Scout monument on Baden-Powell's summit. Weather-beaten lodgepole and limber pines dot the summit area, one of the latter identified by an interpretive sign.

switchback up through pines and firs, heading toward the main crest of the San Gabriels at Throop Peak. An impressive 3540 hours of volunteer labor by Boy Scouts were required to build this trail, which was completed in 1982. About halfway up the trail, lodgepole pines dominate the forest, but keen eyes will spot a few limber pines. Look closely at the needles: lodgepole pines come in bundles of two needles each, while limber pines have bundles of five needles.

Return by way of the trail descending Baden-Powell's northeast ridge. After 40 switchbacks and 3.8 miles of descent you'll reach the large Vincent Gap trailhead. About halfway down the trail, on the 25th switchback corner, a side trail leads about 200 yards east to a dribbling pipe at Lamel Spring.

**ANGELES FOREST**

On the trail—Mount Baden-Powell Traverse

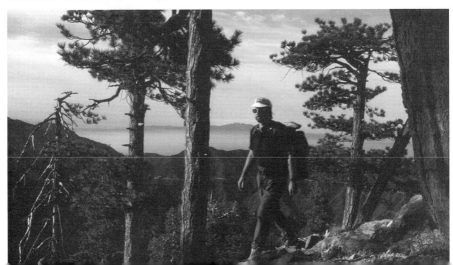

## trip 6  Ross Mountain

| | |
|---|---|
| **Distance** | 13.4 miles round trip, Out-and-back |
| **Hiking Time** | 9 hours (round trip) |
| **Elevation Gain/Loss** | 5500'/5500' |
| **Difficulty** | Strenuous |
| **Trail Use** | Suitable for backpacking |
| **Best Times** | May through November |
| **Agency** | ANF/SGRD |
| **Recommended Map** | USGS 7.5-min *Crystal Lake* |
| **Notes** | Navigation required, moderate terrain, bushwhacking |

see map on p. 308

**DIRECTIONS** From Interstate 15, north of San Bernardino, exit at Highway 138 and turn west. Drive 8.6 miles to Angeles Crest Highway, and turn left. Continue through Wrightwood and Big Pines; stay on Angeles Crest Highway for a total of 15 miles until you reach the large trailhead parking lot at Vincent Gap (mile 74.8 on Angeles Crest Highway).

Isolated and difficult to reach, Ross Mountain stands tall on the divide between the trench-like East Fork San Gabriel River and a shallower but equally steep-walled tributary called Iron Fork. To get there you must first climb Mount Baden-Powell, and then descend 2000 feet down a hardscrabble ridge. Weary peak-baggers have dubbed the mountain "Ross Pit"—you'll know why when it comes time to turn around and return the same way you came.

Starting from Vincent Gap, hike the 40 switchbacks of the Pacific Crest Trail to Mount Baden-Powell's summit (3.8 miles). Once you reach the top, you simply follow the rounded ridge leading south for another 2.9 miles to Ross Mountain's 7402-foot high point.

From the Baden-Powell summit, you swoop down along the eroding south rim of Mine Gulch and reach (1 mile and 1000 feet below) a flat area shaded by stately Jeffrey pines, suitable for camping. Ahead, there are fewer trees, and more chaparral. Short climbs alternate with long, steep, rocky downhill stretches.

According to the register kept on Ross Mountain, only a dozen or so climbers come this way every year. Die-hards have set speed records from Vincent Gap, while others have ascended the mountain by bushwhacking up the south slope from Iron Fork, a very impressive feat indeed.

A panoramic view of the canyons below Ross Mountain may be had by walking 0.2 mile farther to the mountain's south brow. When it's time to return, breathe a long sigh of regret and then tackle the job. The climb back up to Baden-Powell is nearly always a sweaty affair, with a southern exposure all the way and little shade.

## trip 7  Lookout Mountain

| | |
|---|---|
| **Distance** | 4.6 miles round trip, Out-and-back |
| **Hiking Time** | 2½ hours (round trip) |
| **Elevation Gain/Loss** | 2300'/2300' |
| **Difficulty** | Moderately strenuous |
| **Trail Use** | Dogs allowed |
| **Best Times** | October through June |
| **Agency** | ANF/SGRD |
| **Recommended Map** | USGS 7.5-min *Mt. Baldy* |
| **Notes** | Navigation required, moderate terrain, bushwhacking |

see map on p. 308

**DIRECTIONS** Exit the 210 Freeway at Baseline Road on the border between the cities of Claremont and Upland. Go west on Baseline for 0.7 mile, then turn right (north) on Mills Avenue. After 1.1 mile the main road (signed Mount Baldy Road) veers right. Stay on it and drive uphill another 8 miles to Mount Baldy village. Just as you approach the village, turn left on Glendora Ridge Road. Follow it 1 mile to Cow Canyon Saddle, where parking space is available on the left side of the road.

Lookout Mountain, a prominent bump on the south ridge of Mount San Antonio, was named after "Baldy Lookout," a wooden tower constructed there during 1915-16 and used every season until 1927. After being seriously damaged by a windstorm in 1927, the lookout was moved over to neighboring Sunset Peak, where it remained in place until the 1970s.

In the mid-1920s, Lookout Mountain was one of two sites used by Nobel-prize-winning physicist Albert Michelson during a several-year effort to obtain a precise value for the speed of light. Beams of light from a rapidly rotating octagonal prism at "Station Michelson" on Mount Wilson were fired toward "Station Antonio" at Lookout Mountain, where they were reflected back to the prism on Mount Wilson by means of a large concave mirror. The distance between the stations (approximately 22 miles) was obtained with unparalleled precision by

Old Baldy seen from Lookout Mountain

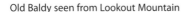

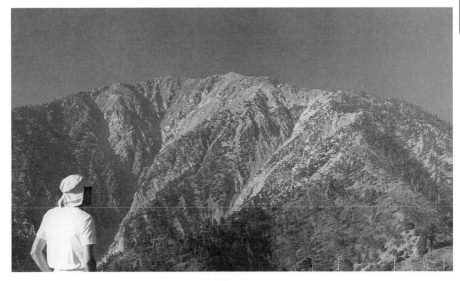

**ANGELES FOREST**

triangulation from a carefully surveyed baseline down in the San Gabriel Valley. The travel time of the light was measured as a function of the rate at which the prism had to turn in order to properly intercept the reflected beam. The round-trip distance divided by the round-trip travel time of the light gave the speed, which as every student knows is close to 300,000 kilometers per second, or 186,000 miles per second (about 670 million miles per hour).

Today Lookout Mountain draws about 100 visitors yearly, many of whom are lucky enough to spot a bighorn sheep or two. A primitive path to the top, unmaintained since the days of the Baldy Lookout, is narrow but still followable.

From the trailhead, walk 0.3 mile north on a gated dirt road to a large clearing. Notice the fire break going north up a steep ridgeline. Climb up that fire break and look for an obscure trail contouring to the left.

The trail curves along a west-facing slope, and at 0.9 mile gains a saddle southeast of Lookout Mountain. It then turns northwest and zigzags up Lookout Mountain's southeast ridge until the ridge becomes too steep, at 1.4 miles. Barely recognizable from now on, the trail traverses the shady northeast flank of the mountain, gains the north ridgeline, and turns south to reach the summit (2.0 miles).

Rusted metal and shards of plate glass are reminders of the old lookout. You'll also find the three in-line concrete pillars, pointing toward Mount Wilson, that supported the large mirror used during the Michelson experiments.

The summit makes a fine spot for a picnic lunch, complete with a great view of Old Baldy looming above and parts of the metropolis below. Since bighorn sheep frequent this area, don't camp on the summit—just come for the day.

## trip 8 Coldwater Canyon Truck Trail

see map on p. 308

| | |
|---|---|
| **Distance** | 10.5 miles round trip, Out-and-back |
| **Hiking Time** | 5 hours (round trip) |
| **Elevation Gain/Loss** | 1600'/1600' |
| **Difficulty** | Moderately strenuous |
| **Trail Use** | Suitable for backpacking, dogs allowed |
| **Best Times** | October through May |
| **Agency** | ANF/SGRD |
| **Optional Map** | USGS 7.5-min *Mt. Baldy* |
| **Notes** | Marked trails/obvious routes, easy terrain |

**DIRECTIONS** Exit the 210 Freeway at Baseline Road on the border between the cities of Claremont and Upland. Go west on Baseline for 0.7 mile, then turn right (north) on Mills Avenue. After 1.1 mile the main road (signed Mount Baldy Road) veers right. Stay on it and drive uphill another 8 miles to Mount Baldy village. Just as you approach the village, turn left on Glendora Ridge Road. Follow it 1 mile to Cow Canyon Saddle, where parking space is available on the left side of the road.

Although wilderness areas do not normally contain maintained dirt roads, Sheep Mountain Wilderness does. Several private inholdings and preexisting mining claims were necessarily included within the boundary of Sheep Mountain Wilderness when it was created in 1984. Coldwater Canyon Truck Trail guarantees access to several private ranches in the Coldwater Canyon area as well as a tungsten-mining operation in Cattle Canyon. The road is open to hikers and equestrians, but not to bicycles (mountain biking is prohibited in all wilderness areas).

Hiking down Coldwater Canyon Truck Trail is one of the easiest ways to maximize your chance of sighting a bighorn sheep in the San Gabriels. Cool or cloudy days are best; sunny days are scorchers most of the year, as you'll be on shadeless south-facing slopes most of the way.

From the trailhead, walk 0.3 mile north on a dirt road to a large clearing. From there, follow the dirt road (the Coldwater Canyon Truck Trail) that contours west, well above Cow Canyon's floor and well below Lookout Mountain's summit. Take note of the fantastically jumbled and contorted exposures of granitic (quartz diorite) and metamorphic (gneiss) rock exposed in the road cuts. Ancient movements along the San Gabriel Fault are responsible. Cow Canyon Saddle marks the eastern terminus of the fault; from there the fault continues almost due west, paralleling Cow Canyon,

lower Cattle Canyon, and the East and West forks of the San Gabriel River.

At 2.8 miles, you reach a saddle on the ridge between Cow and Cattle canyons. Bighorn sheep prints in the road dust reveal this to be a popular crossing point for the agile creatures. Ahead, the road continues crookedly down the falling ridgeline between the two canyons. At a sharp hairpin turn at 4.7 miles, there's a fine view up rubble-filled upper Cattle Canyon toward Bighorn Ridge.

You can keep going all the way to the wide floor of Cattle Canyon (5+ miles), where a seasonal stream makes its way through a barren, boulder-filled wash. Less than a mile ahead (west) down Cattle Canyon, there's a private ranch—no trespassing. You can, however, turn north on a dirt road going about 2 miles up Cattle Canyon. There's a tungsten mine near the road's end.

## trip 9  Cattle Canyon

see map on p. 308

ANGELES FOREST

| | |
|---|---|
| **Distance** | 6.0 miles round trip, Out-and-back |
| **Hiking Time** | 3 hours (round trip) |
| **Elevation Gain/Loss** | 700'/700' |
| **Difficulty** | Moderate |
| **Trail Use** | Suitable for backpacking, dogs allowed, good for kids |
| **Best Times** | September through June |
| **Agency** | ANF/SGRD |
| **Optional Maps** | USGS 7.5-min *Glendora, Mt. Baldy* |
| **Notes** | Marked trails/obvious routes, easy terrain |

**DIRECTIONS** From the community of Azusa, just north of Interstate 210, drive north on the San Gabriel Canyon Road, Highway 39, for 11 miles to East Fork Road, on the right. Continue up East Fork Road 5.2 miles to the intersection of Glendora Mountain Road. Find parking by the roadside anywhere near here.

From Coldwater Canyon to East Fork, Cattle Canyon carves a sinuous course through a gorge impressively flanked by walls abruptly soaring 1000 feet or more. An old dirt road—now a pleasant hiking path—follows the canyon bottom, crossing the alder-lined stream about two dozen times.

The trail starts from the west side of an old bridge on East Fork Road just east of the intersection of Glendora Mountain Road. You can follow the gradually ascending trail through Cattle Canyon as far as 3.0 miles to a locked gate, posted no-entry. The River Forks Ranch and other private

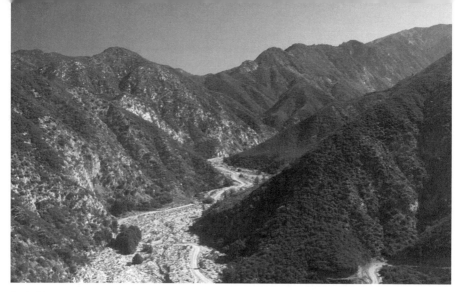

Cattle Canyon

properties in Cattle and Coldwater canyons lie beyond.

This is a great spring or early summer trip. You can go as far as you like, and turn back at any point. The stream flows clear and cool, but not normally so high as to create a hazard when crossing. Streamside vegetation flourishes, and wildflowers dot the sunny flats. The stream and its moist banks are a perfect habitat for a variety of snakes, including rattlesnakes. During the first couple of episodes of warm weather in April or May, you should be wary of the latter, as they are often irritable when they awaken from a long period of hibernation.

## trip 10  Shoemaker Canyon Road

see map on p. 308

| | |
|---|---|
| **Distance** | 5.5 miles round trip, Out-and-back |
| **Hiking Time** | 2½ hours (round trip) |
| **Elevation Gain/Loss** | 900'/900' |
| **Difficulty** | Moderate |
| **Trail Use** | Suitable for mountain biking, dogs allowed |
| **Best Times** | October through May |
| **Agency** | ANF/SGRD |
| **Optional Maps** | USGS 7.5-min *Glendora, Crystal Lake* |
| **Notes** | Marked trails/obvious routes, easy terrain |

**DIRECTIONS** From the community of Azusa, just north of Interstate 210, drive north on the San Gabriel Canyon Road, Highway 39, for 11 miles to East Fork Road, on the right. Continue up East Fork Road 3.3 miles to where you bear left on the paved, dead-end Shoemaker Canyon Road. Continue 1.8 miles to a vehicle gate and parking area.

Known colloquially as the Convict Road, Shoemaker Canyon Road should really be called the Road to Nowhere. The road was part of what was projected to be a 23-year effort to build a highway up along the East Fork canyon to Vincent Gap. (This project was not connected with an earlier road-building effort that included the construction of the famous, stranded "Bridge to Nowhere"; see Trip 11.)

During 1954–69, the county road department, utilizing prison labor, managed to carve out and grade 4.5 miles of new roadway on the canyon wall opposite East Fork Station and Heaton Flat. The project was rendered moribund in 1969 in the face of budget cuts and opposition by conservationists. The creation of Sheep Mountain Wilderness in 1984 finally put to rest, probably once and for all, a project that would have irreparably scarred Southern California's deepest canyon—The Narrows of the East Fork. The enduring legacy of this misdirected road-building effort—massive cuts and fills—will probably be visible on the canyon walls for centuries to come.

Today you can drive the first 1.8 miles of Shoemaker Canyon Road on pavement, then walk the remaining graded-dirt section to reach a pair of tunnels. Beyond the second tunnel there's a great view of the East Fork gorge and its mile-high east wall culminating at 8007-foot Iron Mountain.

From the trailhead, start walking up the unpaved road ahead. After 1.7 miles of walking, you reach the first tunnel, about 400 yards long, completed in 1961. Ahead lies a small abyss—Shoemaker Canyon. It was never bridged; a narrower road contours around it and continues northeast to a second tunnel, about 250 yards long, dated 1964. On the far side of that tunnel, you can veer right and backtrack, circumventing the tunnel by way of an old road bed. There you'll have the best view of the East Fork gorge.

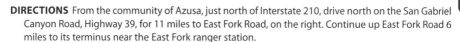

## trip 11  East Fork to Bridge

| | |
|---|---|
| **Distance** | 9.6 miles round trip, Out-and-back |
| **Hiking Time** | 4½ hours (round trip) |
| **Elevation Gain/Loss** | 1000'/1000' |
| **Difficulty** | Moderately strenuous |
| **Trail Use** | Suitable for backpacking, dogs allowed |
| **Best Times** | October through June |
| **Agency** | ANF/SGRD |
| **Optional Maps** | USGS 7.5-min *Glendora, Crystal Lake, Mount San Antonio* |
| **Notes** | Marked trails/obvious routes, easy terrain |

see map on p. 308

ANGELES FOREST

**DIRECTIONS** From the community of Azusa, just north of Interstate 210, drive north on the San Gabriel Canyon Road, Highway 39, for 11 miles to East Fork Road, on the right. Continue up East Fork Road 6 miles to its terminus near the East Fork ranger station.

**B**orn of snow-fed rivulets, the many tributaries of the East Fork gather together to form one of the liveliest mountain streams in the San Gabriels. At The Narrows of the East Fork, the water squeezes through the deepest gorge in Southern California. From the bottom of The Narrows, the east wall soars about 5200 feet to Iron Mountain, and the west wall rises about 4000 feet to the South Mount Hawkins divide.

During the 1930s, road-builders managed to push a highway up through the East Fork to as far as the lower portals of The Narrows. There, an arched, concrete bridge was constructed, similar in style to those that were built in the same era along Angeles Crest Highway. The bridge was to be a key link in a route that would one day carry traffic between the San Gabriel Valley and the desert near Wrightwood. But fate intervened. The great 1938 flood thoroughly demolished most of the road, leaving the bridge stranded far upstream. The next and last attempt to construct a road through the East Fork

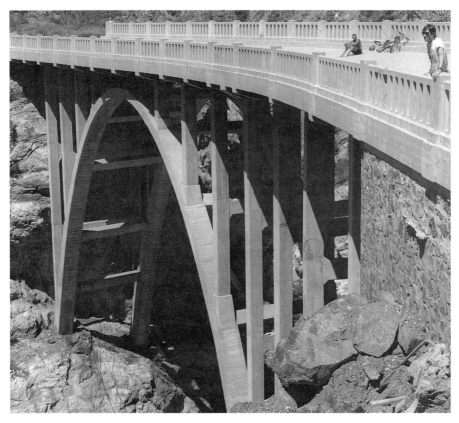

The Bridge to Nowhere

gorge utilized a high-line approach instead (see Trip 10), but that effort was ultimately abandoned as well.

The trek to the old bridge is in the same league as the climb of Old Baldy—an obligatory experience for L.A.-area hikers. On warm summer weekends, hundreds of people walk the trail going up from East Fork Station. A fraction venture as far as the bridge, a leisurely half-day's round-trip hike as long as the water flow in the East Fork isn't too great and swift.

Over the last century or more, gold mining in the East Fork has evolved from a serious business to more of a recreational pastime. Today, claims are being worked around The Narrows area, but mostly it's the fun of playing around in the stream and

catching a bit of color that keeps a number of recreational miners coming back year after year.

There are several creek crossings of ankle- to knee-depth, so wear shoes that you don't mind getting soaked. During parts of winter and spring, high water may render these crossings unsafe.

At the East Fork trailhead, fill out a wilderness permit at the self-issuing register, and then follow the gated service road upstream, high along the right bank, to Heaton Flat Campground, 0.5 mile. Beyond Heaton Flat the road ends, but a well-traveled trail continues up the flood plain. At 2.5 miles, you pass Swan Rock, a cliff-exposure of metamorphic rock branded with the light-colored imprint of a swan.

You can see it best under flat lighting conditions. You're now entering Sheep Mountain Wilderness.

At 3.5 miles, the trail swings abruptly right and climbs about 60 feet to meet a remnant of the old highway. The old road bed carves its way along the east canyon wall, high above what is now a wide, boulder-filled flood plain laced with the meandering, alder-lined stream. The Bridge to Nowhere appears at 4.8 miles, just as the canyon walls start to pinch in. The bridge appears remarkably undamaged after a half

century of neglect, except for its crumbling concrete railings.

The bridge and the area just south of it lie within an island of posted private property. You're allowed passage across the bridge, but please don't stray from the road or the bridge when inside the posted area. From the north abutment of the bridge, a narrow trail contours above the stream, then drops into the lower part of The Narrows. The following trip has more to say about the upper canyon.

### trip 12  Down the East Fork

see map on p. 308

| | |
|---|---|
| **Distance** | 14.5 miles, Point-to-point |
| **Hiking Time** | 11 hours |
| **Elevation Gain/Loss** | 200'/4800' |
| **Difficulty** | Strenuous |
| **Trail Use** | Suitable for backpacking, dogs allowed |
| **Best Times** | April through November |
| **Agency** | ANF/SGRD |
| **Recommended Maps** | USGS 7.5-min *Crystal Lake, Mount San Antonio, Glendora* |
| **Notes** | Navigation required, moderate terrain, bushwhacking |

**DIRECTIONS** *North End:* From Interstate 15, north of San Bernardino, exit at Highway 138 and turn west. Drive 8.6 miles to Angeles Crest Highway, and turn left. Continue through Wrightwood and Big Pines; stay on Angeles Crest Highway for a total of 15 miles until you reach the large trailhead parking lot at Vincent Gap (mile 74.8 on Angeles Crest Highway). *South End:* From the community of Azusa, just north of Interstate 210, drive north on the San Gabriel Canyon Road, Highway 39, for 11 miles to East Fork Road, on the right. Continue up East Fork Road 6 miles to its terminus near the East Fork ranger station.

**B**orn from snow-fed rivulets, the many tributaries of the East Fork San Gabriel River gather together to form one of the liveliest and most remote streams in the San Gabriels. At The Narrows of the East Fork, the water squeezes through the deepest gorge in Southern California. From the bottom of The Narrows, the east wall soars about 5200 feet to Iron Mountain, and the west wall rises about 4000 feet to the South Mount Hawkins divide.

On this epic journey down the upper East Fork, you'll descend nearly a mile in elevation, travel from high-country pines and firs to sun-scorched chaparral, and

cross three important geologic faults—the Punchbowl, Vincent Thrust, and San Gabriel faults. During the course of a single day you could experience a temperature increase of as much as 60°F.

You can do this hike in one incredibly long day with an early start, or you can camp overnight on one of the shaded streamside terraces near the mid-point of the trek. The better camping sites include former trail camps at Fish and Iron forks, and the lower part of The Narrows. Because the route passes through the Sheep Mountain Wilderness, check with the Forest Service to see if you need an overnight permit.

Except at the beginning, navigation on the trip is straightforward—you simply head down-canyon the whole way. Consult a detailed map often if you want to confirm exactly where you are. Heavy runoff after a storm or major snowmelt can create hazardous stream crossings, which is one of the reasons why this trip is only recommended for the late-spring through fall seasons. The other reason is the upper trailhead at Vincent Gap may be unreachable due to snow cover. Contact the rangers for more information about either issue.

The amount of time required to complete the trip can be highly variable due to problems with adverse weather or swift-flowing water, excessive bushwhacking along the banks of the upper river, how heavy your backpacks are, and the hiking ability of the slowest member of your party. This is not a trip for hikers without plenty of successful experience in off-trail wilderness travel.

It's best to have someone drop you off at the starting point on Angeles Crest Highway later pick you up at East Fork Station. That's an 85-mile drive around by way of Interstate 15, Interstate 10, Highway 39, and East Fork Road.

From the parking area on the south side of Vincent Gap, walk down the gated road to the southeast. After only about 200 yards, a footpath veers left, into Sheep Mountain Wilderness. Take it; the road itself continues toward the Bighorn Mine, an "inholding" of privately owned land inside the wilderness boundary.

Intermittently shaded by bigcone Douglas-firs, white firs, Jeffrey pines, and live oaks, the path descends along the south slope of Vincent Gulch. The gulch itself follows the Punchbowl Fault, a splinter of the San Andreas. At 0.7 mile, on a flat ridge spur, look for an indistinct path intersecting on the right. This leads about 100 yards to an old cabin believed to have been the home of Charles Vincent. Vincent led the life of a hermit, prospector, and big-game

hunter in the Baden-Powell/Old Baldy area from 1870 until his death in 1926.

After a few switchbacks, the primitive trail crosses Vincent Gulch (usually dry at this point, wet a short distance below) at 1.6 miles. Thereafter it stays on or above the east bank as far as the confluence of Prairie Fork, a wide drainage coming in from the east at 3.8 miles from the start. You veer right (west) down a gravelly wash, good for setting up a camp. Shortly after, at the Mine Gulch confluence, you bend left (south) into the wide bed of the upper East Fork. For several miles to come, there is essentially no trail. It may take several hours to traverse this stretch, depending on the energy and motivation of your group.

Proceed down the rock-strewn flood plain, crossing the creek (and battling alder thickets) several times over the next mile. The canyon becomes narrow for a while starting at about 5.0 miles, and you must wade or hop from one slippery rock to

Fish Fork Falls

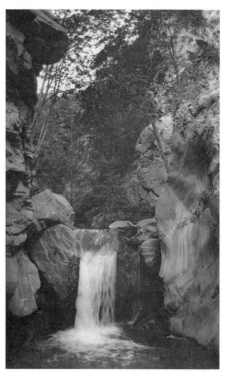

another. Fish Fork, on the left at 7.3 miles from the start, is the first large stream below Prairie Fork.

If you have the time for an intriguing side trip, Fish Fork canyon is well worth exploring. Chock full of alder and bay, narrow with soaring walls, its clear stream tumbling over boulders, the canyon boasts one of the wildest and most beautiful settings in the San Gabriels. About 1.6 miles upstream lies a formidable impasse: There, the waters of Fish Fork drop 12 feet into an emerald-green pool set amid sheer rock walls. A bigger waterfall, inaccessible by means of this approach, lies farther upstream.

Well below Fish Fork, you enter The Narrows. A rough trail, worn in by hikers, traverses this one-mile-plus section of fast-moving water. You'll pass swimmable (if chilly) pools cupped in the granite and schist bedrock, and cross the stream when necessary. Listen and watch for water ouzels (dippers) by the edges of the pools. Old mining trails once threaded the canyon walls here and to the north, but all are virtually obliterated now.

At the lower portals of The Narrows (9.7 miles), you come upon the enigmatically named Bridge to Nowhere. During the 1930s, road-builders managed to push a highway up along the East Fork stream to just this far. The arched, concrete bridge, similar in style to those built along Angeles Crest Highway, was to be a key link in a route that would carry traffic between the San Gabriel Valley and the desert near Wrightwood. Fate intervened. A great flood in 1938 thoroughly demolished most of the road, leaving the bridge stranded.

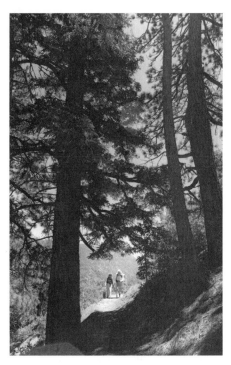

High above the East Fork San Gabriel River

Below the bridge, on remnants of the old road washed out in 1938, you'll run into more and more hikers, fishermen, and other travelers out for the day. At 12.0 miles, Swan Rock—an outcrop of metamorphic rock branded with the light-colored imprint of a swan—comes into view on the right. At 14.0 miles you come upon Heaton Flat Campground. From there a final, easy 0.5-mile stroll takes you to the East Fork Station and trailhead at the end of East Fork Road.

ANGELES FOREST

# chapter 27

# Angeles Forest:
# San Antonio Canyon & Old Baldy

San Antonio Canyon, a yawning gap in the fortress-like south front of the San Gabriels, also serves as the main gateway to the third highest mountain mass in Southern California—Mount San Antonio, or Old Baldy. At 10,064 feet, Baldy's summit looms large over the eastern Los Angeles Basin, the Inland Empire communities of Riverside and San Bernardino, and the western Mojave Desert. It can be seen as far north as the southern Sierra Nevada, and as far south as the Mexican border adjoining San Diego County.

Both San Antonio Canyon and Old Baldy lie astride the Los Angeles-San Bernardino county line. Old Baldy's summit is a county-line bench mark, making it the highest point in Los Angeles County, but not in San Bernardino County. Our coverage of the trails in this chapter includes some that are outside the L.A. County boundary, but we don't include anything east of the divide defined by Cucamonga Peak, the "Three T's," and Mount Baldy Notch, nor north of Old Baldy. You may refer to John Robinson's *Trails of the Angeles* for more on these areas, which are a part of San Bernardino County's share of the San Gabriel Mountains.

The opening of San Antonio Canyon to automobiles, starting in 1908, helped facilitate the rapid development of cabins and resorts in the area. Several hundred cabins dotted the main canyon and its tributaries by the mid 1930s. Camp Baldy—the site of today's Mount Baldy village—grew to become one of the most popular mountain retreats in Southern California. The great flood of 1938, which tore up the whole front face of the San Gabriels, washed away most of Camp Baldy, as well as scores of other cabins that were sited too close to the streams.

The resort era is long-forgotten today, but Mount Baldy (or Baldy Village, as it's known to many residents) remains a viable cabin community. The greater Mount Baldy area, with a population of about 1000, is the second-largest community in the San Gabriels, after Wrightwood.

San Antonio Canyon gets a big influx of skiers and snow seekers during the winter, while a less hectic crowd of hikers and sightseers makes use of the area during the warmer months. In Mount Baldy you can stop by the Forest Service visitor center (Friday through Sunday, 8:30 a.m. to 4:30 p.m.) for the latest on trail conditions, and to obtain permits if needed.

The upper end of San Antonio Canyon includes the Forest Service's Manker Flats Campground and Glacier Picnic Area, as well as a large parking lot for the privately operated ski lift. Backpackers can camp just about anywhere on Forest Service land, subject to the regulations for remote camping.

All trips below require a National Forest Adventure Pass ($5 per day, $30 per year) for trailhead parking.

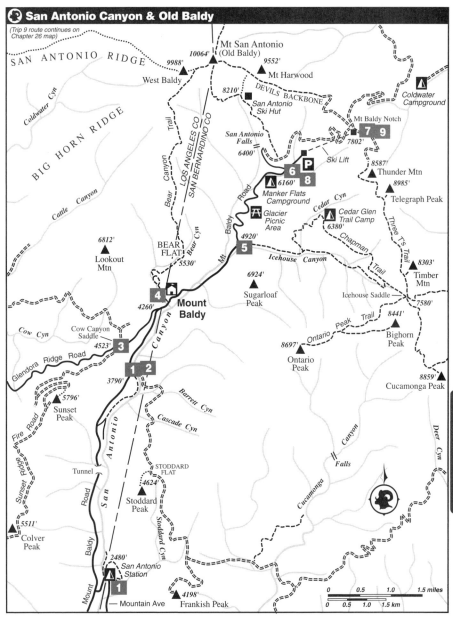

**San Antonio Canyon & Old Baldy**

(Trip 9 route continues on Chapter 26 map)

SAN ANTONIO RIDGE

9988'

10064' ▲ Mt San Antonio (Old Baldy)

West Baldy

9552' ▲ Mt Harwood

Coldwater Cyn

8210' ■ DEVILS BACKBONE

San Antonio Ski Hut

Coldwater Campground

BIG HORN RIDGE

Trail

Bear Canyon

San Antonio Falls
6400'

Mt Baldy Notch
7802'  **7 9**

Cattle Canyon

LOS ANGELES CO
SAN BERNARDINO CO

Baldy Road

**6**
6160' ▲ **8**
P  Ski Lift

8587' ▲ Thunder Mtn

8985' ▲ Telegraph Peak

Manker Flats Campground

Cedar Cyn

Glacier Picnic Area

Cedar Glen Trail Camp
6380'

Chapman

Three T's Trail

6812' ▲
Lookout Mtn

BEAR FLAT
5530'

Bear Cyn

4920'
**5**

Icehouse Canyon

6924' ▲
Sugarloaf Peak

Icehouse Saddle
7580'

8303' ▲
Timber Mtn

**4**
4260'

**Mount Baldy**

Mt Baldy Canyon

8441' ▲
Bighorn Peak

Cow Cyn

Cow Canyon Saddle
4523'  **3**

Glendora Ridge Road

Ontario Peak Trail

8697' ▲
Ontario Peak

8859' ▲
Cucamonga Peak

**1 2**
3790'

Barrett Cyn

Cascade Cyn

San Antonio Canyon

Cucamonga Canyon

Deer Cyn

▲ 5796'
Sunset Peak

Fire Road

Sunset Ridge

Tunnel

STODDARD FLAT
4624' ▲

Stoddard Peak

Baldy Road

Stoddard Cyn

Falls

5511' ▲
Colver Peak

2480'
San Antonio Station

**1**

Mount Baldy Road

Mountain Ave

4198' ▲
Frankish Peak

0    0.5    1.0    1.5 miles
0   0.5   1.0   1.5 km

**ANGELES FOREST**

## trip 1 San Antonio Canyon

|  |  |
|---|---|
| **Distance** | 3.8 miles, Point-to-point |
| **Hiking Time** | 2½ hours |
| **Elevation Gain/Loss** | 100'/1400' |
| **Difficulty** | Moderately strenuous |
| **Trail Use** | Dogs allowed |
| **Best Times** | October through May |
| **Agency** | ANF/SGRD |
| **Optional Map** | USGS 7.5-min *Mt. Baldy* |
| **Notes** | Marked trails/obvious routes, moderate terrain, bushwhacking |

see map on p. 327

**DIRECTIONS** *South End:* Exit the 210 Freeway at Baseline Road on the border between the cities of Claremont and Upland. Go west on Baseline for 0.7 mile, then turn right (north) on Mills Avenue. After 1.1 mile the main road (signed Mount Baldy Road) veers right. Stay on it and drive uphill another 3 miles to Mountain Avenue, where you turn right. Ahead a short distance, enter the parking lot for the San Antonio Ranger Station. The hike ends here. *North End:* The hike begins at the intersection of Mount Baldy Road and the dead-end "Mountain Avenue," which intersects Mount Baldy Road at mile 1.1, 4 miles north of the hike's starting point and 1.3 miles south of Mount Baldy village. (This Mountain Avenue was once connected to the Mountain Avenue near San Antonio Station.)

Over the past century and a half, lower San Antonio Canyon's flood-prone bed has seen the creation and the demise of many a trail, wagon road, and auto road. On this ramble down along the boulder-filled canyon bottom, you'll trace the route of an auto road (now largely obliterated) that, like so many of its predecessors, was built too close to the temperamental stream.

Today's road—Mount Baldy Road—curves along the canyon's west slope, staying a comfortable 200 feet or so above the stream. It is not recommended as a way to "close the loop" on foot for this point-to-point hike because of fast traffic and two narrow tunnels. On the canyon hike itself you must cross the stream several times, so don't go if the water level is too high.

Starting at the upper end, walk south on the old pavement of disused Mountain Avenue. After you bypass a vehicle barrier, the badly deteriorated road bed swings low across the cliff-like face of a promontory called the Hogback. Until 1908 the Hogback, along with a picturesque waterfall in the canyon just below it, were formidable obstacles to travel by man or beast. That year, a toll road suitable for automobiles was pushed through, destroying the falls

in the process. The road was widened and paved in the early 1920s, then badly washed out in the 1938 flood, and then rebuilt again. The final demise came during flooding in 1969; by that time, however, the old road had been rendered obsolete by the straighter and faster Mount Baldy Road, completed in 1955.

At the beginning of the hike, and again 1.4 miles later, you'll pass small hydroelectric power plants, their turbines loudly humming whenever the stream flow allows. These are the descendants of the first power station installed below the Hogback in 1892. It proved to be an efficient but somewhat erratic (because of poor flows in years of drought) source of electric power for communities as distant as Pomona and San Bernardino.

At about 1.8 miles, just below the Mount Baldy Road tunnels, the canyon narrows. Boulder-hopping and bushwhacking are in order, along with some foot-wetting fords. But soon the canyon floor widens and becomes open and sunny, with willows and alders growing along the stream. You can either try to trace pieces of the old road, or stay closer to the stream and travel over the rock-strewn flood plain. During the last mile of the hike you may come upon scores, possibly hundreds, of people out enjoying the sun and the stream, especially if the weather's warm.

Just before the end (3.6 miles) you can climb a bridge abutment to reach a piece of the old road on the east bank. This leads toward San Antonio Ranger Station—the end of the hike.

Behind the station, the Elfin Forest Nature Trail winds for a mile amid typical sage-scrub and chaparral vegetation. It's a worthwhile walk whenever the vegetation is in bloom during the springtime.

## trip 2  Stoddard Peak

| | |
|---|---|
| **Distance** | 6.0 miles round trip, Out-and-back |
| **Hiking Time** | 3 hours (round trip) |
| **Elevation Gain/Loss** | 1100'/1100' |
| **Difficulty** | Moderate |
| **Trail Use** | Suitable for backpacking, dogs allowed |
| **Best Times** | October through May |
| **Agency** | ANF/SGRD |
| **Recommended Map** | USGS 7.5-min *Mt. Baldy* |
| **Notes** | Navigation required, easy terrain |

see map on p. 327

**DIRECTIONS**  Exit the 210 Freeway at Baseline Road on the border between the cities of Claremont and Upland. Go west on Baseline for 0.7 mile, then turn right (north) on Mills Avenue. After 1.1 mile the main road (signed Mount Baldy Road) veers right. Stay on it and drive uphill another 7 miles to the dead-end Mountain Avenue, mile 1.1 on Mount Baldy Road, on the right. This intersection is 1.3 miles south of Mount Baldy village.

**S**toddard Peak's 4624-foot height places it above most of the shaggy, chaparral-covered foothill country, but well below the stony gaze of the western ramparts of the Cucamonga Wilderness. When dusted or spotted with snow, the peak becomes a dichotomous perch between the white-mantled world above and sun-warmed slopes and canyons below. The hike to the top involves mostly road-walking, with a short, rugged stretch near the peak itself.

ANGELES FOREST

Old Baldy seen from Stoddard Ridge

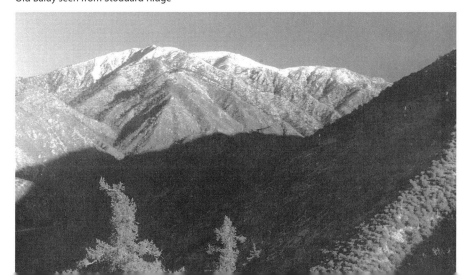

As you set off on the dead-end Mountain Avenue, don't take the old, paved, canyon-bottom road to the south (Trip 1 route), but rather head east on the dirt road that descends past a small hydro-powerplant. Cross San Antonio Canyon's stream and continue curving south, then east on the dirt road as it contours into Barrett Canyon. After passing some picturesque cabins and yapping dogs, you arrive at a locked vehicle gate, 0.8 mile. Bypass it and keep following the road. You climb amid dense oak forest, contour along a sunny slope, curl around steep Cascade Canyon, and then climb gradually to saddle (2.6 miles), where the road begins to descend into the Stoddard Canyon drainage. The gently sloping area adjoining on the east, Stoddard Flat, is suitable for trail camping.

From the saddle, a faint path leads west up through tall brush, and then turns south along the top of a sunny ridge. Proceed 0.4 mile on this path, passing over two false summits, to the true summit of Stoddard Peak as marked on the *Mt. Baldy* topo map. The second false summit you pass over is actually slightly higher than Stoddard Peak.

The ridge falls sharply beyond Stoddard Peak, so there's no need to go on—the view is the best from here. Looking down into San Antonio Canyon, you can see disconnected segments of the old canyon-bottom road, pummeled in the past by floods and slides. Old Baldy, its snow-cap gleaming in winter, dominates the view to the north. To the south, beyond San Antonio Dam (and its usually dry flood-control reservoir), spread the Pomona valley and the Chino Hills. If it's clear enough to see the ocean horizon, you can often see sprawling Santa Catalina Island, plus the low dome of San Clemente Island a little to the left.

## trip 3  Sunset Peak

see map on p. 327

| | |
|---|---|
| **Distance** | 5.8 miles round trip, Out-and-back |
| **Hiking Time** | 3 hours (round trip) |
| **Elevation Gain/Loss** | 1200'/1200' |
| **Difficulty** | Moderate |
| **Trail Use** | Suitable for backpacking, suitable for mountain biking, dogs allowed |
| **Best Times** | October through May |
| **Agency** | ANF/SGRD |
| **Optional Map** | USGS 7.5-min *Mt. Baldy* |
| **Notes** | Marked trails/obvious routes, easy to moderate terrain |

**DIRECTIONS** Exit the 210 Freeway at Baseline Road on the border between the cities of Claremont and Upland. Go west on Baseline for 0.7 mile, then turn right (north) on Mills Avenue. After 1.1 mile the main road (signed Mount Baldy Road) veers right. Stay on it and drive uphill another 8 miles to Mount Baldy village. Just as you approach the village, turn left on Glendora Ridge Road. Follow it 1 mile to Cow Canyon Saddle, where parking space is available on the left side of the road.

The hike to Sunset Peak from Cow Canyon Saddle offers up fine views of the archipelago of high peaks stretching from San Gabriel Wilderness in the west to Cucamonga Wilderness in the east. Mount San Antonio rises from center stage in the north, its bald summit sometimes accented by a brilliant snow cap.

The climb of Sunset Peak is just the beginning of a possible 13-mile, one-way trek along the whole Sunset Ridge (described in earlier editions of this book), which could take you all the way down to the rim of the San Gabriel Valley at Marshall Canyon or Cobal Canyon, an area covered in this edition's Chapter 11. But Sunset Peak alone is an easy-enough destination with a lot of bang for the modest effort of climbing it.

From the parking area at Cow Canyon Saddle, start hiking up the gated fire road on the south side of the road. You gain elevation steadily, accompanied by a mixture of tall chaparral, live oaks, bigcone Douglas-firs, and bigleaf maples. You reverse direction at 1.9 miles, and again at 2.5 miles. Just after the latter switchback, bear left on an old fire break and head southwest straight to the summit (2.9 miles). This worthwhile and fun shortcut, with some easy rock scrambling at the top, saves time and distance over the alternative—a mile of tedious road walking.

Sunset Peak's flat, barren summit makes a fine (but dry) campsite. A fire lookout stood here from the 1920s to the '70s; you'll notice the building's foundation and also the remains of a rainwater collection system.

Much of what lies in view to the south is a large, closed-to-the-public parcel of the Angeles National Forest called the San Dimas Experimental Forest. Much of our current knowledge about fire ecology and erosion in the chaparral plant community has been gained from carefully controlled experiments performed in this outdoor laboratory over the past seven or eight decades.

## `trip 4` **Bear Flat**

see map on p. 327

| | |
|---|---|
| **Distance** | 3.5 miles round trip, Out-and-back |
| **Hiking Time** | 2 hours (round trip) |
| **Elevation Gain/Loss** | 1300'/1300' |
| **Difficulty** | Moderate |
| **Trail Use** | Dogs allowed, good for kids |
| **Best Times** | All year |
| **Agency** | ANF/SGRD |
| **Optional Map** | USGS 7.5-min *Mt. Baldy* |
| **Notes** | Marked trails/obvious routes, easy terrain |

**DIRECTIONS** Exit the 210 Freeway at Baseline Road on the border between the cities of Claremont and Upland. Go west on Baseline for 0.7 mile, then turn right (north) on Mills Avenue. After 1.1 mile the main road (signed Mount Baldy Road) veers right. Stay on it and drive uphill another 8 miles to Mount Baldy village. Look for Bear Creek Road on the left, in the center of the village. Park at or near this intersection.

Barely a mile's walk from the busy little community of Mount Baldy, you can be sitting on a rock, communing with Nature, feet dangling in the sun-and-shade-dappled, crystalline stream of Bear Canyon. With a bit more time and energy, you can climb to Bear Flat, where a binocular sweep of the surrounding hillsides often nets sightings of bighorn sheep.

From the intersection of Mount Baldy Road and Bear Creek Road, in the center of Mount Baldy village, walk up the paved road to its end (0.4 mile), then continue on a dirt trail that soon becomes narrow. Many cabins, in various stages of repair (or ruin), line the way. At one point, a rickety rope-and-plank footbridge serves as the only link between a cabin on one side of the creek and the trail on the other.

Like other inhabited canyons of the San Gabriels, lower Bear Canyon is overrun by non-native ground covers like ivy and vinca, but shaded by magnificent live oaks, bays, and bigcone Douglas-firs.

After crossing the creek twice, the trail divides. Take either path: the right branch climbs up the right slope; the left branch stays low along stream, passing more cabins, before joining the other branch.

After the two paths rejoin, the main Bear Canyon Trail goes by a water tank (part of the town's water supply), switches back, curves around sun-struck slopes, and plunges into a shady oak grove high on the east slope of the canyon. At about 1.7 miles, the trail crosses the stream for the last time. Bear Flat is the bracken-fern-filled, sloping meadow just above this crossing. This is the place to sniff a few spring wildflowers, look for bighorn sheep tracks, and then think about turning back. Beyond this, the Bear Canyon Trail switchbacks up to the south ridge of Mount San Antonio and relentlessly continues all the way to the summit, almost 5 miles away, 4500 feet higher than Bear Flat.

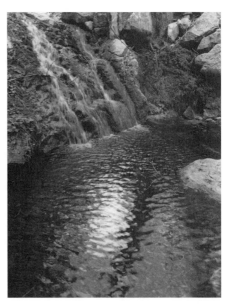

Bear Canyon stream

## trip 5 Cucamonga Peak

| | |
|---|---|
| **Distance** | 12.0 miles round trip, Out-and-back |
| **Hiking Time** | 7½ hours (round trip) |
| **Elevation Gain/Loss** | 4300'/4300' |
| **Difficulty** | Strenuous |
| **Trail Use** | Suitable for backpacking, dogs allowed |
| **Best Times** | May through November |
| **Agency** | ANF/SGRD |
| **Optional Maps** | USGS 7.5-min *Mt. Baldy, Cucamonga Peak* |
| **Notes** | Marked trails/obvious routes, easy terrain |

see map on p. 327

**DIRECTIONS** Exit the 210 Freeway at Baseline Road on the border between the cities of Claremont and Upland. Go west on Baseline for 0.7 mile, then turn right (north) on Mills Avenue. After 1.1 mile the main road (signed Mount Baldy Road) veers right. Stay on it and drive uphill another 9.5 miles to the large Icehouse Canyon trailhead on the right.

Cucamonga Peak's south and east slopes feature some of the most dramatic relief in the San Gabriel range. At 8859 feet, the peak stands sentinel-like only 4 miles from the edge of the broad inland valley region known as the Inland Empire. Go all the way to the top for the view, but don't be too disappointed in case there's nothing below but haze and smog. So much beautiful high country can be seen along the way that reaching the top is just icing on the cake.

Most of the hike lies within Cucamonga Wilderness, requiring a permit for both day and overnight use. Near Cucamonga's summit you'll tackle a steep, north-facing gully that can retain snow into May. Be sure to discuss with a ranger the possible hazards of snow and ice if it's early or late in the season.

From the trailhead, walk past the ruins of the Ice House Canyon Lodge (burned in 1988) and then up along the path that follows the alder-shaded stream. The first couple of miles along the canyon are a fitting introduction to a phase of Southern California scenery not familiar to a lot of visitors and newcomers. Huge bigcone Douglas-fir, incense cedar, and live oak trees cluster on the banks of the stream, which dances over boulder and fallen log. Moisture-loving, flowering plants like columbine sway in the breeze. Some of old cabins along the lower canyon still survive, while others, destroyed by flood or fire, have left evidence in the form of foundations or rock walls.

Old newspaper reports suggest that an ice-packing operation existed in or near Icehouse Canyon during the late 1850s. The ice was packed down San Antonio Canyon on mules to a point accessible to wagons (below the Hogback), whereupon it was carted, as quickly as possible, to Los Angeles for use in making ice cream and for chilling beverages. Whether ice was actually quarried in this canyon or in another, Icehouse Canyon's name is apt enough: cold-air drainage produces refrigerator-like temperatures on many a summer morning, and deep-freeze temperatures in winter.

The Chapman Trail intersects on the left at 1.0 mile. It goes up Icehouse Canyon's north wall, passes Cedar Glen Trail Camp, and contours over to meet the older, canyon-bottom trail. Stay on the latter (Icehouse Canyon) trail; it's about 1.7 miles shorter, it's cooler, and it offers better scenery. At Columbine Spring (2.4 miles, last water during the warmer months), the trail starts switchbacking up the north wall. After passing the upper intersection of the Chapman Trail at 2.9 miles, you continue to pine-shaded Icehouse Saddle, 3.5 miles, where trails converge from many directions. The trail to Cucamonga's summit contours southeast, descends moderately, and climbs to a 7654-foot saddle (4.4 miles) between Bighorn and Cucamonga peaks. Thereafter, it switchbacks up a steep slope dotted with lodgepole pines and white firs.

At 5.8 miles, the trail crosses a shady draw 200 feet below and northwest of the summit. A signed but indistinct side path goes straight up to the summit, 6.0 miles from your starting point in Icehouse Canyon. Return the same way, or take the alternate route, the Chapman Trail, if you'd like a longer but more gradual descent from Icehouse Saddle.

**ANGELES FOREST**

In Icehouse Canyon

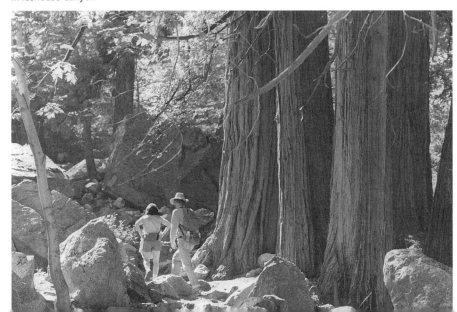

## trip 6  San Antonio Falls

| | |
|---|---|
| **Distance** | 1.2 miles round trip, Out-and-back |
| **Hiking Time** | 1 hour (round trip) |
| **Elevation Gain/Loss** | 250'/250' |
| **Difficulty** | Easy |
| **Trail Use** | Suitable for mountain biking, dogs allowed, good for kids |
| **Best Times** | April through July |
| **Agency** | ANF/SGRD |
| **Optional Map** | USGS 7.5-min *Mount San Antonio* |
| **Notes** | Marked trails/obvious routes, easy terrain |

see map on p. 327

**DIRECTIONS** Exit the 210 Freeway at Baseline Road on the border between the cities of Claremont and Upland. Go west on Baseline for 0.7 mile, then turn right (north) on Mills Avenue. After 1.1 mile the main road (signed Mount Baldy Road) veers right. Stay on it and drive uphill another 12 miles to Manker Flats Campground, 0.5 mile short of the ski-lift parking lot. Parking space can be found on the west side of the divided road, opposite the campground.

At San Antonio Falls, San Antonio Canyon's fledgling stream shoots down a broken rock face, falling a total of about 100 feet in three tiers. With a drainage area of only a few hundred acres, the falls put on a decent show only after a rather big storm or when the snow above is melting at a rapid rate. Three springs in the headwaters of the canyon help keep the falls alive, at a greatly subdued level, after all the snow has melted.

The easy hike to the base of the falls begins on the gated fire road just above Manker Flats Campground. The road, which is closed to all but ski-lift-maintenance vehicles, is thinly paved for the first 0.6 mile. That's just enough to reach a hairpin curve with a good glimpse of the falls to the left.

From the curve, a short but slightly precarious trail contours to the base of the falls, where the plummeting water hits not a pool but a stream bed of broken rock and gravel. If you have small kids, watch them carefully on this trail and near the base of falls to ensure their safety.

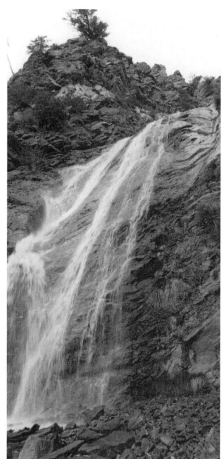

San Antonio Falls

**trip 7**  # Old Baldy—East Approach

see map on p. 327

| | |
|---|---|
| **Distance** | 6.4 miles round trip, Out-and-back |
| **Hiking Time** | 3½ hours (round trip) |
| **Elevation Gain/Loss** | 2300'/2300' |
| **Difficulty** | Moderately strenuous |
| **Trail Use** | Suitable for backpacking, dogs allowed |
| **Best Times** | May through November |
| **Agency** | ANF/SGRD |
| **Optional Maps** | USGS 7.5-min *Mount San Antonio, Telegraph Peak* |
| **Notes** | Marked trails/obvious routes, easy terrain |

**DIRECTIONS** Exit the 210 Freeway at Baseline Road on the border between the cities of Claremont and Upland. Go west on Baseline for 0.7 mile, then turn right (north) on Mills Avenue. After 1.1 mile the main road (signed Mount Baldy Road) veers right. Stay on it and drive uphill another 13 miles to the end of the road, where you enter the parking lot for the Mount Baldy Ski Lift.

No Southland hiker's repertoire of experiences is complete without at least one ascent of Mount San Antonio—Old Baldy. The east approach is the least taxing of the several routes to the summit, but it's by no means a picnic. You start at 7800 feet, with virtually no altitude acclimatization, and climb expeditiously to over 10,000 feet. With easy access, it's beguilingly easy to come unprepared for high winds or bad weather, which although fairly rare, may come up suddenly. Ice, if present, can be a serious hazard as well.

By mechanical means (a car) you can get to the upper terminus of Mount Baldy Road in less than a half hour from the valley flatlands below. Further mechanical means—the Mount Baldy ski lift—carries you to an elevation of 7800 feet at Mount Baldy Notch, where you begin hiking. Although the ski-lift caters mostly to skiers (7 days a week during the winter season), it remains open during the summer season on weekends (9 a.m. to 4:45 p.m.) for the benefit of sightseers and hikers. If it's a weekday, or you don't like being dangled over an abyss, you can always

ANGELES FOREST

Lodgepole pine at timberline, Old Baldy

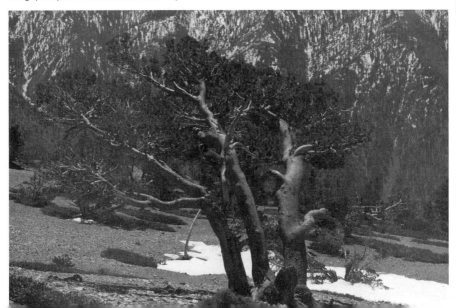

walk up the ski-lift-maintenance road starting from Manker Flats. That option adds 3.6 miles and an elevation change of about 1600 feet both on the way up and on the way down. A lodge at the upper terminus of the lift offers food and beverages.

From Mount Baldy Notch, technically the spot about 200 yards northeast of the top of the ski lift, take the maintenance road to the northwest that climbs moderately, then more steeply through groves of Jeffrey pine and incense cedar. After a couple of bends, you come to the road's end (1.3 miles) and the beginning of the trail along the Devil's Backbone ridge.

The stretch ahead, once a hair-raiser, lost most of its terror when the Civilian Conservation Corps constructed a wider and safer trail, complete with guard rails, in 1935-36. The guard rails are gone now, but there's plenty of room to maneuver, unless there are problems with strong winds and/or ice. Devil's Backbone offers grand vistas of both the Lytle Creek drainage on the north and east and San Antonio Canyon on the south.

The backbone section ends at about 2.0 miles as you start traversing the broad south flank of Mount Harwood. Scattered lodgepole pines now predominate. At 2.6 miles you arrive at the saddle between Harwood and Old Baldy, where backpackers sometimes set up camp (no water, no facilities here). Continue climbing up the rocky ridge to the west, past stunted, wind-battered conifers barely clinging to survival in the face of yearly onslaughts by cold winter winds. You reach the summit after a total of 3.2 miles.

On the rocky summit, barren of trees, you'll find a rock-walled enclosure and a register book that fills up with the names of hundreds of hikers on a fair-weather weekend. Most days you can easily make out the other two members of the triad of Southern California giants—San Gorgonio Mountain and San Jacinto Peak—about 50 miles east and southeast, respectively. On days of crystalline clarity, the Old Baldy panorama includes 90 degrees of ocean horizon, a 120-degree slice of the tawny desert floor, and the far-off ramparts of the southern Sierra Nevada and Panamint ranges, as much as 160 miles away.

# trip 8 Old Baldy—South Approach

see map on p. 327

| | |
|---|---|
| **Distance** | 8.4 miles round trip, Out-and-back |
| **Hiking Time** | 6 hours (round trip) |
| **Elevation Gain/Loss** | 3900'/3900' |
| **Difficulty** | Strenuous |
| **Trail Use** | Suitable for backpacking, dogs allowed |
| **Best Times** | May through November |
| **Agency** | ANF/SGRD |
| **Recommended Map** | USGS 7.5-min *Mount San Antonio* |
| **Notes** | Navigation required, moderate terrain |

**DIRECTIONS** Exit the 210 Freeway at Baseline Road on the border between the cities of Claremont and Upland. Go west on Baseline for 0.7 mile, then turn right (north) on Mills Avenue. After 1.1 mile the main road (signed Mount Baldy Road) veers right. Stay on it and drive uphill another 12 miles to Manker Flats Campground, 0.5 mile short of the ski-lift parking lot. Parking space can be found on the west side of the divided road, opposite the campground.

This route, which makes use of the "ski-hut trail" through upper San Antonio Canyon, is the most varied and interesting of the several ways to reach the top of Old Baldy. The approach is direct and satisfying. The higher you climb, the more rewarding the view, and the greater your sense of accomplishment.

From Manker Flats, walk up the ski-lift-maintenance road 0.9 mile to the unmarked (and easy to miss) ski-hut trail on the left. This junction is 0.3 mile past the sharp hairpin turn opposite San Antonio Falls. The sketchy trail climbs up a rocky slope, then maintains a steep but well-graded ascent high along the east wall of upper San Antonio Canyon. Bigcone Douglas-fir, Jeffrey pine, sugar pine, and white fir trees clothe the slopes, which are accented by blooms of Indian paintbrush, wallflower, and yucca during the late spring and early summer.

Near the last of the big trees, and just below the big, open bowl scooped out of Old Baldy's southeast flank, you arrive at the Sierra Club's San Antonio Ski Hut (2.5 miles). Still in good repair today, the hut was built in 1937 by Sierra Club ski mountaineers who pioneered the then-unfamiliar sport of snow skiing in Southern California. Use of the hut is by reservation only, through the Angeles Chapter of the Sierra Club. Trail campers without reservations are invited to camp in the so-called "Rock Garden" about 200 yards southwest of the hut.

Just beyond the hut, the now-more-primitive trail swings west across a small creek, crosses the Rock Garden, and then switchbacks up the west wall of the canyon. At 3.2 miles, you reach the top of the south ridge of Old Baldy, where you have a fine view down San Antonio Canyon. Continue north along that ridge, following a rocky, primitive trail, 1 mile to the summit.

Normally, the way back down is via the way you arrived. But, if you'd rather not retrace your steps, you could return to your starting point by way of the Devils Backbone Trail, and then either ride the ski lift down or walk down the maintenance road to Manker Flats. With the use of a car shuttle, you could descend the spectacular but foot-punishing Bear Canyon Trail, which loses 5800 feet in 6.4 miles, ending at Mount Baldy village. Or, if you like fast descents down talus and scree slopes, you could walk down to the saddle just west of Mount Harwood, and then drop straight down to the ski lodge 1200 feet below. Sturdy, ankle-protecting footwear is essential for the latter route, which can be recommended only for hikers with an excellent sense of balance.

## trip 9  San Antonio Ridge

| | |
|---|---|
| **Distance** | 14.0 miles, Point-to-point |
| **Hiking Time** | 11 hours |
| **Elevation Gain/Loss** | 4400'/10200' |
| **Difficulty** | Very Strenuous |
| **Trail Use** | Suitable for backpacking |
| **Best Times** | May through November |
| **Agency** | ANF/SGRD |
| **Recommended Maps** | USGS 7.5-min *Telegraph Peak, Mount San Antonio, Mt. Baldy, Glendora* |
| **Notes** | Navigation required, difficult terrain, bushwhacking |

see map on p. 327

**DIRECTIONS** *East End:* Exit the 210 Freeway at Baseline Road on the border between the cities of Claremont and Upland. Go west on Baseline for 0.7 mile, then turn right (north) on Mills Avenue. After 1.1 mile the main road (signed Mount Baldy Road) veers right. Stay on it and drive uphill another 13 miles to the end of the road, where you enter the parking lot for the Mount Baldy Ski Lift. *West End:* From the community of Azusa, just north of Interstate 210, drive north on the San Gabriel Canyon Road, Highway 39, for 11 miles to East Fork Road, on the right. Continue up East Fork Road 6 miles to its terminus near the East Fork ranger station.

**G**et set for a spectacular and extremely challenging traverse along the spine of the San Gabriel Mountains. From the top of Old Baldy, you descend a net elevation of 8000 feet to East Fork San Gabriel River by way of San Antonio Ridge and Iron Mountain. Done in the manner described here (net downhill), the trip is certainly the most tortuous hike of all those included in this book.

My companion and I did the trip in reverse, from East Fork to Baldy, an option open to you if you're a real glutton for punishment. One of our rewards, besides the aerial-like views, was the sighting of a large herd of bighorn sheep. Some 25 sheep scooted over a rocky saddle on San Antonio Ridge as we watched in amazement from a hundred yards away.

You begin with the standard approach to Old Baldy's summit by way of the Mount Baldy ski lift and the Devils Backbone Trail. Remember that during the non-snow-skiing season the lift operates on weekends and holidays only, starting at 9 a.m. If you're making this a one-day hike (practical only around the summer solstice when the days are long) be sure you're at the lower station of the lift by 9 a.m. If you're backpacking the route, an internal-frame pack with a

compact and narrow profile will save you much grief. External-frame packs tend to get entangled in the brush. Do check with the Forest Service to make certain there is access to the ski lift and to both the start point the end point of this trip.

Start your journey by riding the ski lift up to Mount Baldy Notch. From the notch, take the maintenance road to the northwest that climbs moderately, then more steeply through groves of Jeffrey pine and incense cedar. After a couple of bends, you come to the road's end (1.3 miles) and the beginning of the trail along the Devil's Backbone ridge, featuring severe dropoffs and spectacular vistas both north and south.

The backbone section ends at about 2.0 miles as you start traversing the broad south flank of Mount Harwood. Scattered lodgepole pines now predominate. At 2.6 miles you arrive at the saddle between Harwood and Old Baldy, where backpackers sometimes set up camp (no water, no facilities here). Continue climbing up the rocky ridge to the west, past stunted, wind-battered conifers barely clinging to survival in the face of yearly onslaughts by cold winter winds. At 3.2 miles you reach the Old Baldy's 10,064-foot summit, where you'll find a rock-walled enclosure and a register

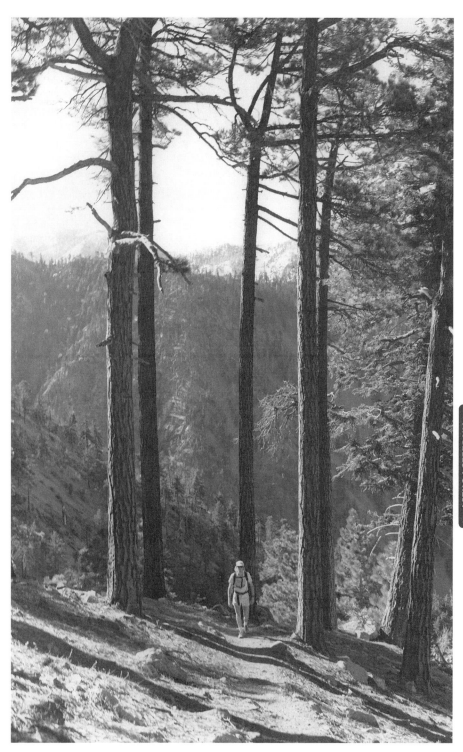

On the Ski Hut Trail

book that fills up with the names of hundreds of hikers on a fair-weather weekend.

From Old Baldy's summit, proceed west to 9988-foot West Baldy (3.7 miles). From there you can visually trace the rounded San Antonio Ridge in the distance as it curves gradually left and finally becomes a serrated spine leading to Iron Mountain's summit. Based on what you can see, estimate how long it will take you to walk over to Iron Mountain—then multiply that figure by at least two.

From West Baldy, you descend through talus and timberline *krummholz* (stunted, almost prostrate trees) and then through taller trees to the first saddle in the ridge at 5.2 miles (7772'). On the undulating ridge ahead, you travel through sparse groves of timber and thickets of snowbrush, a low-growing but very thorny variety of ceanothus. The topo map shows trails connecting several old mines in the upper Coldwater Canyon drainage to the south, but mines and trails alike have been unused for decades.

At a low point in the ridge west of peak 7758 (7.0 miles) some hand-and-toe rock climbing begins on a savage-looking arête

to the west. This is your last chance to reconsider and turn back. Consider that only about 40 percent of your total effort has been expended so far. The mile-long traverse to Iron Mountain ahead is by far the most taxing stretch on the whole trip.

Work your way over and around pinnacles of upthrust rock on the arête, mostly a slow process of stepping over or bashing through low chaparral. Bighorn sheep tracks may guide you. Take great care not to pull on or otherwise dislodge blocks of rock; many seem to be delicately balanced and poised to tumble. Also make sure that no two climbers are in the same "fall line." Ropes are of practically no value here as much of the rock is too crumbly to be used as an anchor. While you're on this tense stretch, try to relax occasionally and enjoy the dizzying vistas into the precipitous Fish Fork canyon on the north and the more gentle Coldwater Canyon drainage on the south.

When you finally reach Iron Mountain's 8007-foot summit (7.9 miles), you'll find a register in a red can appropriately labeled BIG BAD IRON. In it, a scribe has written "Through

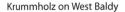

Krummholz on West Baldy

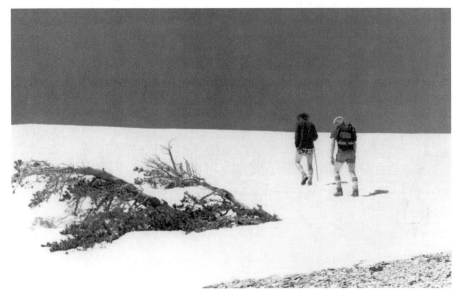

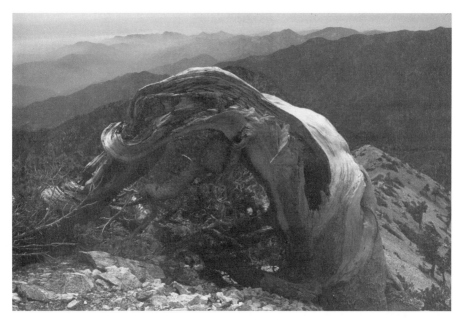

Wind-battered lodgepole pine near Old Baldy

bad chaparral and stinging nettle; to do Big Iron you need pants of metal . . ."

Most climbers do Iron by way of the south ridge, easier than the way you came, but tortuous (and torturing) all the same. Take a long breather on top and revel in the view. Some nice camp or picnic sites can be found amid the scattered pines just below the summit.

When it's time to leave, head down the south ridge on a rather-well-beaten but occasionally very steep climbers' path. Huge yuccas, some with a thousand slender daggers, grow uncomfortably close to the path. Keep your speed down lest you slide into one of them. A couple of pine- and-fir dotted flat areas on the way down offer a chance to rest and cool off. At a 4582-foot saddle (10.3 miles) you come upon the comparatively well-maintained Heaton Flat Trail, which zigzags southeast up a hill, gaining about 150 feet, then descends, more or less steadily over the next 3 miles, to Heaton Flat. From there, walk out on the service road to the trailhead at East Fork Station.

ANGELES FOREST

# chapter 28

# Santa Catalina Island: Avalon

From high points on the mainland, Santa Catalina Island is often seen either floating over a blanket of fog like a mirage, or rising boldly from the surface of the sea. The island, third largest of the several Channel Islands strung along the Southern California coast, lies only 19 miles at its closest point from the Palos Verdes peninsula. It's the only Channel Island with a town of any real size, and the only one catering to large numbers of tourists.

"Catalina" stretches 21 miles in length and up to 8 miles at maximum width. A half-mile-wide isthmus called Two Harbors separates the 6-mile-long northwestern end of the island (called the West End) from the larger southeastern part. The town of Avalon and Avalon Bay snuggle into an eastern corner of the island, protected from the prevailing winds which come out of the west and northwest. Avalon experiences the same almost-frost-free climate as the most even-tempered areas of the Southern California coastline, and enjoys what is probably the cleanest air of any populated area near the Southern California coastline.

For most of this century, Catalina was owned by the Wrigley family (of chewing-gum and Chicago Cubs fame), whose interest in developing the island as a vacation destination was mostly limited to the Avalon area. Catalina's interior remained largely off-limits to tourists until the creation of the Catalina Island Conservancy in 1972, whose function is to preserve and protect the wild landscape and biological diversity of the island. Today 86 percent of the island is owned by the Conservancy, and is open to light recreational use.

The languid pace of life on Catalina Island reflects its aloofness from the often frantic business of living on the Southern California mainland. A weekend visit there is truly relaxing, whether you choose to lodge in Avalon or prefer to rough it at one of the several campgrounds spread around the island's coast and interior.

Why is Catalina included in this book on Los Angeles County hikes? Because it lies within the county's jurisdictional boundary, and because so many L.A.-area residents vacation there. Of the million or so visitors to the island per year, many engage in hiking and mountain biking. To do that it's necessary to obtain a free permit for hiking (or a $20 two-day or $65 annual permit for mountain biking) from the Catalina Island Conservancy office in Avalon.

Ferries to Catalina depart from terminals at Marina del Rey, San Pedro, Long Beach, and Newport Beach. The trip takes about an hour and costs about $70 per round trip. Helicopter flights are available from Long Beach and San Pedro. Lodging in Avalon ranges from $75-per-night cottages to $400-plus bed-and-breakfasts. For more information, including information on camping, hiking permits, and bicycling permits, the following two websites and phone numbers are most useful: Catalina Island Conservancy, www.catalinaconservancy.org, (310) 510-0143; and the Catalina Chamber of Commerce, www.catalinachamber.com., (310) 510-2595.

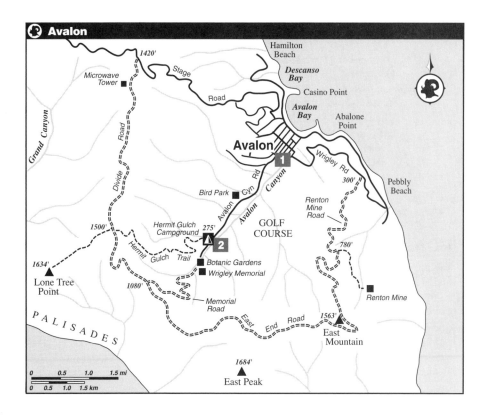

In this chapter and the next, we profile four of the best hikes on Catalina—two in this chapter in the Avalon area, and two in the next chapter originating from Two Harbors.

Avalon Harbor

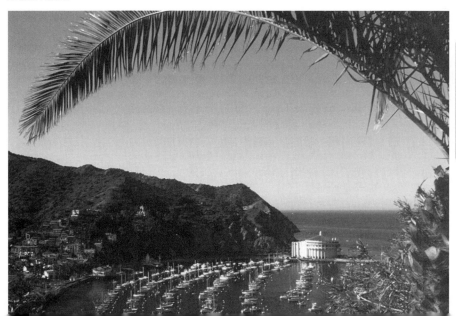

# trip 1  East Mountain

| | |
|---|---|
| **Distance** | 8.5 miles, Loop |
| **Hiking Time** | 5 hours |
| **Elevation Gain/Loss** | 2000'/2000' |
| **Difficulty** | Moderately strenuous |
| **Trail Use** | Dogs allowed |
| **Best Times** | October through June |
| **Agency** | CIC |
| **Optional Map** | USGS 7.5-min *Santa Catalina East* |
| **Notes** | Marked trails/obvious routes, easy terrain |

see map on p. 343

**DIRECTIONS** The assumed starting point is Clemente Avenue and Wrigley Road (aka Mount Ada Road) on Avalon's south edge, about 4 blocks from the middle of town.

On certain crystal-clear days (most common between November and March) this "grand tour" of the eastern end of the island affords an ever-changing panorama of the blue ocean, San Clemente Island to the south, and the snow-capped summits of the San Gabriel Mountains on the mainland.

The route takes you up along gently graded paved and dirt roads to East Mountain, a broad summit area marking the last gasp of the island spine before it falls eastward into the ocean. No matter what the time of year, beware of the sun. You'll be climbing along the lee side of the island, fully exposed to morning and midday temperatures easily 20 degrees higher than along the immediate coastline. Bring lots of water and don't forget your shade hat either.

Mountain bikers, who are only allowed on the "primary" road system of the island, can utilize a longer loop variation on the hikers route described here. They are allowed to use Renton Mine Road, East End Road, Divide Road, and Stage Road—a considerably longer route.

Starting off on paved Wrigley Road you swing around the high ridge overlooking Avalon Bay, enjoying picture-postcard-perfect views of boats at anchor and of the famous round Casino building on the bay's far side. The distinguished edifice on the right at 0.5 mile is The Inn on Mount Ada, now a bed-and-breakfast, but formerly

the Wrigley family home. The home was designed to take advantage of the sunrises and sunsets visible from its commanding perch.

Go right at 1.3 miles on Renton Mine Road; the paved road descends left toward a power plant at Pebbly Beach. A gradual ascent takes you to another junction, 2.7 miles, where you make another right on East End Road. On the slopes hereabouts, notice the St. Catherine's lace, a type of buckwheat endemic to the dry slopes of the island. The flower clusters on this large (up to several feet high) shrub can spread as wide as a foot, with a creamy white color fading to rust in the fall.

After curling around East Mountain, East End Road proceeds due west along the ridgecrest, with spectacular views north down to Avalon Bay and south over the sparkling waters to San Clemente Island. You'll notice that thick accumulations of chaparral coat the north-facing slopes, while the sunnier, south-facing slopes are much more parched and brown. Drought-resistant prickly-pear cacti grow abundantly on the ridgecrest and down along the drier slopes.

At 6.8 miles, you'll veer sharply right on Memorial Road. Some easy walking down this dirt road takes you along a cool, north-facing slope covered by tall and luxuriant (by mainland standards) growths of scrub oak, manzanita, and toyon. At the bottom of the hill you come upon Wrigley Memorial, a 130-foot-tall edifice built as a memorial to chewing-gum magnate William Wrigley, Jr., who purchased the island in 1918.

The famed botanic gardens started by Wrigley's wife (Ada Wrigley) in the 1920s lie just below the monument. Distinguished by a virtually frost-free climate, the gardens are home to an extensive array of native Southern California plants, as well as exotics from distant corners of the world. Once beyond the garden gates, 1.4 miles of road-walking down Avalon Canyon will take you back to Avalon.

## trip 2  Lone Tree Point

| | |
|---|---|
| **Distance** | 5.5 miles, Loop |
| **Hiking Time** | 2½ hours |
| **Elevation Gain/Loss** | 1500'/1500' |
| **Difficulty** | Moderate |
| **Trail Use** | Dogs allowed, good for kids |
| **Best Times** | October through June |
| **Agency** | CIC |
| **Optional Map** | USGS 7.5-min *Santa Catalina East* |
| **Notes** | Marked trails/obvious routes, easy terrain |

see map on p. 343

**DIRECTIONS**  Start hiking at Hermit Gulch Campground, a 1.5-mile walk, golf-cart-ride, or taxi up Avalon Canyon Road from Avalon.

This popular springtime hike starts from Hermit Gulch Campground and loops over the main divide of the island overlooking Avalon. The highlight is a side trip over to Lone Tree Point, which commands an unparalleled view of the cliff-like Palisades falling sheer to the ocean. You'll encounter a couple of very steep grades on the old fire break leading to Lone Tree Point, so be sure to wear running shoes or boots with a studs or lugs to ensure plenty of traction. Small children would need some assistance on that stretch.

Bison, boar, deer, and goats have all been introduced on the island at one time or another. Efforts to eradicate the feral goats, whose impact on the island's vegetation were extreme in some areas, have been successful.

Lone Tree Point

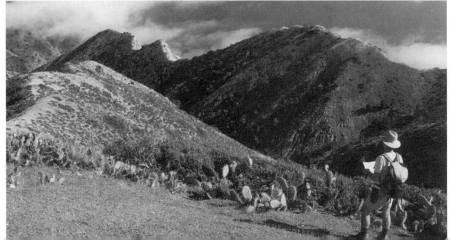

SANTA CATALINA

On this hike and across the island today, you'll commonly see bison and deer. Also, keep an eye on the sky for bald eagles. The Catalina Island Conservancy is attempting to restore bald eagle populations in an effort to displace invasive golden eagles, which have had a tendency to prey on the rare native Santa Catalina Island fox.

From Hermit Gulch Campground, follow the narrow but distinct trail up the ravine to the west (Hermit Gulch). Before long you leave the trickling stream in the canyon bottom and begin a twisting ascent up along a shaggy slope. Red monkey flower, shooting star, and lupine dot the trailside and adorn small clearings amid the tangles of chaparral. After a 1200-foot gain (1.5 miles) you meet Divide Road, a fire road following the eastern spine of the island. Most of the elevation gain for the hike is now behind you.

Turn right, walk a few paces, and then climb the steep embankment to the left. Ahead you'll see an old fire break heading southwest, up and over several rounded, barren summits. Continue for 0.7 mile or more, passing over the peaklet designated Lone Tree on most maps. That's where you'll find the best view of the ocean and shoreline. Sometimes you can gaze south over the shore-hugging fog and spy the low dome of San Clemente Island, some 40 miles across the glistening Pacific. During the best visibility you can trace the mainland shoreline down as far as San Diego, and also spy the long crest of the Peninsular Ranges—the chain of mountains running through Riverside and San Diego counties into Baja California.

After taking in the visual feast, backtrack to Divide Road. From there you can loop back to the starting point via a somewhat longer but more gradually descending route. Head south down Divide Road for 0.8 mile, then veer left on Memorial Road. Easy walking down this dirt road takes you down to Wrigley Memorial, through the botanic gardens, and finally to Hermit Gulch Campground, a short distance down Avalon Canyon Road.

# chapter 29

# Santa Catalina Island: Two Harbors

If the popular Avalon area is too crowded for you, try Two Harbors, a quintessential "sleepy village." Camping, hiking, backpacking, water sports, and wildlife-watching are the norms here.

In addition to a small lodge and cabins in tiny Two Harbors itself, hillside campsites abound at Little Fishermans Cove Campground just east of town. The more remote Parsons Landing Campground is accessible by way of a 7-mile road (see Trip 1 below).

Two Harbors is served by ferry from San Pedro and Marina del Rey, and by helicopter from Long Beach and San Pedro. For more information, including information on camping, hiking permits, and bicycling permits, the following two websites and phone numbers are most useful: Catalina Island Conservancy, www.catalina conservancy.org, (310) 510-0143; and the Catalina Chamber of Commerce, www. catalinachamber.com., (310) 510-2595.

If you're camping and plan to cook your own meals, be sure to ask about the availability of firewood, charcoal, or stoves at either campground. (Stove fuel is not allowed on the ferry boats that serve the island.)

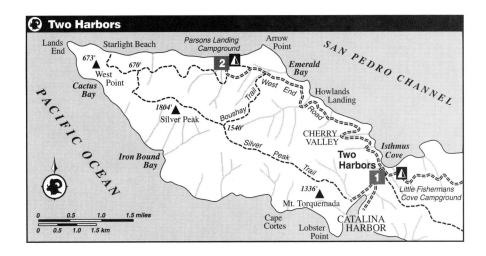

## trip 1  Parsons Landing

|  |  |
|---|---|
| **Distance** | 14.0 miles round trip, Out-and-back |
| **Hiking Time** | 6 hours (round trip) |
| **Elevation Gain/Loss** | 900'/900' |
| **Difficulty** | Moderately strenuous |
| **Trail Use** | Suitable for backpacking, suitable for mountain biking, dogs allowed |
| **Best Times** | All year |
| **Agency** | CIC |
| **Optional Maps** | USGS 7.5-min *Santa Catalina North, Santa Catalina West* |
| **Notes** | Marked trails/obvious routes, easy terrain |

see map on p. 347

**DIRECTIONS** The hike begins at the small community of Two Harbors.

Parsons Landing is not only the site of a small beach and a spacious camping area; it is also the home of one of the best examples of native Southern California grassland. Gray-green after winter rains, bleached gray during drought, the perennial grasses here have found the right combination of fine-grained soil, soaking winter rains, desiccating summer drought, and the absence of heavy grazing by domestic animals in the past.

The native grasslands of Parsons Landing are only one example of the botanical richness and diversity of the north slope of Catalina's West End. This side of the island has not been so damaged by feral animals, such as goats, whose populations multiplied too rapidly in the past. The chaparral and oak-woodland habitats here look healthy. On the sheltered, north-facing slopes (especially at Cherry Valley) you'll find plenty of the native Catalina cherry, a large shrub or

Above Parsons Landing

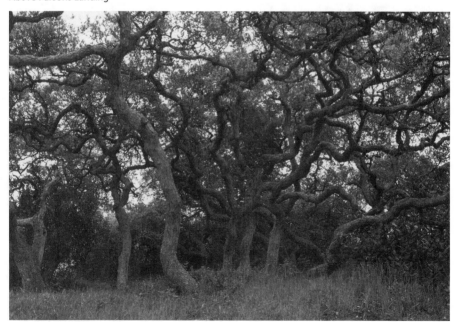

tree (up to 45 feet tall) displaying spike-shaped clusters of white flowers during the spring. Its dark, red fruits resemble large black cherries.

The hiking route from Two Harbors to Parsons Landing sacrifices the economy of straight-line travel for ever-changing scenic delights. Covering an air-line distance of only 3.5 miles in 7 walking miles, the gently graded road hugs the shoreline, swinging around every ravine and canyon along the way.

The trip is most rewarding, and not at all exhausting, if you can spend a night at Parsons Landing Campground. From there, if you're ambitious, you can loop around the island's west end—see Trip 2 below. Some travelers like to use mountain bikes to get to Parsons Landing, then travel farther on foot into areas where bikes are prohibited.

From Two Harbors, head for the road clearly etched onto the steep, dry slope west of Isthmus Cove. At 1.5 miles, the sinuous course of the road takes you on a long detour into Cherry Valley. Over the next few miles you'll pass several Scout or organizational camps and private marinas.

At about 6.2 miles, past Emerald Bay, you come to an intersection: the Boushay Trail goes left; you stay right. After another 0.5 mile, where the road bends left (southwest) you continue going straight (west) on a trail through grassland to the scattered camp and picnic sites of Parsons Landing. Try the boulder-backed picnic area close to the water's edge.

## trip 2  Silver Peak & Starlight Beach

| | |
|---|---|
| **Distance** | 10.5 miles, Loop |
| **Hiking Time** | 5½ hours |
| **Elevation Gain/Loss** | 1700'/1700' |
| **Difficulty** | Moderately strenuous |
| **Trail Use** | Dogs allowed |
| **Best Times** | October through June |
| **Agency** | CIC |
| **Optional Map** | USGS 7.5-min *Santa Catalina West* |
| **Notes** | Marked trails/obvious routes, easy terrain |

see map on p. 347

**DIRECTIONS** The hike is assumed to begin at Parsons Landing Campground.

This hike to the highest point on the west end of Catalina, 1804-foot Silver Peak, introduces you to the wild and often wind-swept windward edge of the island. Spectacular views are the norm most of the way.

Assuming you're starting the hike at Parsons Landing Campground (see Trip 1), go back toward Two Harbors to the point where the Boushay Trail (an old fire road) takes off, up-slope to the south. The old road's winding course takes you 2 miles along chaparral-coated slopes and a ridgeline to a junction with the Silver Peak Trail—a fire road traversing the spine of the island's west end. Here, amid brick-red soils and rock outcrops, you get your first glimpses of the west end's dry and heavily eroded south-facing slopes falling precipitously to the blue and emerald ocean below.

Just over a mile west of the Boushay Trail, Silver Peak Road passes about 100 feet below Silver Peak's nearly barren summit. You can scramble up through a sparse grove of Catalina ironwood trees and reach the top for an all-inclusive panorama. San Nicolas and Santa Barbara islands can be seen to the west on many days. Very rarely, Anacapa, Santa Cruz, and Santa Rosa islands off the coast of Santa Barbara, as well as the mainland shoreline west of Ventura, can be seen in the northwest. Quite often, especially in spring and summer, there's nothing to see at all, as you may be wreathed in low clouds scudding over the island's spine.

Past Silver Peak, the fire road (now nothing more than a wide bulldozer track) swings sharply downhill, beginning a sometimes very sheer descent down the wind-buffeted ridgeline to the west. After descending a total of about 1100 feet, you reach a T-intersection. You'll return to Parson's Landing on the road to the right. But first make the side trip left down to Starlight Beach, one of the most isolated and wild stretches of Catalina's coastline. You'll have to scramble a bit in the end to reach the rocky shore, where the ebb and flow of the waves dance over rock-dimpled sand. On clear days you can clearly see the low dome of the Palos Verdes peninsula some 20 miles across the San Pedro Channel, and it's hard to believe such a serene and beautiful place as Catalina's northwest shore can exist so close to the L.A. metropolis.

Climb back up to the T-intersection and return to Parsons Landing on the road that contours and lazily drops across steep, north-facing slopes. Each ravine you cross harbors a mini-forest of tangled oaks and chaparral. By the late afternoon, the often-misty atmosphere of the morning may have turned transparent, rendering the waters of the San Pedro Channel down below a deep azure.

Starlight Beach

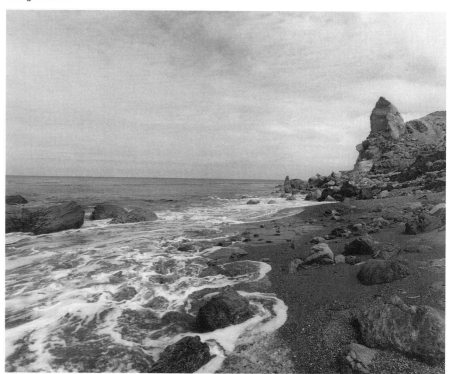

# Best Hikes

## BEST BEACH HIKE

**Point Dume to Paradise Cove** (Chapter 1, Trip 1). During lowest low tides, the Point Dume coastline offers up the finest array of tidepool life in the county.

## BEST SUBURBAN HIKES

**Paradise Falls** (Chapter 3, Trip 2). A glorious waterfall hidden in an intimate little gorge.

**Santa Clarita Woodlands** (Chapter 5, Trips 9-11). Lush woods and trickling streams, just beyond the San Fernando Valley.

**Placerita Canyon** (Chapter 6, Trip 2). A quiet, woodsy retreat only a few minutes away from San Fernando Valley.

**Ben Overturff Trail** (Chapter 11, Trip 2). Serene and pristine canyon country, just uphill from the San Gabriel Valley.

**Marshall Canyon Trail** (Chapter 11, Trip 6). Hike through two of the best-preserved canyons of the San Gabriel foothills.

**Will Rogers Park** (Chapter 12, Trip 1). Ocean and city lie at your feet on this island of open space on L.A.'s west side.

**El Prieto Loop** (Chapter 20, Trip 1). Follow a trickling stream along a deeply shaded Front Range canyon on the edge of Altadena.

**Millard Canyon** (Chapter 20, Trips 8, 9). A deep, shady cleft graced by a small stream and a 50-foot waterfall, barely 10 minutes' drive from the edge of the Pasadena suburbs.

## BEST MOUNTAIN HIKES

**The Grotto** (Chapter 15, Trip 6). Here, the primeval mountain and canyon country of the Santa Monica Mountains survives intact.

**Hoegees Loop** (Chapter 21, Trip 2). The riparian splendor of the Front Range (San Gabriel Mountains) at its best.

**Cucamonga Peak** (Chapter 27, Trip 5). From shady brook to high mountain crest, Cucamonga offers a complete mountain experience.

**Old Baldy** (Chapter 27, Trips 7, 8). An obligatory climb, 10,064-foot Old Baldy is the highest point in the San Gabriel Mountains as well as in Los Angeles County.

## BEST CANYON HIKES

**Lower Solstice Canyon** (Chapter 13, Trip 9). Alongside a trickling stream, enjoy some of the county's finest oak woodlands.

**Zuma Canyon** (Chapter 14, Trips 1, 2). Big-scale canyon country within a small-scale mountain range.

**Big Santa Anita Canyon** (Chapter 21, Trips 3-5). A shady wonderland of cascades, pools, and streamside greenery.

**East Fork San Gabriel River** (Chapter 26, Trips 11, 12). The East Fork has carved out the granddaddy of Southern California canyons, a mile deep as measured from the top of the east wall.

**Icehouse Canyon** (Chapter 27, first part of Trip 5). An easy mile or two up the tumbling Icehouse stream takes you to tall-timbered canyon recesses.

## BEST WATERFALLS AND SWIMMING HOLES

**Monrovia Canyon Falls** (Chapter 11, Trip 1). Easy hike along a densely shaded canyon stream, ending at a 40-foot cascade.

**Fish Canyon Falls** (Chapter 11, Trip 3). A real payoff in the end when you discover a magnificent 100-foot cascade.

**Escondido Falls** (Chapter 13, Trip 12). By far the best waterfall in the Santa Monica Mountains.

**Trail Canyon Falls** (Chapter 19, Trip 2). A beautiful and unexpected find tucked amid the chaparral country of lower Big Tujunga Canyon.

**Royal Gorge** (Chapter 20, Trip 4). Features a deep, chilly pool fed by a small waterfall.

**Sturtevant Falls** (Chapter 21, Trip 3). A scenic attraction for more than a century. Popular and easy to reach.

**Devils Canyon** (Chapter 24, Trips 2, 3). Two waterfalls in the middle canyon present a impassable barrier for hikers. Deep pools in the lower canyon are accessible (with difficulty) from canyon mouth.

**Cooper Canyon Falls** (Chapter 25, Trip 1). A small but beautiful cascade in a sublime, High Country setting.

**San Antonio Falls** (Chapter 27, Trip 6). Dependably impressive when swollen with snowmelt during spring and early summer. A very easy walk to the base.

## BEST VIEW HIKES

**Top of the Peninsula** (Chapter 2, Trip 1). Features a stunning panorama of ocean and islands on clear, winter days.

**North End Traverse** (Chapter 7, Trip 3). Spectacular vistas of San Fernando Valley and all the basin-bordering mountain ranges.

**Mount Lee** (Chapter 8, Trip 2). A top-of-the-city view in every direction from over the HOLLYWOOD sign.

**Topanga Overlook** (Chapter 12, Trip 7). Unbelievably spacious views of Santa Monica Bay and the ocean.

**Sandstone Peak** (Chapter 15, Trip 7). This volcanic outcrop crowning the Santa Monica Mountains overlooks the ocean, Channel Islands, and much of Los Angeles and Ventura counties.

**Inspiration Point** (Chapter 20, Trip 12). Summon up the energy to go an extra mile to Panorama Point, where there's an even better perspective of the L.A. megalopolis below.

**Jones Peak** (Chapter 21, Trip 8). A quick, hard climb into the Front Range (San Gabriel Mountains), yielding an ever broader view of coastal and urban L.A.

**Twin Peaks** (Chapter 24, Trip 5). Some of Southern California's most wild and inaccessible terrain lies directly below these crags.

**Mount Baden-Powell** (Chapter 26, Trip 5). Its 360-degree view encompasses mountains, deserts, and the ocean.

**Cucamonga Peak** (Chapter 27, Trip 5). The peak's prominent southern exposure offers an unparalleled, panoramic view of both the L.A. Basin region and the Inland Empire.

**Lone Tree Point** (Chapter 28, Trip 2). The pseudo-Hawaiian vista atop Catalina's east end includes eroded palisades and the green- and blue-tinted ocean.

## BEST HISTORICAL WALKS

**Old Stagecoach Road** (Chapter 5, Trip 3). Trace the notorious "Devil's Slide" segment of a 19th-Century stage road linking Northern California with Southern California.

**Pico Canyon** (Chapter 5, Trip 12). Roll the clock back a century and appreciate Southern California's early oil-drilling industry.

**Mount Lowe Railway** (Chapter 20, Trip 11). Follow the path of more than 3 million passengers who rode rails into the sky on the Mount Lowe Railway.

## BEST WILDFLOWERS

**Vasquez Rocks Natural Area** (Chapter 6, Trip 5). A convergence of three plant communities here yields a plethora of blooms during wet years.

**Eagle Rock Loop** (Chapter 12, Trip 8). A broad range of wildflowers characteristic of the Santa Monica Mountains is represented here.

**Lookout Loop** (Chapter 13, Trip 2). Good displays of meadow wildflowers.

**Charmlee Wilderness Park** (Chapter 15, Trip 4). Wildflowers characteristic of grassland, chaparral, and oak woodland habitats.

**La Jolla Valley & Mugu Peak** (Chapter 16, Trip 2). The giant coreopsis in La Jolla Canyon is especially noteworthy.

**Devil's Punchbowl** (Chapter 25, Trips 7-9). Flora from both mountain and high desert areas are represented here.

# BEST AUTUMN COLORS

**Placerita Canyon** (Chapter 6, Trips 2, 3). Willow, sycamore, cottonwood, bigleaf maple, and California walnut trees contribute various shades of yellow and rust.

**Serrano & Big Sycamore Loop** (Chapter 16, Trip 4). Big Sycamore Canyon, in particular, is touted as the finest example of sycamore savanna in the California State Park system.

**Liebre Mountain** (Chapter 18, Trip 1). The golden leaves of the black oak, a common tree in these northern reaches of L.A. County, put on a fine autumnal show.

**Down the Arroyo Seco** (Chapter 20, Trip 3). Brightly colored sycamores and maples contrast with the somber browns and greens of the oaks and the chaparral.

**Bear Canyon** (Chapter 20, Trip 7). Alders, sycamores, and maples line the narrow floor of this canyon.

# BEST BIRD AND WILDLIFE WATCHING

**Cheeseboro Canyon** (Chapter 4, Trip 6). At dawn and at dusk, deer, bobcats, and coyotes roam the oak-dotted hills and canyon floor. Birds of prey patrol the skies.

**Lost Cabin Trail** (Chapter 13, Trip 2). The trail probes an area set aside for special protection within Malibu Creek State Park

**Vetter Mountain** (Chapter 22, Trip 2). Birds and animals typical of yellow-pine forests are found here.

**Coldwater Canyon Truck Trail** (Chapter 26, Trip 8). Bighorn sheep are often seen crossing the fire road that serves as the trail into Cow Canyon.

**Blue Ridge Trail** (Chapter 26, Trip 2). Birds and animals typical of lodgepole-pine forests are found here.

**Santa Catalina Island** (Chapters 28, 29). Wildlife on the island includes deer, boar, and bison.

# Recommended Reading

## Los Angeles Area Outdoor Guidebooks

Benti, Wynne, *Favorite Dog Hikes in and around Los Angeles,* Spotted Dog Press, 1995.

Brown, Ann Marie, and Sheer, Julie, *Moon Take a Hike Los Angeles*, Avalon Travel Publishing, 2006.

California Coastal Commission, *California Coastal Access Guide*, 6th ed., University of California Press, 2003.

McAuley, Milt, *Hiking Trails of the Santa Monica Mountains*, 6th ed., Canyon Publishing Company, 1998.

McKinney, John, *John McKinney's New Day Hiker's Guide to Southern California*, Olympus Press, 2004.

Robinson, John W. and Christiansen, Doug, *Trails of the Angeles: 100 Hikes in the San Gabriels*, 8th ed., Wilderness Press, 2005.

Schad, Jerry, *101 Hikes in Southern California*, 2nd ed., Wilderness Press, 2005.

Schad, Jerry, *Top Trails Los Angeles*, Wilderness Press, 2010.

Schaffer, Jeffrey P., et al., *The Pacific Crest Trail, Southern California*, 6th ed., Wilderness Press, 2003 (Includes log and maps of the Pacific Crest Trail in Los Angeles County.)

Stone, Robert, *Day Hikes Around Los Angeles*, 4th ed., Day Hike Books, Inc., 2003.

## History and Natural History

Bakker, Elna S., *An Island Called California*, University of California Press, 1984.

Bailey, H.P., *The Climate of Southern California*, University of California Press, 1966.

Belzer, Thomas J., *Roadside Plants of Southern California*, Mountain Press Publishing Company, 1986.

Hall, Clarence A., *Introduction to the Geology of Southern Califronia and its Native Plants*, University of California Press, 2007.

Mallan, Chicki, *Guide to Catalina and California's Channel Islands*, 5th ed., Moon Publications, 1996.

McPhee, John, *The Control of Nature*, Noonday Press, 1990.

Munz, Philip A., and Lake, Diane, *Introduction to California Spring Wildflowers of the Foothills, Valleys and Coast*, University of California Press, 2004.

Munz, Philip A., et. al., *Introduction to California Mountain Wildflowers*, revised ed., University of California Press, 2003.

Peterson, P. Victor, *Native Trees of Southern California*, University of California Press, 1966.

Raven, Peter H., *Native Shrubs of Southern California*, University of California Press, 1966.

Robinson, John W., *The San Gabriels, Southern California Mountain Country*, Golden West Books, 1977.

Robinson, John W., *The San Gabriels II, The Mountains from Monrovia Canyon to Lytle Creek*, Big Santa Anita Historical Society, 1983.

Robinson, John W., *Mines of the San Gabriels*, La Siesta Press, 1973.

Robinson, John W., *Mines of the East Fork*, La Siesta Press, 1980.

Rundel, Philip W., and Gustafson, John Robert, *Introduction to the Plant Life of Southern California*, University of California Press, 2005.

Saunders, Charles F., *The Southern Sierras of California* (abridged edition), Big Santa Anita Historical Society, 1984.

Schoenherr, Allan A., *A Natural History of California*, University of California Press, 1995.

Sharp, Robert P., *Coastal Southern California* (geology guide), Kendall/Hunt Publishing Company, 1978.

Sharp, Robert P., *Geology Field Guide to Southern California*, William C. Brown Company, 1972.

Sharp, Robert P. and Glazner, Allen F., *Geology Underfoot in Southern California*, Mountain Press Publishing Company, 1993.

Thrall, Will, ed., *Trails Magazine*, L.A. County Dept. of Recreation, Camps & Playgrounds, 1934-39; 1941.

Nature Study Guides published by the Nature Study Guild: *Pacific Coast Tree Finder*, *Pacific Coast Bird Finder*, *Pacific Coast Fern Finder*, *Mammal Finder*.

## Maps and Map/Brochures

U.S. Geological Survey 7.5-minute topographic quadrangles (complete coverage of Los Angeles County).

Los Angeles Sheet, Bouguer Gravity Map, 1974, California Division of Mines and Geology. (This map supersedes the 1:250,000 scale Los Angeles geologic map on which it is based.)

Geologic Map of the San Bernardino Quadrangle, 1:250,000 scale, California Division of Mines and Geology, 1986.

Santa Monica Mountains and Rim of the Valley Corridor Park Lands, Santa Monica Mountains Conservancy. (A map and guide to public recreation and open space lands surrounding Los Angeles.)

Tom Harrison Maps. (Tom Harrison publishes a series of waterproof topographic maps of hiking locales throughout the Santa Monica Mountains and the Angeles National Forest.)

Map and Guide of Griffith Park. (This new relief-shaded map of the park trails is available at the park.)

Angeles National Forest recreation map/brochure, 1995.

*San Gabriel Mountains*, Wilderness Press, 2005. (This topographic trail map, included with the book *Trails of the Angeles*, is also sold separately.)

*Trails of the Simi Hills*, Wilderness Press, 2007. (Shaded relief recreation map of the Simi Hills.)

Catalina Conservancy Visitor Map & Guide.

# Local Organizations

The three largest private environmental organizations in Los Angeles County are listed here. Scores of other organizations or groups, including Internet-organized hiking groups, can be found by way of Internet searches.

**Sierra Club, Angeles Chapter**
3435 Wilshire Blvd #320
Los Angeles, CA 90010
(213) 387-4287

(The Angeles Chapter, with nearly 60,000 members, has 13 regional "groups," numerous standing committees, and several special activities sections. Its outings program offers over 4,000 hikes and backpack trips each year, the majority of them in Los Angeles County. All outings are published in a three-times-yearly schedule distributed free to members and also available for purchase at outdoor equipment stores. More information can be found at **www.angeles.sierraclub.org.**)

**Audubon Society, Los Angeles**
7377 Santa Monica Blvd.
Los Angeles, CA 90046
(323) 876-0202

**The Nature Conservancy, Los Angeles**
(213) 327-0104

# Agencies & Information Sources

Angeles National Forest (Supervisor's Office)
701 N. Santa Anita Avenue
Arcadia, CA 91006
(626) 574-5200

Angeles National Forest,
Los Angeles River District (ANF/LARD)
12371 N. Little Tujunga Canyon Road
San Fernando, CA 91342
(818) 889-1900

Angeles National Forest,
Santa Clara/Mojave Rivers District (ANF/SCMRD)
28245 Avenue Crocker, Suite 220
Valencia, CA 91355
(661) 296-9710

Angeles National Forest,
San Gabriel River District (ANF/SGRD)
110 N. Wabash Ave.
Glendora, CA 91740
(626) 335-1251

*Note:* The above offices are open weekdays only. On weekends you can call or visit the following Forest Service visitor facilities:

> **Chilao Visitor Center**
> Angeles Crest Highway
> La Cañada, CA 91011
> (626) 796-5541

> **Grassy Hollow Visitor Center**
> Angeles Crest Highway
> Wrightwood, CA 92397
> (626) 821-6737

> **Mount Baldy Visitor Center**
> Mount Baldy Road
> Mount Baldy, CA 91759
> (909) 982-2829

Catalina Island Conservancy (CIC)
(310) 510-2595

City of Rancho Palos Verdes (CORPV)
(310) 544-5260

City of Sierra Madre (COSM)
(626) 355-5278

Charmlee Wilderness Park (CWP)
(310) 457-7247

Clairemont Hills Wilderness Park (CHWP)
(909) 399-5460

Conejo Recreation and Parks District (CRPD)
(805) 495-6471

Devil's Punchbowl Natural Area (DPNA)
(661) 944-2743

Eaton Canyon Natural Area (ECNA)
(626) 398-5420

Griffith Park (GP)
(323) 644-2050

Glendale Parks and Recreation (GPR)
(818) 548-2000

Henninger Flats Fire Station (HFFS)
(626) 794-0675

Los Angeles City Recreation & Parks Dept. (LACRPD)
(323) 913-7390

Los Angeles County Dept. of Parks and Recreation (LADPR)
(213) 738-2961

Leo Carrillo State Park (LCSP)
(818) 880-0363

Los Padres National Forest
Ojai District (LPNF/OD)
(805) 646-4348

Malibu Creek State Park (MCSP)
(818) 880-0367

Monrovia Canyon Park (MCP)
(626) 256-8282

Mountains Restoration Trust (MRT)
(818) 591-1707

**National Park Service** (NPS)
**(Santa Monica Mountains National Recreation Area)**
401 West Hillcrest Drive
Thousand Oaks, CA 91360
(805) 370-2301
(*Note:* ask about their free, quarterly publication that lists  guided hikes and other events held in the Recreation Area)

**Placerita Canyon Park** (PCP)
(661) 259-7721

**Point Mugu State Park** (PMSP)
(818) 880-0363

**Palos Verdes Estates Shoreline Preserve** (PVESP)
(310) 378-0383

**Puente Hills Landfill Habitat Preservation Authority** (PHPA)
(562) 945-9003

**Royal Palms Beach** (RPB)
(310) 305-9546

**Rancho Simi Recreation and Parks District** (RSRPD)
(818) 584-4400

**Santa Monica Mountains Conservancy** (SMMC)
(310) 858-7272
The conservancy's website **www.lamountains.com** features a comprehensive list and links to all L.A.-region parks and outdoor recreation areas.

**Santa Monica Mountains National Recreation Area** (see "National Park Service")

**Santa Susana Pass State Historic Park** (SSPSHP)
(310) 455-2465

**Topanga State Park** (TSP)
(310) 455-2465

**Vasquez Rocks Natural Area** (VRNA)
(661) 268-0840

**Wildwood Canyon Park** (WCP)
(818) 238-5440

**Will Rogers State Historic Park** (WRSHP)
(310) 454-8212

# About the Author

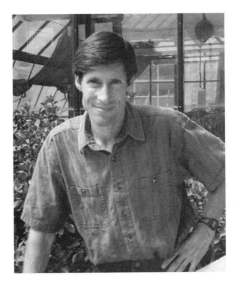

Jerry Schad's several parallel careers have encompassed interests ranging from astronomy and teaching to photography and writing. He teaches astronomy and physical science at San Diego Mesa College, and currently chairs the Physical Sciences Department there.

Schad has run or hiked many thousands of miles of distinct trails throughout California, in the Southwest, and in Mexico. He is a sub-24-hour finisher of Northern California's 100-mile Western States Endurance Run, and has served in a leadership capacity for outdoor excursions as close as Southern California and as far away as Madagascar. More information can be found at Schad's website: **www.skyphoto.com.**

BOOKS BY JERRY SCHAD

*50 Southern California Bicycle Trips*
*101 Hikes in Southern California*
*Adventure Running*
*Afoot & Afield Los Angeles County*
*Afoot & Afield Orange County*
*Afoot & Afield San Diego County*
*Back Roads and Hiking Trails: The Santa Cruz Mountains*
*Backcountry Roads and Trails: San Diego County*
*California Deserts*
*Cycling Orange County*
*Cycling San Diego*
*Physical Science: A Unified Approach*
*Top Trails Los Angeles*
*Trail Runner's Guide San Diego*

# Other Southern California Books from Wilderness Press

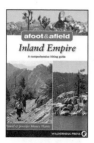

## Afoot & Afield Inland Empire

Over 200 memorable hikes in the mountains and deserts of Riverside and San Bernardino counties, including parts of the Angeles and San Bernardino national forests, Santa Rosa and San Jacinto Mountains National Monument, the Palm Springs area, Joshua Tree National Park, Mojave National Preserve, plus dozens of trails in urban and regional parks.
ISBN 978-0-89997-462-0

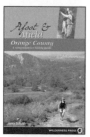

## Afoot & Afield Orange County

In 87 hikes in the parks, preserves, designated open spaces, and public lands surrounding Orange County's densely populated coastal plain, this book provides fresh inspiration for trips along the coast from Huntington Beach to San Clemente, in the rugged Santa Ana Mountains, and through the foothills from Anaheim to the Santa Rosa Plateau Ecological Reserve.
ISBN 978-0-89997-397-5

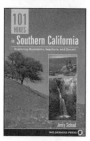

## 101 Hikes in Southern California

The book that proves there's more to SoCal than theme parks and strip malls. From the San Gabriel Mountains to the Anza-Borrego Desert and everywhere in between, this guide offers an incredible selection of exciting trips covering scores of hidden places just beyond the urban horizon.
ISBN 978-0-89997-351-7

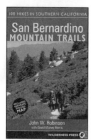

## San Bernardino Mountain Trails

The classic guide to three mountain ranges in Southern California: the San Bernardinos, the San Jacintos, and the Santa Rosas. Covers 100 of the best hikes in these mountains; includes a separate foldout sheet map.
ISBN 978-0-89997-409-5

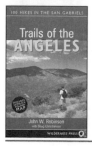

## Trails of the Angeles

The authoritative volume to hiking in the San Gabriel Mountains includes 100 classic trips in the Angeles National Forest. The hikes range from one-hour strolls to challenging two-day backcountry trips. Comes with a separate foldout sheet map.
ISBN 978-0-89997-377-7

For ordering information, contact your local bookseller or Wilderness Press, www.wildernesspress.com